THE Vaginal Birth After Cesarean Experience

THE Vaginal Birth After Cesarean Experience

Experience

Birth Stories by Parents and Professionals

Lynn Baptisti Richards & Contributors

FOREWORD BY MICHEL ODENT

BERGIN & GARVEY PUBLISHERS, INC.
MASSACHUSETTS

In order to protect the personal and political privacy
of the contributors of this book, some of the names
and settings have been changed.

First published in 1987 by
Bergin & Garvey Publishers, Inc.
670 Amherst Road
South Hadley, Massachusetts 01075

789   987654321

Printed in the United States of America

Library of Congress Cataloging-in-Publication Data

The Vaginal birth after cesarean (VBAC) experience.

Includes bibliographies and index.
1. Cesarean section—Miscellanea.
2. Natural childbirth—Miscellanea.
3. Midwives—Miscellanea.
I. Richards, Lynn Baptisti.
[DNLM: 1. Cesarean Section—popular works.
2. Labor—popular works.
WQ 150 V126]
RG761.V34 1987 618.4   87-15107
ISBN 0-89789-119-8 (alk. paper)
ISBN 0-89789-120-1 (pbk.: alk. paper)

*This book is dedicated to my children, Gabriel, Zachary and Elijah,
who have been the source of my growth and have made this book possible.*

*Thank you to all those who have contributed
their stories, thoughts and feelings to this book.
Special thanks to my husband, Harlan, my parents,
and my friends, Barbara, Kathleen, Cindy and Nancy,
for all their patience, love, support and hard work.*

Contents

Foreword
MICHEL ODENT, OB/GYN   xi
Letter to Lynn
NANCY WAINER COHEN   xiii
Preface   xv
Introduction: *Special Care Nursery—A Fictionalized Account*   xvii

PART I: Out of the Wombs of Mothers

1. **VBAC: New and Untested?**
   LYNN BAPTISTI RICHARDS   3

2. **Forty Years Ago in France**
   ALICE PATRICK   4

3. **VBAC Comes to America:** *Thirty Years Ago in Maine*
   MURIEL MOORES   5

4. **The Myth of High Blood Pressure**
   KAREN LACASSE   9

5. **"Remember, You Have a Small Triangular Pelvis"**
   PAT KOWALEK AND SARAH MARKOWITZ   14

6. **Abandoned for Being Too Recalcitrant**
   ANDREA KELLY-ROSENBERG   19

7. **My Baby, My Body:** *A Ward of the State?*
   GINA DISNEY   25

8. **Disco Birth**
   CAROLYN ANDERSON   34

9. *Herpes Absolution*
   PAM MORRISON   34

10. *Laying the Bugaboo of Uterine Rupture to Rest: VBAC after*
    Four Cesareans
    MARY JO CAMILLUS   43

11. *VBAC Triplets*
    MEG WESTON   51

12. *Home Alone for Four Days of Labor*
    DIANE WIRKKALA   57

13. *Turning Around More Than 180 Degrees*
    ED AND MARIA ANDERSON   61

14. *What a Difference Support Can Make!*
    GINA AND RICHARD BERQUIST   71

15. *You Could Have Died*
    KARYN AIKIN   86

16. *From ICU to Empirical Midwifery*
    APRIL ALTMAN   89

17. *Twice a Cesarean: The Birth of Onna Chunaha*
    ALICE JORDAN   101

18. *The Movement Continues*
    JUDY AND ALLEN TWIST   108

19. *How I Became a Feminist*
    KAREN DIESSEL   122

20. *My Brother—I Felt Like I Had Known Him All My Life:*
    A Child's Perspective
    THE TAYLOR FAMILY   141

21. *Sexual Abuse and Letting Go*
    BARBARA   144

22. *Having a Vaginal Cesarean*
    LINDA STELLA ZENTNER   153

23. *Be Thankful For Your Baby, No Matter How She Was Born!*
    BARBARA CULLIGAN   161

24. *"I Came Up and Up to Your Head, and I Touched You"*
    JUDY GARVEY   173

PART II: Out of the Hands of Practitioners

25. *Defining Complication*
    KAY MATTHEWS, FAMILY NURSE PRACTITIONER, NURSE-MIDWIFE,
    DOMICILARY MIDWIFE   185

26. *VBAC Training, 1947–1950*
    IRWIN KAISER, OB/GYN   186

27. *Classical VBAC*
MITCH LEVINE, OB/GYN 187

28. *Mandatory Labor after Previous Cesarean*
KENNETH MCKINNEY, OB/GYN 187

29. *A Perfectly Round Head*
KAY MATTHEWS, FAMILY NURSE PRACTITIONER, NURSE-MIDWIFE, 189
DOMICILIARY MIDWIFE

30. *Once a Cesarean, Never a Cesarean*
IRWIN KAISER, OB/GYN 191

31. *Expert Witness*
KAY MATTHEWS, FAMILY NURSE PRACTITIONER, NURSE-MIDWIFE, 191
DOMICILIARY MIDWIFE

32. *Talking Women into VBAC*
KENNETH MCKINNEY, OB/GYN 192

33. *A Five-Hour, Second Stage VBAC*
THERESE DONDERO, C.N.M., AND GERRIANNE BODD, R.N.C. 193

34. *Saving the Doctor's Wife*
STEVEN MELTZER, OB/GYN 197

35. *The Effect of Malpresentation on Vaginal Birth*
KENNETH MCKINNEY, OB/GYN 199

36. *Breech VBAC Without Pelvimetry*
LEO SORGER, OB/GYN 200

37. *Natural Protocol for Breech Birth*
MICHEL ODENT, OB/GYN 202

38. *Obstetrical Training for Breech Delivery*
IRWIN KAISER, OB/GYN 203

39. *Prophylactic Cesarean for Herpes Disputed*
OB/GYN NEWS 203

40. *Repeating Indications??*
LEO SORGER, OB/GYN 204

41. *My Favorite Story*
MITCH LEVINE, OB/GYN 205

42. *Two Out of Three Ain't Bad!*
PIXIE WILLIAMS, M.D. 207

43. *Commitment to VBAC*
KENNETH MCKINNEY, OB/GYN 212

44. *By the Skin of Her Teeth*
ALEXANDRA PAYTON, MIDWIFE AND BARRY GOLDIN, OB/GYN 215

45. *The Spitting Image of His Father*
ANASTASIA HOLMES, MIDWIFE 223

46. *Knockout*
PHYLLIS MALONEY, R.N., C.C.E. 225

47. *Everything You Didn't Do*
CINDY DUNLEAVY, MIDWIFE   227

48. *Completely Unscathed*
LEO SORGER, OB/GYN   228

49. *Dispelling the Final Naivete*
ISABEL ANDREWS, MIDWIFE   229

50. *Failure*
THREE MIDWIVES   237

51. *From Marshmallow to Monster*
KATHERINE HUGHES, VBAC EDUCATOR, LABOR COACH, MIDWIFE   240

52. *VBAC as Triumph*
LEO SORGER, OB/GYN AND BARBARA BROWN-HILL, VBAC
EDUCATOR AND BIRTH ATTENDANT   249

Glossary   253
Resources   265
Indexes   275
Opening: A Photographic Essay
    following page   177

Foreword

by
MICHEL ODENT,
OB/GYN

This book is supposed to be a book about vaginal birth after cesarean. As a matter of fact it is much more than that. Many mothers who give birth normally, with their own hormones, after a previous cesarean, have something in common. They have reached a high degree of awareness. This experience turns them into campaigners for alternatives to the current obstetrical practices. They rediscover authentic midwifery. They feel—they know—that midwifery should not be part of the institution of medicine. Instead, the institution of medicine should be at the service of midwives and women. This book lets us understand that one cannot disassociate topics such as VBAC and authentic midwifery.

It is not by chance that the most favorable places to engender a new awareness are countries where submission to technology is most deeply rooted, such as the U.S.A. and Canada.

The reappearance of authentic midwifery deserves to be studied and understood as one of the most significant sociological phenomena of the end of the twentieth century.

Because this phenomenon originates from subjective experiences, one must first listen to mothers before beginning other kinds of research. This is why the book proposed by Lynn Richards is so important. It is necessary as a basic document.

Letter to Lynn

Your manuscript arrived this week just as we were leaving for vacation. I tucked the pages in the carry-all and have just spent the last two days, on and off, reading. I remember your working title, the one that spurred you on: *Very Beautiful and Courageous.* How appropriate that I read it here by a lake, next to the mountains. It is so grounding, so beautiful, so open, so connecting here. I found your words to be the same.

Of all the beautiful and courageous women out there, dear friend, you stand, in my mind's eye and in my heart, tall, lovely, loyal, and brave (and I don't even know if ever you were a Girl Scout!). I am so happy that this book is out of your heart—where it was born lovingly and lived wisely and adventurously—and on to pages for others to see. It is time that others knew that you, too, breathed "VBAC" from the very moment your cesarean was done (and your spirit cried "No!") and that every subsequent breath echoed "VBAC, VBAC, VBAC. . . ."

I remember our first meeting; it was in 1975. We knew within an instant that we were sisters in this work, twins, feverishly and frantically looking for each other in a sea of then mostly unconscious "cut-me-open, it's-all-right-with-me, I-don't-care" moms. We knew within that same instant that we were friends, old friends *and* new friends.

We have spent many hours together over the years, our paths intertwined. How we have talked and laughed, and, oh, how we have cried. I watched your metamorphosis—first from cesarean mother to VBAC mother, then from music teacher into childbirth educator, and then from a woman birthing her child at home with only her four year old present (*only?* we should all be blessed with such wonderful, calm, supportive birth attendants!) into a midwife. I don't need to remind you of the many personal, interpersonal, and political challenges you faced. Thanks to the women—and to God—there were always a victory and a joy sprinkled in along the way (and always when these were most necessary, don't you think?).

While others began to join the VBAC movement and do their work, you, Lynn, were doing just about the most important VBAC work of all—assisting cesarean women as they birthed their VBAC babies. While many other midwives were buckling under political and administrative pressures and kowtowing to doctors' orders, you were in homes calming moms and waiting patiently for yet another VBAC babe. While others were yelling "high risk!" to VBAC couples, you were gently teaching these couples how low risk they really could be. And while others were looking into technology, you were looking into your heart and soul. I want the whole world to know the hours, days, toils, tears, sweat, and love you have given to VBAC.

Your book inspired me. I felt braver and more courageous just reading it. (Women who are pregnant these days need to be courageous, don't they, for they face an inordinate amount of prejudice, manipulation, fear, and ignorance at just about any hospital maternity unit on the continent. You have gleaned so many Truths about birth, not the least of which is the knowing that the women who birth freely must be protected and honored and that these women are the most beautiful and courageous of all. You have always known that if it weren't for these women, we could lose Birth for all, and you have used your Light, your breath, your heart, and your hands to preserve the blueprints.

Your presence in my life, Lynn, your support for me, your love and understanding for VBAC have been invaluable. What a gift you have been all these years. What a contribution you have made to birthing families, and what a blessing you have been to so many babies. This book, as an extension of you, is a gift to the planet. Simply stated, my friend, you are a VBAC affirmation. Even more simply, I love you.

[signed]   *Nancy Wainer Cohen*

Preface

This book is written from the heart, and is meant to speak to the heart. Of course, many subjects that are addressed in this book are both medical and psycho-spiritual in nature, and thereby require both intellectual and emotional understanding.

However, as this book does not hope to "prove" the safety of Vaginal Birth After Cesarean (VBAC) or even the absoluteness of any scientific question, it does not offer powerful scientific documentation as its source of truth. Statistics are not the only method of seeking truth. This book has chosen to seek truth primarily through the experience of life and birth.

The scientific studies that do and do not support the theories espoused in this book are readily available. This book encourages us to look up any unfamiliar terms, to read further childbirth literature, and attend workshops for parents and professionals (glossary and a list of workshops appear at the end of the book). We can then go to our nearest medical library to look up the subject(s) of our choosing in the *Index Medicus* (the readers' guide to medical journals), which lists reports of all the current research. Through our own research we will gain power in knowing that medical information is not privileged to the few who wear white coats, but is available to all of us who are willing to take the responsibility to do our own research and draw our own conclusions. In order to grow, we must each do this work for ourselves.

This is a book about growth—growth in birth and growth in our lives. Within these pages are experiences which cannot be analyzed with the mind alone, theories which cannot be studied by science or proven by statistics. As Bernie Seigel, M.D. writes in his book, *Love, Medicine, and Miracles:*

Statistics rarely alter deeply held beliefs. Numbers can be manipulated to make bias seem like logic. Rather than dwell on statistics, I now concentrate on individual experiences. To change the mind one must often speak to the heart . . . and listen. Beliefs are a matter of faith not logic.

Truths are the gifts of life's experiences, to be discovered by each of us alone. This book does not hope to espouse all truths. But rather the purpose and hope of this book is to become a catalyst for each of us to find the truth within ourselves. In sharing the birth and life experiences of so many who have traversed the path of VBAC we may share not only in their process of seeking a Vaginal Birth After Cesarean, but share as well in the process of deepening the awareness of ourselves as Very Beautiful and Courageous souls.

Introduction

Special Care Nursery:
A Fictionalized Account

Gregory, almost two hours old, had still not been seen or touched by either of his parents. He had spent his quiet-alert period being poked and prodded, staring into fluorescent lights above his lonely isolette in the special care nursery. As he began to feel hungry and tired, his tiny whimpers grew to frantic screams. Perhaps there was no one for him.

Gregory had left a warm secure world of incomparable closeness. He had lived within love itself, within his mother's being, surrounded by the sounds and sensations of her body, constantly in tune with her energy, her every thought and feeling.

During labor, he had begun to prepare for his world to change, to leave this closeness, to come into another closeness. The labor was slow, as slow as he and his mother had needed it to be to enable them to let go of the old closeness, to come into the new one.

Gregory had begun a journey on a path which, though difficult at times, seemed perfect and time-tested. With each contraction, his small body had curled into position, seeking the path that his mother was opening to him through her cervix. With each contraction, the path had become more clear, his position more secure. And perhaps because of his growing clarity and security, he could endure the ever-mounting awesome power that surrounded him. Carefully, slowly, listening intently, every nerve ending in his head grew more acutely tuned to the sensitive job of navigating the bony pelvis.

Suddenly sharp pain lanced his scalp. (The insertion of the internal fetal monitor lead.) Confusion. Had he taken the wrong path? He wiggled to find a way to stop the pain. But with each contraction, the mounting pressure intensified the wound. He could no longer allow his nerves to be so keenly aware. He had to shut down the pain. And in so doing, he shut down his ability to perceive the best course to navigate the narrow channel.

Gregory felt afraid, and so did his mother. He could always tell when she was afraid—her heart would pound faster, and everything around him felt tight and unyielding. The stronger contractions pushed his sore head against a rigid cervix. What had begun perfectly and lovingly, now seemed all wrong, desperate, and lonely. A peaceful passage had become a perilous fight for survival.

Gregory suddenly felt his mother's body bump and thump. She rolled around, then bump, she had jumped off something. Then another jump and she was back on something else. Then they were moving fast on wheels, almost as fast as in the car. the ride stopped, and his mother's belly became very tight around him. He heard her scream (as the epidural needle was placed in her back). "Don't worry, Mom, you'll be all right. I'll be coming out soon, and then you'll feel better," he tried to tell her.

Suddenly, Gregory's ability to fight, his very awareness of life itself soon waned. His sensitivities slowly faded. He could feel himself drifting somewhere between life and death. (The effect of anesthesia and analgesia). He could hear his mother's screams. Something terrible must

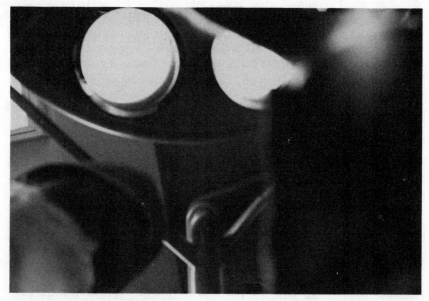

Gregory's first view of the world

Dr. Steven Meltzer photograph

be happening. (The operation was begun with incomplete anesthesia.) His mother, too, seemed to be drifting far away, out of touch. (When the epidural "failed" she had been given general anesthesia.) "Don't go away, Mother." It was closeness with her that he most feared losing.

Suddenly, his world felt invaded. Something grabbed his sore head, twisted, and pulled hard through a new hole. No tunnel, no path, just a hole in the very place that had held him so close within his mother. A rush of icy cold air stung in his chest. Brilliant white lights blinded his sensitive eyes. Loud noises blared in his heretofore muffled ears. Another hard pull . . . his neck wrenched . . . he squirmed in the vast, cold space. A scream of terror. Where was she—his mother?

Perhaps the new world he had come to knew no closeness, no love, no mother. For two hours he waited for her, his eyes searching for hers, his ears listening for those familiar sounds of her body—her heart, her breath, her voice. He longed for her touch. He wanted to be held close.

A pain grew in his belly. Suck. Suck. He needed to suck. He needed his mother. Did she not hear his cries? Did she not care? Was there no longer a mother? Exhausted and in despair, he slept.

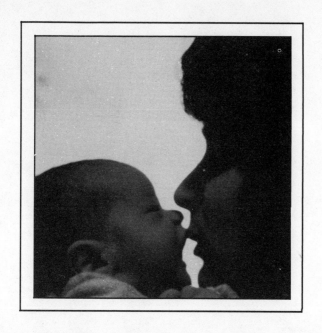

P · A · R · T

I

Out of the Wombs of Mothers

1

VBAC: New and Untested?

LYNN BAPTISTI RICHARDS

According to the medical journal articles from this country VBAC appears to be a new and even somewhat frightening possibility. One article even cites the stress upon the physician as a factor for consideration in making the decision as to whether or not to allow such a dangerous and innovative procedure. (Of course, the stress upon the mother in undergoing major abdominal surgery simply because she had done so previously was never mentioned.) Clearly, VBAC has been considered new territory to be explored.

On the other hand, in Europe, Asia, and Africa, VBAC is a long-standing tradition. VBAC has been studied and documented in foreign research for years. VBAC in Europe is not a rarity. It is simply expected. However, many American doctors have been closing their eyes to this "foreign" research, as if American women were somehow "different." Could it be that the uteri and vaginas of American women are inherently weaker than their European, Asian, or African counterparts? Could it be that in Africa, Asia, or Europe the previously scarred uterus could be so entrusted with safe delivery of their babies through their vaginas, yet in America the previously scarred uteri are internal bombs about to explode if labor would be allowed to occur? "WHAT A DIFFERENCE AN OCEAN MAKES!!" as Bonnie Donovan, author of *The Cesarean Birth Experience* once remarked.

For many years in Europe, the VBAC guidelines for safety did not include continuous monitoring and IV; in-house anesthesiologist and obstetrician; limitations of size, number, and position of the fetus. The guidelines simply indicated a hospital birth. VBAC fear was negligible, intervention was negligible, and most VBAC attempts ended with healthy vaginal births.

3

2

Forty Years Ago in France

ALICE PATRICK

COMMENTS: *How long have European women been having VBACs, so unmonitored, so unintervened, so successfully? Alice Patrick, now in her late seventies, grandmother of a VBAC mother, and a VBAC mother herself writes of her uncontroversial births, which took place more than forty years ago in France.*

ALICE: I had a vaginal birth (VBAC) in 1933. My two previous pregnancies had been difficult. The first, when I was sixteen or so, was a forceps delivery and the baby subsequently died. My second pregnancy, about a year or so later, was a cesarean, with a classical incision.

My last pregnancy, however, was the easiest of them all. I worked right up until I went into labor. I didn't have what they call prenatal care. In France, at that time, we didn't know what such a thing meant. When I began to have labor pains, I went to a hospital run by nuns. They were midwives by necessity.

I remember one nun saying that my baby was coming out at a hundred miles per hour. She was so fast! One young nun was whispering to her superior that she had never delivered a woman before, and was scared. The elder nun replied that she had to start sometime! But I remember thinking, "Why did she have to start with me?"

My daughter was born after a very short and relatively painless labor. I don't remember exactly how much she weighed, but I think it was eight or nine pounds. I stayed in the hospital about eight days, which was the custom then. This upset me, as I wanted to go home badly.

I never saw a doctor before or after the birth, and the thought of not having a vaginal birth never occurred to me or worried me in the least.

3

VBAC Comes to America: Thirty Years Ago in Maine

MURIEL MOORES

COMMENTS: *The European tradition of VBAC moved to America when doctors who had been trained in Europe subsequently moved to America, bringing with them their own standards. Muriel Moores of Fairfield, Maine, now a grandmother, writes of her cesarean and VBAC births (the VBAC with a foreign-trained physician).*

MURIEL: My due date was October 10, 1947. On October 11th, I started hemorrhaging and was taken to the hospital and prepped, but no labor happened. Dr. Marston, my family practitioner, packed my vagina to stop the bleeding.

COMMENTS: *In those days most vaginal bleeding (other than the normal bleeding of the menses or lochia) was handled with vaginal packing. Vaginal packing is done by inserting more and more sterile gauze into the vagina until finally it is packed tightly. This creates pressure on the bleeding vessels which slows and eventually stops the bleeding.*

MURIEL: I was examined by three or four doctors. However, none of them ever told me anything about what they had found. After three days in the hospital I was sent back home. Doctor Marston came to my house to visit me a few days later. He said that he and the surgeon had conferred, and had decided to do a cesarean because the baby was breech.

On October 23, 1947, the doctors performed the cesarean section at the Redington Hospital in Skowhegan, Maine. I had sodium pentathol as I refused to have a spinal.

COMMENTS: *Spinal anesthesia in those days was in its infancy. Since the greatest risk in any surgery is from the anesthesia, Muriel preferred the anesthesia that was more "proven" in effectiveness and safety.*

MURIEL: I had never been in the hospital before. I had never heard of a cesarean birth before mine. I was afraid they would start my incision before I was asleep, so I tried to keep talking as long as I could.

I had a beautiful baby girl named Rosemary Ann. My baby weighed about six pounds and ten ounces. I saw my baby about four hours after the operation. She took one look at me and threw up. After I healed, my scar ran from my navel to the top of my pubic hair line.

COMMENTS: *At that time, almost all cesareans were done with classical (vertical) incisions.*

MURIEL: Having a cesarean made me feel that I couldn't do anything right. As was usual at that time, I was in bed for ten days after my cesarean. You get so tired and weak when you're in bed all that time. I was mad at the nurse because she wouldn't let me stay up for more than five minutes. So I dangled my legs over the edge of the bed when she wasn't looking. I did what I felt like doing.

Years later my sister, who is a nurse, looked up my records at the hospital. She told me that my cesarean wasn't done for breech. It was a placenta previa.

COMMENTS: *In all likelihood, the doctors had determined that Muriel had a placenta previa when she arrived at the hospital hemorrhaging. It has been long known in the practice of obstetrics that any painless vaginal bleeding near term pregnancy could indicate a probable low-lying placenta or placenta previa, which means that the placenta is either partially covering or fully covering the opening of the cervix. When the cervix begins to dilate, the woman begins to bleed. If the placenta is only low-lying, and not completely covering the cervix, sometimes a vaginal delivery is possible. However, if it is a complete previa (completely covering the cervix), the lives of both the mother and the baby are at risk with cervical dilatation.*

In those days, when presented with a choice between cesarean and vaginal birth, most physicians chose vaginal birth as being the less risky of the two choices. Therefore, although even a low-lying placenta does present a risk, the physician hoped that he could avoid the more risky procedure of cesarean delivery. What was once considered to be a very high risk procedure (cesarean), is now commonplace, and is often thought of erroneously as "risk-free birth."

It is probable that the many exams done by the doctors those first three days Muriel spent in the hospital were done to determine whether or not the placenta was simply low-lying or a full previa. Without the use of sonagraphy, manual determination of this condition is done by attempting to engage the fetal head. If the head cannot drop into the pelvis, then the placenta is completely blocking the descent, and therefore is a full previa.

Since Dr. Marston clearly knew that Muriel had a placenta previa, why did he tell her she needed to have a cesarean for a breech? He probably wanted to protect her from fear. Maybe he didn't want to explain to her about placenta previa and all the risks associated with it. Perhaps he believed that if she knew it would only make her more afraid, more difficult to deal with as a patient. He wanted to keep his patient calm.

MURIEL: I was mad that the doctor hadn't told me the truth. At the time I only knew there was a complication, and I trusted the doctors to take care of it. I didn't understand then that the patient has the right to ask questions. The doctors didn't seem to feel the need to take the time to explain. They seemed to feel, "Why bother to explain? You're too dumb to understand, anyhow!" But the doctor should let the patient know what is going on. The doctor should talk **to** us, not over our heads.

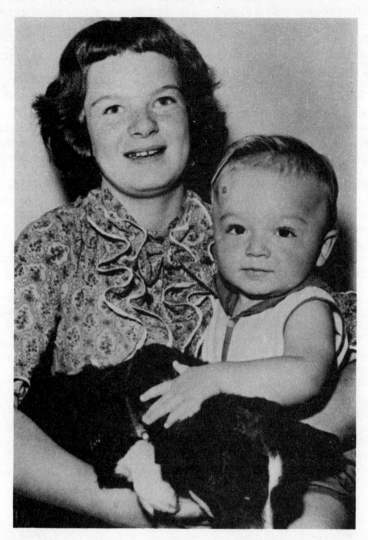

Rosemary Ann Moores (13), born by cesarean, and James Michael Moores (1½), VBAC, in 1961

Eleven years and nine months after my cesarean I had a beautiful baby boy, named James Michael, who weighed 7 lbs. 15 oz. My new doctor, Dr. Andrew Szendey, said I could have a vaginal birth or a cesarean. It was up to me. I chose to have a normal birth if possible. The doctor told me he wanted me to go to the hospital as soon as anything started happening so that he could stop labor if necessary.

On July 14th at about 1:00 in the afternoon, my water broke and my girlfriend proceeded to take me to the hospital, eighteen miles away. We finally made it, after having to change a flat tire on the way. I was fine, but my girlfriend was a nervous wreck.

I was prepped and waited, and then I waited some more. A nurse would stop in every half hour or so to see if I was having any pains yet. Finally after supper, when asked if I was having labor pains yet, I said, "No, just cramps, like I was going to start my period." The nurse checked. I was having contractions and didn't even know it! I had heard how awful labor pains were, but all I had were just a few mild cramps.

I was all dilated and ready at 9:30 that evening, but he was a stubborn little guy (and still is) and he wasn't born until 2:10 in the morning of the fifteenth. I was bearing down as hard as I could.

I saw my baby as soon as I got back in my room and was settled in. Then the head nurse came in to see me. She said, "Didn't you have a section here a few years ago? Did your doctor know that?" She was quite disgusted that Dr. Szendey would let me go into labor and have a natural birth after a cesarean!

I was glad to have had a natural birth. It gave me a good feeling, knowing I was a normal woman and could do something right. I felt like a complete woman after having a natural birth.

COMMENTS: *In 1959, Muriel Moores had a VBAC after a classical cesarean. She had no monitor, no IV. Although she pushed for more than four and a half hours, her scar did not rupture. Neither she nor her baby died. She had a painless labor because no one made her feel that she should be afraid. She birthed her own baby, and felt better about herself and her newborn baby.*

Muriel's doctor's guidelines about VBAC were the ones he had brought with him from Europe where VBAC is routine and common. Today the American College of Obstetricians and Gynecologists (ACOG) have constructed such rigid guidelines that Muriel Moores would not be given any choice about how she could deliver her next baby. She would have to have another cesarean. When we consider the "advancement" of modern obstetrics and its ability to handle the emergencies in childbirth, it is absurd that nearly thirty years ago it was easier for Muriel to have a VBAC than it would be today.

4

The Myth of High Blood Pressure

KAREN LACASSE

KAREN: Eight years ago my son Mark was born vaginally after a fairly normal eighteen hour labor. Four years later we were expecting our second child. Dick and I attended Lamaze childbirth classes in my last trimester. Our instructors had talked about cesarean births, mentioning that 30 percent of all pregnancies ended with a cesarean birth. Dick and I were unconcerned. Since I had delivered vaginally the first time, we felt sure I would this time also.

My second pregnancy was somewhat normal, except for a slight increase in my blood pressure, and my obstetrician was not overly concerned. I feel that the reason for the high blood pressure was my excessive weight gain of eighty pounds. I was just one of those women who feel that being pregnant is the perfect opportunity to take advantage of all the forbidden foods that I would not normally eat in excessive amounts. Although I ate three well balanced, nutritious meals each day, it was between meals when I would eat anything that was sweet.

COMMENTS: *Contrary to popular belief, high blood pressure in labor is usually not an effect of weight gain in pregnancy. Though it is true that obese people tend to have higher blood pressure (because of the increased capillary venous pressure necessary to pump blood through such an expanded system), dangerous high blood pressure in pregnancy or labor is usually a direct effect of insufficient nutrition or increased stress rather than an effect of weight gain itself. Getting adequate nourishment and discovering sources of tension and methods of stress-reduction are generally the best methods of avoiding dangerous high blood pressure in pregnancy or labor.*

KAREN: I started labor, with a bloody show, on June 5, 1978, at around 4:00 P.M. At 7:00 P.M., the contractions were five minutes apart, so a nervous Dick and I made the one mile trip to the hospital.

At around 9:00 P.M. a nurse began taking my blood pressure every five minutes. Now, I was becoming nervous. The doctor arrived in the labor room an hour later and told Dick and I that he was going to do a cesarean section. He said he was concerned that my baby may be in danger because of my "high" blood pressure (150/90). I was fully dilated and had just had the urge to push, but I was afraid that my baby's life was at stake. I was in no position to argue. I did not know what a high, low, or even normal blood pressure was. So I trusted my doctor. Minutes later, I was wheeled away to the operating room.

9

COMMENTS: *Had Karen been better informed, she might have had more power in the decision-making process about how she could safely deliver her baby. All of us should know the guidelines for blood pressure—what is normal, what is high, what is low, what is borderline. In addition, we should have a sense of our normal baseline blood pressure. We should know the possible causes of blood pressure changes and what we can do to change our blood pressure. If Karen had realized that her pressure of 150/90 was not truly high, but rather a borderline pressure, and that anxiety and excitement can cause the blood pressure to rise, she might have been able to find a way to help herself to relax and lower the pressure, enabling her to safely complete the birth process herself.*

KAREN: I awoke four hours later in excruciating pain. I did not think about the baby, only how horrible I felt. Someone finally told me that the baby was a 10-pound healthy boy, but I was too concerned about myself to care.

Four hours later, I was brought to the maternity floor. Finally, ten hours after the cesarean with a stomach pump through my nose, intravenous in my hand and a hole in my belly, I met my new son Nathan. My first reaction when I saw him was that the nurse had given me the wrong baby. Nathan had black hair, while Mark's had been blonde. He had brown eyes, Mark's were blue. And he had very large ears. Dick convinced me that Nathan was ours, as he had seen him right after he was born.

COMMENTS: *Is this baby really mine? Recently, a law suit has been invoked by a thirty-five-year-old man who discovered that the woman who he had called "mother" for his whole life was not really his mother. The hospital had mixed up the babies! The only guaranteed method of preventing this mix-up is to be fully awake at the birth of the baby, and not permit the baby to leave your arms for the duration of the hospital stay!*

KAREN: Two days later, I developed an infection (from the cesarean) which caused me to have a fever of 103 degrees for the next three days. I was perspiring profusely from the fever and at the same time receiving very painful injections in my bottom to clear up the infection.

COMMENTS: *Post-operative infection occurs in 40% of all cesareans. Luckily, Karen was not separated from her baby. However, many hospitals routinely separate mothers from their babies if the mothers become febrile (develop a fever). These mothers not only lose the initial bonding period with their infants immediately after birth, but also lose contact with their babies for the duration of their postcesarean infections as well. The irony of this policy is that postcesarean infections are not infectious diseases—they cannot be transmitted from the mother to the baby. The relationships of mothers and babies are once again being invaded and compromised because of erroneous routine hospital procedures.*

KAREN: After a seven-day stay in the hospital, Nathan and I went home. I felt totally depressed and useless. I did not have the energy or strength to do anything. I detested the feeling of helplessness. I did not like depending on others to do what I had considered to be my responsibilities. So, three days after I left the hospital I began to force myself to take back my household responsibilities.

COMMENTS: *Often cesarean mothers feel the need to challenge themselves. Their sense of their ability to function as women and mothers has been threatened by the cesarean. Their birth experiences have left them feeling as less than whole strong people. Hence, they must prove themselves by challenging themselves to "self-sufficient recovery," which may actually be dangerous to their health and safety.*

KAREN: I concluded that I would never have another cesarean birth, ever. One year after Nathan's birth, I was unexpectedly pregnant again. I was delighted. I had read about VBAC in the past year and hoped that someday I would be able to end my childbearing years with a satisfying birth experience.

I vowed not to gain as much weight as before because I did not want any obstacles to stand in the way of my having a successful VBAC. However, despite my efforts, I still gained seventy pounds.

As I grew I interviewed doctors. The excuses ranged from fear of rupture because of the previous infection to probable death. I was very discouraged.

Dick became a little concerned that I still did not have a doctor. "Karen," he said, "I think that you should give in and have another cesarean." I then informed him that I would deliver the baby at home alone rather than go through that hell again.

As a last resort, I called Dr. Smith at the Strong Maternity Center which is located in a big old victorian house in Strong, Maine. Dr. Smith's receptionist informed me that Dr. Smith delivers his VBAC patients at Franklin Memorial in Farmington, Maine (a 40-mile round trip for me) as an extra precaution. Since he is a general practitioner and cannot perform surgery, a surgeon is always present at these deliveries.

After Dr. Smith examined my previous medical records, he commented that a blood pressure of 150/90 was not high enough to warrant a cesarean.

COMMENTS: *In most cases where true hypertension is associated with other signs of preeclampsia, (such as protein in the urine, excessive swelling, headaches, dizziness, blurred vision, etc.) before a cesarean is done, magnesium sulfate is usually infiltrated via an IV in order to attempt to control the rising pressure. It would seem that the doctor who had ordered the previous cesarean was either ignorant or had other motivations for doing the cesarean.*

KAREN: Dr. Smith examined me the following week and told me that he thought my chances of delivering my baby vaginally were excellent, considering my good health and determination.

DR. CHRISTOPHER SMITH: Karen LaCasse was a very good candidate for VBAC. She had delivered vaginally previously. She had a supportive husband and family. And she had had an easy straightforward first stage of labor.

KAREN: Dr. Smith convinced Dick that I was not going to die, and that he felt quite confident that I would have a short uncomplicated delivery.

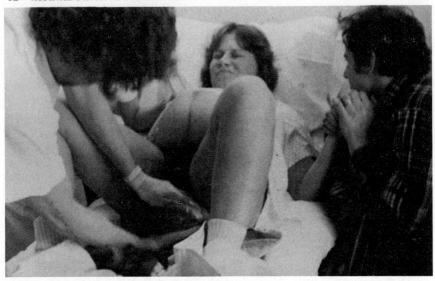

Jesse's head is out, and the cesarean scar can't be mistaken.

On March 11, 1980, I awoke at 2:00 A.M. with what felt like Braxton Hicks (pre-labor) contractions. By 6:00 A.M. contractions were regular and 7 minutes apart. We rushed out to begin our half-hour drive.

DR. CHRISTOPHER SMITH: In Karen's case there were no nervous family members or tremulous nurses.

KAREN: Dr. Smith arrived minutes later. After he examined me, he assured me that my blood pressure was normal for a laboring woman (140/90). Everything was going to be okay.

KAREN: At about 10:00 A.M. I had the urge to push. It was then that I felt my first twinge of fear. I thought about the half of one percent chance of my uterus rupturing and felt that if it was going to do so, then now would be the time.

COMMENTS: *Though it is often thought that pushing is the most likely time for a uterus to rupture, statistically the most likely time is during the last month of pregnancy, prior to labor.*

KAREN: When Dr. Smith told me to go ahead and push, I instantly forgot all my worst fears and concentrated on pushing out my baby. The nurse then asked Dr. Smith if I was going to deliver in the delivery room and his reply was simply, "What's wrong with her delivering right here?" So, 10 minutes later, after an easy 8-hour labor, our third son, Jesse, was born. He weighed 9 lbs. 4 oz., and measured 23 inches long. Dick was elated. Dr. Smith hugged me, and told me that I had done beautifully.

DR. CHRISTOPHER SMITH: Certainly there will be difficult times, but fortunately there will be Karen LaCasses to balance the trying labors.

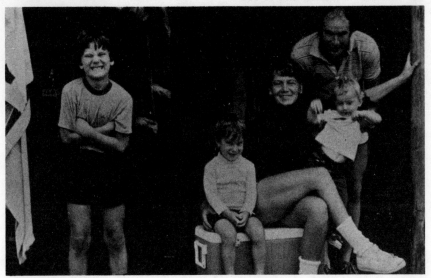

The LaCasse family

KAREN: I felt great, and was very much in love with my new beautiful baby. Jesse nursed right away and I had him with me for the rest of the day.

While I love my three boys equally, I always tend to relate to the events of Jesse's birth with so much excitement and enthusiasm. My cesarean birth of Nathan was not a pleasant experience. Afterwards, many well-meaning family and friends told me how lucky I was to have a healthy baby, but I still felt that I had somehow been cheated from not being able to deliver him vaginally. Of course, the end results of my vaginal and cesarean births were the same. But the feelings of incompetence and anger were so deep, that after Jesse's birth I felt satisfied and complete, and better able to justify the events of Nathan's birth.

5

"Remember, You Have a Small Triangular Pelvis"

PAT KOWALEK AND SARAH MARKOWITZ

PAT: My desire to have a VBAC began as soon as I awoke from my cesarean. Somehow I felt immediately that my cesarean wasn't necessary, and in the months to come, I couldn't be convinced otherwise.

My first step towards having a VBAC was to change doctors because the one who did the cesarean would not even consider a VBAC. After speaking to friends and visiting several doctors, I decided upon a group of four doctors. That was a mistake from the start. Dealing with such a large number of different personalities was a problem. Each doctor had his own ideas but defended his partners. Although they said they'd "attempt" a VBAC, things would have to go according to their narrow criteria.

I often asked the doctors for the names of patients who actually had a VBAC. They brushed me off and told me to ask the nurse (who couldn't remember).

Eight months passed. I was getting nervous. I had no one to talk to who had had a VBAC. I knew plenty of women who had had cesareans, but they were all satisfied with their cesareans, and even went back for seconds!

After reading *Silent Knife*, I started making phone calls. Through the underground network I found Lynn's VBAC classes. I must say her first class was an eye opener. One VBAC mother told her story. I felt that I had finally found what I was looking for (and more)—women who were planning VBACs or women who had already successfully had them!

When David and I left Lynn's class that night we felt overwhelmed. We knew we had lots of work cut out for us. The weeks that followed were very busy with classes, private sessions, lots of reading, and soul-searching.

SARAH (Lynn's apprentice): I first met Pat a month and a half before her due date. She was upset about her doctors, but was really afraid to make another change. Pat was trying to decide where to have her baby. She felt unsafe about giving birth in the hospital. She felt unsafe at home, as well. She couldn't see any any other alternative. We met and discussed the option of laboring at home and going to the hospital shortly

14

before the birth of the baby. Pat remained indecisive and unsure about going to the hospital throughout the remainder of the pregnancy, a feeling that continued throughout the labor. Pat needed the security of knowing the technology was available to her on a moment's notice, but she greatly feared the misuse of the technology by the doctors in the hospital.

Pat and I spent a lot of time together examining the issue of whether to stay with the group of doctors or to change practitioners. We searched for a way that she could have her needs met. As Pat's requests were continually ignored, refused, or responded to inconsistently among the group of doctors, she became more and more panic-stricken.

We spent a lot of time affirming that it was her right to have her needs met, and that she could trust herself to know what she and the baby needed in order to move through her labor. We worked to help her to view the doctors as her employees, rather than to see herself as their patient.

PAT: The next big step was finding a new doctor and deciding what kind of birth we wanted. Time was running out. It was my due date and I still did not have a doctor I could trust. On Friday I called Dr. Stone to make an appointment to meet him on Monday. I really felt comfortable with him. He was not threatened by our requests, and he told me if I needed him over the weekend that I could call him. I felt reassured.

SARAH: Since Pat had stated her needs to have a secondary labor support person, Dr. Stone wanted to meet me. I telephoned him to set an appointment for our meeting, and he took my name and phone number.

PAT: I was examined by Dr. Stone Monday morning, April 16. I was then about a week overdue. He told me there was no cervical change, and I shouldn't expect to go into labor for awhile. He gave me a chart to start recording fetal movement. I was only half listening. As I was walking to my car after my visit my water broke. At 3:00 P.M. contractions began. David came home from work.

SARAH: Pat called me informing me that labor had started. I told her to call me back when contractions were closer. Later she called again and wanted me to come to her home to check her.

PAT: The next several hours went by quickly.

SARAH: I arrived and Pat was only 3 centimeters, but she was dealing with her contractions as if she were in very active labor. I got her up out of bed and suggested eating and walking. Since I felt it would be a really long time, I told her I was going home and that I would come back when she needed me in a couple of hours. I felt ambivalent about leaving Pat. In retrospect, though, this was the best thing I could have done for her. Pat had to find a way to deal with her labor on her own, to trust her own body and her own ability to birth this baby. I could not do it for her.

PAT: At 8:00 P.M. we called Dr. Stone, and the service said that Dr. Scanlon was on call.

SARAH: I had been home less than an hour when David called and asked me to return. When I returned Pat was in active labor, and was about 6 centimeters dilated.

PAT: David and I were walking around the block at about 11:00 P.M., squatting during contractions.

SARAH: Pat's labor was progressing very quickly, but she did not want to move to the hospital. However, she did not seem to feel safe at home, either.

PAT: I had to decide where to have my baby. I felt reluctant to go to the hospital, since Dr. Scanlon was on call. I had met him only once, and I wasn't impressed. However, at about 1:00 A.M. we finally decided to go to the hospital. I can remember the crazy outfit I wore—a white tee shirt, a corduroy jumper, no underwear, sneakers and socks.

Sarah was wonderful. She never pitied me once. Whenever I complained about pains she just said, "That's good, good baby pressure." David was great, too. He went through every contraction with me and kept me going. By the time we got to the hospital, he sounded like a Sarah clone.

COMMENTS: *Good labor support is not sympathetic. Good labor support is not feeling for the person, wishing you could take away their pain. Good labor support is letting them know that the pain and pressure they are experiencing are positive, normal, and natural feelings that MUST HAPPEN if the labor is to complete itself with the blossoming forth of a baby through the woman's own power.*

PAT: They put the fetal heart monitor on once when I arrived. The nurse asked me to urinate but I couldn't. I hadn't urinated since about 10:00 P.M. Nevertheless, they proceeded to give me two IV's.

COMMENTS: *Though it is of the upmost importance to remain hydrated during labor (one of the functions of the IV), it is also extremely important to empty the bladder. Having a distended bladder can interfere with the progress of labor, as the distended bladder can actually prevent descent of the baby. In addition, having a distended bladder during pushing can cause bladder damage either temporarily or permanently. Therefore, as Pat had been drinking throughout the labor as well as openly in the hospital and had not urinated at all during that period, the bladder should have been checked and possibly catheterized before running any further fluids via IV. In this case, the IV fluids themselves carried a potential risk of causing further problems.*

PAT: The staff was amazed at how far along I was.

SARAH: The resident came in, examined Pat and said she was fully dilated. Then the chief resident came in, examined her, and said she was fully dilated. Then about 15 minutes later Dr. Scanlon came in.

PAT: He examined me and told me, "My, but you DO have a triangular pelvis. How large was your last baby? Well, this baby is much larger." He then told me to start pushing.

SARAH: It was very obvious to me that Pat had made wonderful progress, but that she was not going to be given much opportunity or much time to push this baby out. The nursing staff was very cooperative in letting me in as a labor support person, and also in not interfering with what Pat needed.

SARAH: I suggested squatting to Pat. She proceeded to squat on the bed. Her pushing was ineffective.

PAT: I was pushing my bottom down into the mattress.

COMMENTS: *At this point in labor, many women push ineffectively, as it takes time for them to learn to respond to their body's signals about letting the baby come down.*

PAT: Dr. Scanlon criticized the way I was pushing, saying I was wasting a lot of energy. At one point, four people were telling me "the correct way to push"—Dr. Scanlon, the nurse, David and Sarah. I filtered everyone out except David and Sarah. I tried lying down, but I didn't like that. I suppose I already had it in my mind that I wanted to squat. At this point, Dr. Scanlon remarked, "Remember, you have a small, triangular pelvis," and left the room. I remember thinking that he would do a cesarean if things didn't progress.

We then moved to the floor—Sarah behind me and David on the floor below.

SARAH: It was very important for me to position myself behind Pat. I did not want it to appear to the hospital that I was infringing upon their territory, nor did I want to raise political questions about my usual role in birth as a lay midwife in a state where lay midwives are clearly outlawed.

PAT: I was pushing and David said he saw the head. He told me to touch it.

SARAH: Dr. Scanlon was standing in the doorway and the nurse was changing the bed. Both the nurse and the doctor were aware that Pat was squatting on the floor. However, Pat was not aware that the doctor had been in the doorway throughout the time she was pushing.

PAT: Suddenly, I saw Dr. Scanlon's feet coming through the doorway of the labor room. Even though the head was crowning I was afraid that Dr. Scanlon still might do a cesarean. So, I pushed really hard, and whoosh! Eric was born, all at once, at 3:13 A.M. I was surprised to see him so fast! David caught him and I immediately said, "It's a boy!" I was very happy and excited. I almost felt drunk.

Dr. Scanlon began screaming, "Get the baby!", and Eric began to cry. I knew everything was all right. David went to the delivery room with Eric. I got up onto the table, and they wheeled me to the delivery room. Eric was covered with a lot of blood and they were cleaning him up. My placenta came out easily, and then Dr. Scanlon examined my scar.

SARAH: Pat had sustained a fourth degree tear through her rectal sphincter.

PAT: As Dr. Scanlon sewed me up, he said that my tearing wasn't necessary, and that I had gotten blood on his mocassins. But I was so happy that I didn't pay much attention.

COMMENTS: *Dr. Scanlon was absolutely correct. Pat's tear had been sustained unnecessarily. Had he not attempted to undermine her confidence in her ability to birth her own baby, had he not subtly threatened her with a cesarean if progress were not rapid, she absolutely would not have sustained such a deep tear. Her fear of having a cesarean caused her to blast her baby out! Blasting the baby out causes tears. When mothers are given the space to simply follow their own bodies' cues as to when and how much to push (especially when they are in an upright position such as squatting), the babies are usually born smoothly with little or no tearing.*

Unfortunately Dr. Scanlon blamed squatting for the tears. He blamed Sarah for the tears. He even threatened to press charges against Sarah, but of course he had no grounds for charges. He could not see that the attitude he brought with him into the birthplace had triggered deep and powerful fears causing the woman to tear herself wide open to avoid being cut by his knife!

PAT: Initially, I felt anger toward Sarah and David for letting me push so hard once Eric's head had crowned. But I know now that it was my own fear of another cesarean that made me push so hard.

David and I were very happy and excited about our birth. I'm sure they're still talking about us at that hospital. And Eric will probably grow up to be a football player some day with those shoulders!

A few months after Pat delivered her baby squatting on the floor, another pregnant woman took a tour of the delivery suite there. She asked the nurse quite innocently (never having heard the story of Pat's birth), "Can I squat to deliver?" The nurse looked aghast and replied, "Well, we've had a lot of problems here with squatting"

Pat, David, David John (3), and Eric (8 mos.) Kowalek, Christmas 1984

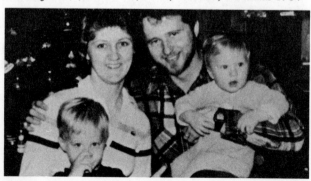

6

Abandoned for Being Too Recalcitrant

ANDREA KELLY-ROSENBERG

ANDREA: This story is very, very precious to me. It is like part of my flesh, or a child. It is a sacred gift I offer you. I did not know that the story of this birth would grow to have such significance to me. Its significance grows and changes with time, and I feel it will continue to do so. Because of its preciousness to me, I find I cannot tell you all of it. It is not an issue of confidentiality, it is a matter of possessiveness—I still feel too possessive, too attached to my story to give it all away yet, like a baby who is too young to be left with a sitter.

My Cesarean Birth—Noah

I had Noah by lower-segment cesarean section after 17 hours of pitocin-induced labor (beginning labor with an artificial hormone), following ruptured membranes (the membranes which contain the amniotic fluid surrounding and protecting the fetus have been ruptured). The diagnosis was cephalo-pelvic disproportion (CPD).

COMMENTS: *Cephalopelvic disproportion (CPD) is a relative diagnosis indicating that this particular baby's head is supposedly too large for this particular mother's pelvis at this particular time.*

ANDREA: Noah's apgars were 7 and 9, and he weighed 7 lbs. 12 oz. Initially I was delighted to be rescued out of the horrendous pitocin contractions that did nothing to dilate me (I stayed at 4 centimeters for 10 hours). However, by two months post partum I was beginning to have nagging doubts. When I expressed them to my obstetrician, he told me, "The real reason we have so many cesareans now is because you middleclass dames don't want to put up with the pain of labor." That did it I was a medical establishment heretic as well as a radical feminist from that day forward.

The emotional pain surrounding my cesarean was tremendous. The feeling of total lack of control, of having my power stolen from me, the pain of being separated from my husband, Rob, and then from Noah, and the condescension and lack of understanding I received from most people, was almost too much to bear. I spent many sleepless nights during those early months, crying—wishing, it had all been so different.

19

I had good experiences mothering Noah, but I think that was because I belonged to a wonderful new mothers' support group. Otherwise I think the lack of confidence I felt because of the cesarean experience would have contributed to a disastrous post partum.

I first heard about VBAC from a Nancy Wainer Cohen article that a friend gave me. I was elated and challenged by it. I wanted another child but I never could have put myself through that horror show of cesarean section again, at least not without giving my body a good solid chance to prove itself under ideal conditions.

I started to look for a birth attendant before I conceived, for I was unwilling to conceive without knowing I could have what I needed—a natural, unmedicated, untechnological labor. I had a few false starts. One family practitioner looked at me like I was from Mars; another said that his "ass would be grass" if he took on a technically "high risk" situation like mine. The homebirth midwife here declined to accept me as a client. And the next-most-natural-and-respectful birth attendant was Linda, my midwife. She had to get special permission to take me on. I believe I was her first VBAC. At first even she was skeptical and I had to talk her out of my CPD diagnosis from my previous cesarean. She was not one for routine IVs or monitors, two things I desperately didn't want. So I got pregnant.

COMMENT: Shortly before the onset of labor with her second pregnancy, Andrea wrote me this letter:

Dear Lynn,
    I write this with a certain amount of self-consciousness that is overcome by my loneliness. I don't know any other VBAC mothers! NOT ONE!
    I know a couple of cesarean mothers waiting in the ranks to see how I do (a rather uncomfortable position—I am a test case for them). I can support them in their interest in a VBAC, but they are little support for me in my uncertain moments.
    My husband is a total and wonderful support. He has educated himself to the hilt, and is the only person I trust absolutely and completely for the total letting-go of labor. But he is a man, and I have long ago accepted the separation between us that is determined by our bodies. What I mean is, he can never completely know what it is to be pregnant, be in labor, have a cesarean, or nurse a baby.
    Except for Rob, all along I have had to talk people into a natural VBAC. My labor support person initially thought I was nuts, though she's totally on the bandwagon now, after much effort on my part. My friends love me, and know how important a VBAC is for me, and so out of their love have been supportive. But I can tell they are worried and skeptical, too, and besides they just aren't VBAC mothers.
    YOU ARE THE ONLY VBAC MOTHER I KNOW. Period. And as things get down to the wire and I look at what's behind and what's ahead, I feel incredibly lonely for another VBAC mother—not just a VBAC mother, but one who wants to take responsibility for her own birth, who's not willing to be hooked up to the machines and take her chances with the

doctors. *As far as I can tell, I am the first woman in the Portland area to have this sort of VBAC—the other VBACs I have heard about have been fully mechanized affairs, though still "successful."*

I have been so occupied with the work of creating my own birth, of preparing myself in all ways, of preparing Noah, that the loneliness of this position didn't hit me until a few days ago, after I put the polishing touches on my birth letter.

I remember thinking about setting up a support group when I first was contemplating VBAC. But as a working mother (running a nursery school) it just seemed like too much to take on—especially since I didn't know how much real support I would get. I thought I might end up giving more support than I would get. I don't regret this decision , but nevertheless I find myself feeling very alone-in-the-struggle right now.

My VBAC Birth—Laura

Laura weighed 7 lbs. 4 oz. with apgars of 7 and 9. The length of my labor was: 5 hours at home, the last 3 fairly hard; 10 hours in the hospital, all of it wimpy and frustrating; then, following a night of morphine-induced rest at the hospital, 10 final hours of good hard labor resulting in (at last!) the happy event. I don't just say "35 hours of labor" since I think that gives a very false impression of how things really went.

The two major problems with my labor were that my fear of the hospital weakened my contractions, and my midwife didn't really have faith that I could deliver vaginally. She thought my lack of progress during day one of my labor was because something was indeed wrong with my pelvis, whereas I knew that I was tense because of the hospital. The irony was that her negativity made me get even more tense, and slowed my labor even more; my lack of progress made *her* even more doubtful and we got into a terrible vicious circle. I was horribly discouraged—I *knew* I could have that baby, and I was very angry that I had not planned a homebirth, even though I couldn't find a midwife who would do it at home.

Fortunately, the obstetrician on call was more positive. She suggested at a point when I just about wanted to throw myself out the window, that I take a shot of morphine and go to sleep, and see if things would pick up in the morning. At first I was suspicious, but what she said made sense, so I did it. Rob went home to be with Noah, and our friend and labor coach, Marla, went home, too.

I didn't sleep at first. My contractions stopped, and I felt a pleasant rush of relaxation from the morphine, so I was able to think clearly. At first I thought, well, I'm going to be another cesarean. How am I going to deal with that? I knew the cesarean was not going to be a medical necessity, but was a result of my midwife and the hospital getting me so up tight. But still, for about the first hour of my thinking, it seemed inevitable to me.

Then something changed. I don't know how or why. I was NOT going to have a section! I simply was not. How was I going to get people off my back, then, long enough to get my labor re-going? I thought about this for awhile, as I listened to obstetricians condescend to women in labor down the hall. The answer come to me all at once—I won't let anyone examine me. They can listen to the baby, but they can't examine me every two hours. If no one knows how much progress I've made or failed to make, they can't shake their heads in that discouraging, negative way that makes my contractions weaken. I'll give myself the day (I decided), until 5:00 P.M., as long as the baby is OK, to get my labor to show some strength.

After I had made this decision, and rehearsed confrontations with my midwife a few times in my mind, I did fall asleep for a few hours. A contraction woke me up at 4:00 A.M. and by 7:00 A.M. I was working fairly hard. I brushed my teeth, washed my face, and started over.

I had to fight hard to have my own way. When I did let my midwife examine me, at 9:00 A.M. I was still 4 centimeters. She did her headshaking bit again, and said I'd need a pressure catheter and perhaps pitocin.

COMMENTS: *When a woman's labor has been arrested (without progress) for several hours in active labor, judicious use of pitocin can often stimulate contractions enough to complete the dilatation. Pitocin is a chemical simulation of the hormone oxytocin which is secreted by the woman's body during labor. Pitocin is usually administered via IV because it can be most carefully controlled when administered in this manner. Pitocin is a powerful drug. Although it can be of significant assistance when definintely indicated, it also carries significant risks to both the mother and the fetus. Misuse of pitocin may cause uterine rupture as well as fetal distress. Usually a pressure catheter is inserted into the womb of the mother via her vagina to measure the strength of the contractions, and an internal monitor is attached to the scalp of the baby to monitor the baby's heart rate while pitocin is administered.*

However, pitocin is often misused. The key words are "arrest of active labor." We must first define whether or not this woman's labor was ever truly active labor. Usually a woman who is not yet 5-6 centimeters dilated is not yet in active labor. She can be having what appears to be very strong contractions yet still be in the inactive phase of her labor. Since the inactive phase is more frequently subject to interferences, the labor can be easily shut down by environmental or psycho-spiritual disruption. Therefore, what appears to be "arrest of labor" can actually be "disruption of labor." Often the key is to discover the cause of the disruption and ameliorate the problem as quickly as possible.

ANDREA: I put my foot down at that point—no pressure catheter, no pit, no more exams til 5:00 P.M. My midwife got pretty angry. That was hard. I wanted her to remain an ally, and it was hard to lose her.

She turned me over to the obstetrician on call. This one was a male doctor. He was not nearly as positive as the woman the day before, and was wholly obnoxious. I refused to let him examine me, and I refused to let him manipulate me by telling me I was compromising the baby's life. I told him I thought he was manipulating me, and of course he wanted nothing at all to do with me after that. This was at about 10:30 A.M., and from then until the birth we were really pretty much on our own.

Rob went out and recruited a nurse to listen to Laura's heartbeat every half hour for us. While I rested between contractions, it occurred to me suddenly that we were without medical supervision. We had been abandoned as too recalcitrant. I felt a quick fright at this. Then I thought, the alternative is a pressure catheter and pitocin, and that was so entirely unacceptable to me that I felt the courage to go on.

When I began to have the urge to push at about noon, I weakened my position on exams and Marla went to get the midwife to examine me. I was 5 centimeters, and Laura had moved down to about +1 station. At 1:00 P.M. I was nine centimeters and +3 station.

COMMENTS: *Stations approximate the descent of the baby through the mother's pelvis. The landmarks of the pelvis which define stations are the ischial spines which are palpable by the practitioner in the transverse (side to side) axis of the pelvis, approximately midway between the pelvic brim (top of the pelvis) and the outlet (bottom of the pelvis). Since the ischial spines are said to be the most narrow part of the woman's pelvis, once the baby has passed through the spines, the possibility of cephalopelvic disproportion is said to be dispelled.*

Just as dilatation is approximated in centimeters, so are the stations approximated in centimeters. If the presenting part is at the level of the ischial spines (midway through the pelvis) it is said to be at 0 station. If the baby is still approximately 2 centimeters above the landmark of the ischial spines, it is said to be at − 2 station. If the baby hs already passed through the spines and is now 3 centimeters below them, it is said to be + 3 station. Minus 5 station is defined as a head not yet into the pelvic brim, and + 5 station is crowning.

ANDREA: At 1:45 P.M. Laura was born. People have asked me how I knew my pelvis was large enough when I stayed again at four centimeters for so long, as with my first labor. In one sense I didn't know. But I wanted to give my body a fair shake—to labor without IV, monitor, and the negative atmosphere that I knew would keep me from birthing a baby. But in another sense I knew absolutely that I could birth that baby—it was just this very strong intuitive knowledge.

I had the things that were important to me—an unmedicated, un-hooked-up-to-the-machines delivery, no routine pitocin afterward, and constant contact with the baby and Rob afterwards. We had made arrangements with a supportive pediatrician that Laura not be sent to the nursery after birth, but be "check-in" at our bedside. She never left my sight.

Interestingly, the things that I felt less strongly about, I consistently didn't get—for example, the midwife did an episiotomy which I doubt was necessary, but that wasn't a huge issue to me. Then, there were the wrong assumptions that I had made—that the midwife would let the cord drain before cutting it. She didn't—she had my husband cut it right away. I think Laura's apgars would have been better if this had been delayed. The biggest mistake I made, that I would warn women against, is that I assumed my midwife would do certain things that she didn't do, so I didn't check them out beforehand. If I had to do it again, I would make absolutely NO assumption. None. I would check *everything* out, at least 2 or 3 times, while making eye contact.

But all in all, I was very happy with the birth. It is I feel my greatest accomplishment to date—I did much emotional and spiritual preparing for it, and it paid off. It was a tremendous growth experience, and made me feel very very powerful. I think I would tell other women who want a VBAC that you have to want it very badly. And you have to know, intuitively, exactly what you need to birth a baby. If that's a 3-piece band playing "Jingle Bells," — fine, trust that, and figure out some way to get it. I needed space and time, and I got it, and it worked. It was a beautiful and deeply spiritual experience.

COMMENTS: *When we fully accept our own aloneness in life, we come to terms with ourselves, with life and death, and push past that undefinable "something" into a consciousness far greater than we have experienced before in this life. Without Andrea's willingness to "do it alone," to "be alone," she might never have reached what she defined as "a beautiful and deeply spiritual experience."*

ANDREA: Whenever I face another difficult endeavor, I wish I had a nickel for every time I've moaned, "This is just like the VBAC. I feel so ALONE!" I now realize that in all of life, feeling alone is a normal and necessary result of taking on a large piece of work, not some kind of symptom of aberration or unacceptability.

My Home VBAC—Anna Augustine

ANDREA: I had a wonderful birth, though unusual. I poked along for 35 hours to get to 5 centimeters, sleeping between contractions, and eating now and then. The midwife finally broke my water, and Annie was born 49 minutes later! This was all at home!

7

My Baby, My Body: A Ward of the State?

GINA DISNEY

Gina: My labor with my first baby began with the rupture of membranes in the middle of the night. I went to the hospital the next morning without contractions. After we arrived, meconium was discovered in the fluid.

COMMENTS: *Meconium is the baby's first bowel movement. Usually, the baby does not pass meconium until after it is born. However, if the baby has been stressed, the anal sphincter may relax thus releasing the meconium prematurely. Although the presence of meconium in and of itself is not a complication, it may be an indicator (not an absolute diagnosis) of possible or potential fetal distress.*

GINA: Because of the meconium I was admitted to the hospital to be monitored even though I was only 3 centimeters dilated. After I was hooked up to the monitor my husband, Ricky, paid more attention to the bleeping machine than he did to me!

The doctor started IV pitocin, saying, "It's good to have an open vein in case of emergency." But I thought I was only having a baby!

COMMENTS: *Though the presence of meconium staining does indicate possible stress, and therefore the need to closely monitor the well-being of the baby (in my opinion, not necessarily with an electronic monitor), and even the need to get the labor moving, the use of pitocin at this time is actually contraindicated when a baby is already in questionable distress. Unfortunately, most medically trained practitioners are not aware of, or are not open to, other methods to induction that might be less stressful to both the mother and the baby. Going for a walk, taking a shower, a castor oil/herbal induction, an enema, talking about fears of labor would all be possible methods of induction far less stressful than pitocin to both mother and baby.*

GINA: The next examination was the first time I heard the words cesarean section. "What? No, not me. I took care of myself! Not me! It was supposed to be one of those other women, not me!" I was told to calm down. Hysterics were not going to help anyone or anything.

Following a set of x-rays and the insertion of the internal monitor, the doctor came in and examined me again. I was three to four centimeters dilated. He said, "The x-rays show that you have a borderline pelvis. It measures 9.5. If the baby is of low birth weight, say 6 or 7 pounds, you could possibly pass it. "Pass it? We weren't talking about a kidney stone. People "pass" kidney stones. Women give "birth" to babies! If the baby is over seven and a half pounds, you will have a very hard delivery. There is the possibility of brain damage, and possibly death since the pelvis may not be large enough to accommodate and let the baby's head through. I'm suggesting now a cesarean. It's safe, fast and the only alternative at this point."

I still couldn't believe it! I asked for more time. He looked at the clock and gave me one hour to "get the baby down" and left. This man was talking death. This was supposed to be birth . . . life. What woman and man in their right mind would refuse surgery when you truly believed your baby's life was in danger?

COMMENTS: *When doctors speak to laboring women about the possibility of death or brain damage to the unborn baby, the doctor knows that the parents will agree to anything he then suggests (usually a cesarean). Whether or not the doctor actually is consciously manipulating the parents' decision, they remain powerless unless either they themselves have pursued the study of midwifery or they have the support of another midwife or professional labor support person. The woman cannot refuse all interventions simply because they are interventions. For there are times when interventions are actually necessary for the health of the mother and/or the baby. Such decisions must be made through knowledge not ignorance.*

GINA: Ricky and I discussed it and came to the conclusion that maybe we were being unreasonable. The doctor was probably right.

I was crushed! What about my Lamaze birth? What about me? I had never been cut open before.

Who had the answers? It was up to me to ask the questions and do research. I thought I had prepared myself by attending childbirth classes. I have since learned that childbirth classes are not enough. You have to explore all the alternatives yourself. It was my responsibility and I hadn't done it. I wasn't nearly as informed as I should have been, or thought I was.

COMMENTS: *Taking responsibility for our births (investigating all the possibilities and making decisions that are right for us) removes birth from the realm of fantasy and dreams, and places it clearly within reality. Often it is not until our dreams have been destroyed that we are willing to actually WORK to have a positive birth.*

GINA: Ricky and I signed to have the cesarean. I cried. How could Ricky be proud of me? How could I be the world's greatest Lamaze student? I hadn't even used any breathing techniques yet! How could this happen to me?

COMMENTS: *Gina's desire to be "the world's greatest Lamaze patient" created a pressure to perform that made her labor and birth a test of her abilities rather than a process through which she would flow and grow. Such pressure to do labor "right" can create deleterious effects on a woman's natural release in labor. When we feel those pressures to perform within ourselves, we may need to ask ourselves, "Who do we really need to be proud of us, to love us, to respect us—our husbands,*

our mothers, our fathers, ourselves?" When we find a way to love ourselves
regardless of how we may give birth to our babies, we give ourselves the freedom
to let go of controls and give birth.

GINA: At 8:14 P.M., our 8 lb. 12 oz. baby girl was born by cesarean. She
didn't really cry, she just kind of hung there as she was held up for us
to see. A great feeling of pride and love came over me. She was so
beautiful! So pink and bald and fat! I was so happy, I cried. I looked
back at Ricky and said, "Isn't she beautiful?" He just stared at me. His
eyes were smiling, but I didn't see his lips to know for sure. I couldn't
see underneath the surgical mask.

The nurses wrapped up our Gillian in a blanket and gave her to her
daddy. I couldn't hold her since my hands were strapped down. I nuz-
zled her as Ricky held her next to my face. She smelled so good and
felt so soft. She still hadn't really cried all that much. She kind of whimpered, and stared right in our faces. I remember saying to Ricky, "Gee
that wasn't so bad. I really hadn't felt a thing."

Ricky was told at 11:00 P.M. that he had to leave. It was the first
time in our five years of married life that we wouldn't be sleeping
together. I was very lonely and scared once he left. I was especially
missing my baby. I had her underneath my heart for the past nine
months and all of a sudden we were separated. I felt very empty inside.

And then, without any warning, the pain was excruciating! It felt
like my abdominal area was being pierced by hot irons. I started to get
nervous. I went to ring for the nurse, and realized I had no call bell. I
was put into a room with two other women. As there was no bed available,
they just pushed me up against a wall and left me on the stretcher bed.
I didn't want to wake the other women so I lay there for a couple of
minutes just waiting for someone to pass by. It seemed like an eternity
and finally a man (I guess it was a new father going back to his wife in
labor), passed by. I yelled to him, "Would you please get a nurse for
me?"

About five minutes later the nurse arrived. I said, "I'm starting to
feel a lot of pain. Could you please get me my doctor?" She said the
doctor had left and that she would see what he had ordered. "Left?
How could he leave a patient immediately after surgery? I thought they
had to stay to make sure you were all right." The nurse laughed when
I said that to her. She said, "That only happens on TV!" She came back
later with a pill. I couldn't sleep at all. The pain continued to worsen.
I called for a nurse again, and she said she'd get me something a little
stronger.

The next morning I awoke and immediately wanted my daughter.
My husband arrived with a bouquet of beautiful flowers, and we spent
the rest of the day with our daughter. I was happy and believed what
we did was right.

It was not until a few months later that I started to doubt that I really
needed a cesarean. I read all I could about cesareans and VBAC. I
learned that what was once a life-saving procedure was becoming routine. Then, I went to hear Lynn Richards speak about cesareans. I didn't

even know this woman and it was as if she knew one of the most intimate parts of my life! Everything that she said happens, happened to me. Everything that she said cesarean mothers feel, I felt.

I realized that I had put my faith and my trust in my OB rather than myself and my body's ability to open up and bring forth my child. It happened and I couldn't change it, so I had to accept it. I did, but I swore next time it would be different.

We started looking for a doctor. One doctor agreed to do a VBAC, but wanted to "set a date for surgery anyway." I just walked out on him. Others were supportive, but didn't think my chances were good. Their words were "not a good candidate." Some asked me why I would want to put myself through such an ordeal, since most attempts fail anyway. I heard it all! I was really getting discouraged.

Finally, I found a doctor I liked (Dr. Smith). When I interviewed him, we talked about my first birth, my feelings about it, and what I expected of him as a doctor. He did a pelvic exam to see the approximate size of my pelvis, and he told me it was an adequate pelvis. I left his office feeling very at ease and confident.

However, he had an associate (Dr. Jones) who wasn't as supportive of VBAC. Every time I saw him, he reminded me about my alleged CPD (cephalo-pelvic disproportion—see glossary), and the fact that I only had a 50-50 chance. He was just so negative.

In my 6th month, Dr. Jones wanted me to have a glucose tolerance test (a blood test to screen for diabetes). I asked him, "Why?" He said there had been a "sugar show" in my urine that morning (a Monday after a long weekend of cake, cookies, etc.), and that my first child was 8 lb. 12 oz., which he considered to be large. I had a history of diabetes in my family, so he just wanted to do this as a precaution. The test did not seem to be necessary to me. I didn't have any problems with my health with my first pregnancy; I had gained sixty pounds with Gillian, and only twenty-eight with my second; and all the women in my family had had big babies (between 7 and 11 pounders).

On my way home from my appointment I bought urine test sticks to test my urine myself everyday. In the month that followed, sugar had spilled lightly only twice. I decided not to have the test. When I didn't show up for the test, I was asked to sign a statement that I was informed of all the effects of diabetes on a pregnant lady and her baby.

COMMENTS: *Gina's attempt to take full and complete responsibility for the decisions surrounding this pregnancy was evidenced by her decision to test her own urine, and make a decision based upon her knowledge and the results of the tests. Urine test sticks can be purchased and used by anyone who can see variation in colors, comparing the results on the stick with the chart on the bottle. Gina did not blanketly refuse the test without attaining further knowledge. She refused the more complex test after doing successive simple urine tests.*

In my experience as a midwife, however, I do feel that it is possible (not necessarily probable) that Gina was marginally diabetic. Had she been my client, I would certainly not have recommended the glucose tolerance test, but might have recommended the less-invasive glycosolated hemoglobin and a serum glucose.

Although in order to have an accurate reading, all of these tests must be done following an over-night fast, the glucose tolerance test requires that the woman follow the fast with a heavy sugar load. In my opinion, a heavy sugar load following a fast could be dangerous to anyone, most especially a pregnant woman who is possibly diabetic.

However, since diabetes in pregnancy (even marginally) can create complications for mother and/or baby, without question I certainly would have worked with Gina on her diet. Dietary changes can often assist in the balance of blood sugar levels, thus preventing the complications which can occur with the consistently high blood sugar levels of diabetes.

GINA: At one prenatal visit I was really down and depressed. When Dr. Smith came in, he examined me and he said he could tell by my eyes that I wasn't doing well. I told him I was starting to doubt myself and my decision. Since the baby was my main concern, I just really wanted what was best for him/her. I had attended a VBAC seminar and I realized that I was scared to death of having another cesarean and of having a VBAC. He assured me that what I was doing was right and that I would have a beautiful, healthy baby.

Part of my doubts had stemmed from the attitudes of my family and friends. Their negativity affected me strongly. Except for a few loyal friends and my husband, everyone told me, "You're crazy to put yourself through all that pain for nothing. After all, you're going to end up sectioned anyway and the baby could die." Didn't these people realize that maternal mortality following cesarean delivery is much greater than maternal mortality following a vaginal birth? That infection is a common occurrence of cesarean mothers and babies? That, if I opted to have my baby "by appointment," he/she could be taken from me before he/she was ready? That pneumonia and lung/respiratory disease among cesarean babies is very high? How could anyone choose major surgery over at least trying a VBAC?

At my last office visit two days before I went into labor, I was 3 centimeters dilated and the baby was at "0" station [had descended to the level of the ischial spines in the mid-pelvis]. I thought that was terrific. I figured all systems were go.

When I went into labor, Dr. Smith was out of town. He had told me prenatally, that even if he wasn't on call, he would still attend my birth. But he wasn't there! I had a cup of herbal tea, got myself together and decided it would be okay.

My membranes ruptured at 4:00 A.M. At 6:15 we arrived at the hospital. The contractions were 3 minutes apart, lasting 90 seconds. When Dr. Jones came to examine me, I was 5 centimeters and the baby was still at "0" station. He gave me some time to get the baby down, (now where had I heard that before?) or else! I refused the fetal monitor and the IV. I insisted on a comfortable chair. I didn't care if they had to go to the Chief of Staff's office to get one!

One hour later I was seven centimeters dilated and the baby was at "0" station. Dr. Jones said "Gina, you're not doing well. I have office hours at noon today. Make up your mind. I'll be back at 8:00." Not doing well? I thought I was doing great. I had really dilated, something I hadn't done the first time around. The baby was still high but he could drop at the last minute.

COMMENTS: *Actually, for this stage in labor, the baby was not unusually high. Many babies remain at or even above the level of the ischial spines (0 station) until after the mother begins active pushing.*

GINA: I felt I was not even going to think about having a cesarean at this point. During all this, the contractions were one on top of the other and lasting a long time. The pain was excruciating! I would think a contraction was going down and immediately another peak would arise. This can't go on much longer. The baby had to have come down!

COMMENTS: *Back to back contractions and double peaking contractions are a sign of nearing the end of the first stage of labor.*

GINA: Dr. Jones came back in at 8:00 and told me I was being totally irrational and uncooperative in continuing with labor. He proceeded to tell me every horror story you could imagine. I told him to get out. He got another doctor for a second opinion. Doctor Brown came in and said I was 8 to 9 centimeters dilated and the baby was high for this point in dilation. He felt the baby was around 9 pounds, and after looking at my previous records, he concluded that he didn't think I would deliver vaginally.

COMMENTS: *Gina's labor was progressing quickly and well. There was absolutely nothing medically wrong with her or her baby. This scene was a power play, designed to undermine Gina's ability to birth her own baby. The doctor had a belief system which he needed to maintain—that women who have had previous cesareans for CPD (cephalo-pelvic disproportion) cannot possibly birth their own babies. He needed to stop Gina from dispelling his beliefs. He needed to dispell her faith in herself!*

GINA: I was really confused. Dr. Jones felt the baby to be around 7 pounds. Dr. Brown said 9 pounds. I was secretly hoping Dr. Jones was right.

Dr. Brown suggested I walk a bit to see if that would help. By then my body was full of pins and needles. I couldn't even stand, much less walk.

COMMENTS: *Dr. Brown was probably right. If she had gotten up and walked around, the head would probably have "come down." But Gina needed more than a simple suggestion. She needed a professional labor support person, someone knowledgeable in alternative approaches to obstetrics to give her the knowledge, confidence, and support she needed to complete her labor.*

GINA: I had withstood, thus far, more than 2 hours of transition. I was shaking, vomiting, freezing, and crying. My husband sent the doctors on their way and gave a good tongue lashing to one of them. He came back in and massaged my legs, got me a heated blanket, and washed up. Things felt better and looked better.

At 10:00 A.M. I was faced by the doctor and the hospital administrator telling me that if by 11:00 A.M. I hadn't decided to sign the cesarean papers, they would have a court order to deliver my (?) child by cesarean section. At this point I broke down. After all the reading and practicing I did, I never looked into the legal aspects of cesarean. We didn't know how to fight it.

COMMENTS: *Cases of court-ordered cesareans now stand on record in this country—one in Georgia, and one in Colorado, according to the Hastings Center Report, June 1982. In both of these cases the doctors had argued that without surgical delivery (cesarean) the fetus would die. However, in both cases the doctor's predictions were questionable.*

In the Georgia case (indication—placenta previa; see glossary), the woman's family petitioned the Georgia Supreme Court to stay the order for the cesarean, and a few days later, "the woman delivered a healthy baby without surgical intervention."

In the Colorado case (indication—fetal distress, see glossary), the baby was delivered by cesarean nine hours after the doctor had reported "distress" based upon the monitor tracings, and sought the court order because of the woman's refusal of surgery. The physician reported that he was surprised that the outcome was not poor—the baby was still healthy nine hours after diagnosis of fetal distress. He added, "The case simply underscores the limitations of continuous fetal heart monitoring as a means of predicting neonatal outcome."

Both cases underscore the fact that a pregnant woman's right to refuse surgery is slipping away. According to the Hastings Center:

> Do we really want to restrain, forcibly medicate, and operate on a competent refusing adult? . . . It encourages an adversarial relationship between the obstetrician and the patient, and gives the obstetrician a weapon to bully women he views as irrational into submission. Attempts at vaginal deliveries after cesarean, for example, may fall victim to such a rule. . . . It seems wrong to say that patients have the right to be wrong in all cases except pregnancy—in that case, why should only doctors have the right to be wrong?

The time for women to take action, to avoid losing their rights to informed consent in childbirth is now.

GINA: At 11:33 A.M., our 9 lb. 4 oz. son was delivered by cesarean. When they took Richard out of me I couldn't believe the size of him. He looked 3 months old! He was so fair—so different from his sister! The pediatrician said we could dress him and send him out to help the Jets! He was beautiful!

The next day I saw Dr. Smith. I wanted to yell at him. I wanted to ask sarcastically how his weekend was. I didn't get a chance because as soon as he came in he said he couldn't believe I put up with transition as I did. He didn't want to know how I was doing physically, he wanted to know how I was doing emotionally since he knew how much I didn't want to have a cesarean. I told him I couldn't believe that Dr. Jones was going to get a court order. Then he said to me, "If you were on a plane, would you tell the pilot how to do his job?" In other words I was being reprimanded for not obeying my almighty doctor. Anyway, who is the pilot in a birth? I say, "The woman is the pilot." The doctor is there in case of an emergency to intervene in life threatening situations.

The doctor's excuse for the cesarean was that my baby was tied up in the cord and that his head measurement was 14-3/4 inches. Who knows how it would have turned out, but I felt I had no choice. My unborn child was a ward of the state. Believe it?!

COMMENTS: *Without a doubt, Gina was faced with a labor intervention that few of us have ever considered—a court order to have a cesarean!*

Though it is probably true that by 10:00 A.M. the morning of her labor, Gina was without much bargaining power within the confines of the hospital, she might have maintained her power over her own body had she seen the writing on the wall, and made different decisions earlier.

What were the first signs that trouble was brewing? Dr. Jones was never supportive of VBAC! In her desperate search for a doctor, any doctor, who would support her decision to have a VBAC, she became so enamored with Dr. Smith's understanding and caring, that she dared not change doctors because of a "personality rift" with her favorite doctor's partner. She attempted to have a guarantee that the "good doctor" would be there. That might have seemed the perfect solution. But when he was not there for her when she went into labor, did she have to accept the "bad doctor"?

Though many times women have cesareans because they feel they have no choice, in reality we are never without a choice. What were Gina's choices?

1. She could have called a professional labor support person to come to her house to help her labor at home, then move to the hospital once the baby had moved down sufficiently that vaginal birth would be imminent.
2. She could have called her supportive friends to come to her house while she labored at home, and then go to the hospital.
3. She and her husband could have stayed at home alone until she felt birth was imminent, or just had the baby by themselves.
4. She could have decided to go to the hospital to "test the water" with Dr. Jones, being wary and having another plan in mind if he proved to be unsupportive to her labor and VBAC plans. Then when she found him to be intransigent in his opinion that she would need another cesarean, regardless of her wonderful progress in labor, she could have signed herself out of the hospital, enacting upon her secondary plan before the court order could have been obtained.

Gina unfortunately made the choice to accept a person as her birth attendant whom she knew to be negatively disposed toward her birth plans. Of course, she could not have known beforehand to what lengths this doctor would go in order to remain in power over her.

However, Gina's story should be a warning to all pregnant women— if you and your doctor/midwife (or their partner) are at odds prior to the labor, do not under any circumstances accept him/her as your birth attendant. *Always be prepared within yourself to have your baby by yourself, if need be!* Place the trust, first, in yourself and your baby; and secondly, only, in the professionals whom you have hired to assist you.

And what of the integrity of the "good doctor," Dr. Smith? He clearly knew what Gina needed and wanted. He even promised he would give it to her. He reneged on his promise. Was it not his responsibility to let her know he would be out of town? Did he have no intention whatsoever to be there for her, regardless of who was on call?

When push came to shove, the day after the birth, did Dr. Smith support Gina, or his partner, Dr. Jones? Well, we might say he appeared to support Gina. He wanted to know how she was feeling. Like a good daddy, he had to prove how much he loved her. He had to keep her loving (trusting) him. But to him, his partner had been right. To him he had to defend his partner under all circumstances, regardless of his decisions. To him his partner had had the right to abuse this woman, to sexually disempower her, to "rape" her by forcing an unwanted and unnecessary cesarean upon her. I wonder how sincere all of his "understanding and support" could have been. Or was he, too, baiting her, waiting for the moment when he could prove his ultimate control of the birth? How could she ever trust him again?

Yet, many of us are lured into trusting and returning to that same doctor again. Rather like an abused child or a battered wife, we hope that if we are only "good enough next time" that our daddy-doctor will treat us better. We love our doctors and remain loyal to them regardless of how cruelly we have been treated, because we are desperately in need of their love. But how many of those doctors who are so loved by us would even know our names if they met us walking down the street?

The relationship is out of balance. We all want to be loved and taken care of, but when we are grown up enough to be mothers having babies, we need to be grown up enough to realize that we really do life and birth on our own. Then, and only then, will we be able to choose to accept love and support without desperation, to have truly equal relationships with our birth attendants.

GINA: I gave it my all. I really labored for my son. I wouldn't trade that for anything, except maybe a vaginal birth! I needed to feel what it's like to push my own baby out of my own body. When I hear friends say what it had felt like to actually not be able to hold the urge to push, I actually get jealous! I've not yet felt that feeling. I don't care if it burns, hurts, rips, or anything else. I want to feel it, too!

8

Disco Birth

CAROLYN ANDERSON

One autumn afternoon while driving, I heard the most remarkable news story on the radio. A woman in labor had been admitted to one of the New York metropolitan area hospitals. The staff insisted on an IV and a monitor. She refused. She signed herself out of the hospital, and went to a local discotheque where she danced through her contractions. A little while later, she went into the women's room, and there she birthed her baby. She returned to the dance floor, her baby in arms, to finish the last dance.

9

Herpes Absolution

PAM MORRISON

The Birth of Erin

PAM: When I became pregnant with my first baby, I was extremely concerned about how my herpes might affect my unborn baby. We were living in West Virginia at the time, but moved back to New York specifically because I wanted to be taken care of by doctors who would have the latest information about herpes management.

However, I did not plan to have a cesarean. I planned on having a natural birth. During my pregnancy, I placed cesareans in the back of my mind. After all, that wasn't the way to do it right. One out of four women had sections. I didn't want to be that one. Looking back I think if cesarean prevention had been discussed in my childbirth classes, it might have been different.

COMMENTS: *Even when childbirth educators include cesarean prevention in their classes, cesarean prevention for herpes is rarely discussed. Most practitioners and educators don't realize that there may be ways to prevent herpes outbreaks. And many do not realize that the protocols for safety with herpes are not based upon conclusive studies, but rather are based upon a lack of knowledge of the etiology (causes) of neonatal herpes and its possible devastating outcomes.*

PAM: Two and a half weeks prior to my due date, I had what appeared to be an active genital herpes lesion. Even though no herpes cultures were done, my doctors decided to perform a cesarean. Since I knew prior to the birth that a cesarean was going to be performed, I wanted to be as prepared as possible. At the suggestion of my childbirth educator, I met with a woman who had had three cesareans. We spent several hours discussing the procedures of the operation. Under the circumstances, I tried to be as knowledgeable as possible in the limited time I had.

Before I went into labor, the lesion healed. However, no cultures were done to determine whether or not herpes was still active in my vagina or on my cervix. But my doctors still planned to do a cesarean.

COMMENTS: *Pam's doctors ascribed to the most common theory that the herpes virus continues to be communicable 2 to 3 weeks after an outbreak. So therefore, even though there were no active lesions at the time of labor, the doctors felt compelled to do a cesarean.*

PAM: I was allowed to go into labor, and for that I was excited. It was bad enough having to have a section. At least my baby could be born at its own time, not according to a doctor's schedule.

My 9 lb. 1 oz. girl was born by cesarean. My husband, Keith, was present for the entire procedure, and all the people in the OR were supportive. They all focused on the birth, and the doctor was describing every step. Keith saw everything. From the incision to the birth of the baby was only minutes. I cried, and couldn't stop crying because I was so relieved that my baby was out of me "disease-free."

COMMENTS: *As with many other mothers who have herpes, Pam had been so thoroughly frightened by dire medical predictions that even though she had followed the advice of her doctors (having a possibly unnecessary cesarean), she still feared that her baby would contract a fatal case of herpes. Her fears were not totally unwarranted, however. Studies at the Disease Control Center in Atlanta have shown that some babies born by cesarean to PREVENT herpes have still contracted neonatal herpes.*

PAM: I was thrilled to see my daughter's beautiful face. But I didn't get to hold Erin in the OR. Keith held her in the OR and I was glad that at least he got to bond with her. But looking back, I feel ripped off.

COMMENTS: *Father-centered cesareans (cesareans where the father participates in the birth and bonds with the baby instead of the mother) have now become "the rage" in operating rooms across the country. Mothers are supposed to be grateful that their husbands are mothering their babies, while they lie like lumps of lard on their backs with their hands tied as if they were being crucified.*

Often months later when the woman's feelings of being ripped-off surface, her husband has great difficulty in understanding what she feels she has lost.

For the most part, although the mother's cesarean experience may be radically different from the birth she had envisioned, the father's experience has not been altered significantly from the experience he expected to have if his baby had been born vaginally. He feels, "the birth was perfectly fine—what is she complaining about?" Father-centered cesareans are not healing cesarean wounds. Father-centered cesareans may be creating marital schisms which are at best difficult to heal.

Though I would never advocate that fathers should be denied participation at a cesarean and immediate contact with the baby, these experiences must not be denied to the mother. These experiences are her birthright as a woman, regardless of the method of delivery!

PAM: Erin was put in isolation (separating her from everyone— including me) to "prevent the event of herpes." I asked to see Erin all day long, but wasn't allowed to see her until late that night. The nurse made me get out of bed and sit in a metal chair to hold her. I still had no feeling in my legs. It took forty five minutes to get out of bed into that damn chair. When they finally gave me my baby, I didn't even want her. They even made me wear sterile gloves when I held her. I felt totally defeated. The only saving grace in my relationship with my daughter was nursing. No matter what opposition I faced at the hospital, when I left she was all mine.

COMMENTS: *Pam's experience in "preventing the event of herpes" in the hospital demonstrates the medical paranoia and lack of understanding about herpes. Did the hospital staff truly expect that everything that Pam touched would be contaminated with herpes? She didn't even have an active lesion anywhere on her body at the time of birth!*

Hospitals don't ask anyone with a cold sore or canker sore (oral herpes lesions) on their mouths to wear a sterile cover for their mouths or wear sterile gloves while handling their babies. It would seem to me that it would be far more likely for a baby to get herpes from their parents' (or nurses' or doctors') oral lesions than from their mother's genital lesion. Perhaps they should do daily smears of the mouths of every hospital staff person before they are permitted to enter the maternity floor, especially since more than 80% of the population of the United States has some form of herpes!

Since herpes is not a one-time-only disease, attempting to isolate a mother from her baby to prevent the baby from contracting herpes is a ridiculous solution. Eventually, the mother is going to take her baby home. She will be the primary caretaker, and will not be wearing sterile gloves for the rest of her child's life!

In some of the more prominent hospitals in the country, herpes contamination is prevented not by isolation of the mother from her baby, but by obligatory 24-hour rooming-in—isolating the mother and baby together! Sounds like it might even be to your advantage to have herpes(?) They'll never take your baby back to the nursery to give him sugar-water!

PAM: I had Erin in a Catholic hospital. The priest wouldn't even come in the room to give me communion. The hospital stay was a horror— only reinforcing guilt and totally finishing the job of taking away any remaining self-confidence, self-respect, and dignity I had as a woman and mother. How dare I have a baby when I was a diseased person! These feelings remained inside of me for months.

COMMENTS: *If we took a survey about the most guilt-producing shameful fear-inducing condition a person in American society today could contract, I'm sure herpes would be second only to AIDS. The media and medical model have together succeeded in frightening and manipulating people into believing that everyone who has herpes is a bad person—that the only way for anyone to contract genital herpes is through illicit sexual contact.*

In my experience in counseling women with genital herpes in pregnancy, the overwhelming majority contracted the disease within a monogamous relationship, often through oral sex, at a time in their life of high stress, either physically or emotionally. Isn't it time to throw off the chains of accusations and guilt, and help everyone to understand how to deal with herpes?

PAM: Postpartum recovery was a lifetime—mainly because of how I felt about myself. Having a new little person in your life is an adjustment that no amount of preparation can ready you for—your entire center of being is altered forever. Adding that responsibility to the recovery from the operation, I felt like a baby trying to take care of a baby.

My feelings of self-worth and sexuality were pretty much shot to hell after this birth experience. I felt that I had failed as a woman. I was that one out of four! It took months to even feel any sexual desire. I know that the libido is naturally lower when you are nursing. But the section certainly robbed me of my positive feelings about myself. When a woman sees her pubic hair completely shaven, an incision that is freshly healing, stretch marks and a saggy stomach—well, needless to say she doesn't feel sexy or feminine!

COMMENTS: *Often women who have just experienced a cesarean find that their sense of self-worth and their sexuality has just been reduced to zero. Not only is their sexual desire nil, they may actually experience pain with intercourse. The vaginal pain can be very perplexing to their husbands, and even to their doctors. They reason, "The baby didn't come out of her vagina, so she has no reason to feel any pain there." On the contrary, if a woman has experienced much emotional pain especially regarding her birth and sexuality, if she feels a deep loss at not having been able to push out her own baby through her own vagina, her vagina may become a holding place for her emotional pain, which then translates into physical pain. Help a woman to deal with her frustrations about her birth, and you may find a re-emergence of her sexuality.*

PAM: Because Keith and I believed we had made the best choices for Erin's birth, I never connected any of these feelings with the section. I just believed I was going through a real rough adjustment. I joined a mother's center, but still didn't feel comfortable sharing the real reason for my cesarean—herpes. I told everyone I met I had had a cesarean for CPD (cephalo-pelvic disproportion). Not until I became pregnant again did my feelings about my cesarean surface, and I knew there had to be a better way to give birth.

COMMENTS: *Often the adjustment to motherhood does not leave much room for processing our own feelings about ourselves and our birthing experiences. Sometimes we set aside our feelings unconsciously for our own survival. Sometimes we set aside our feelings because we are afraid to deal with them, or have no support for dealing with them—everyone expects us to be happy because we have a healthy baby! But eventually, as with any difficult experience, our feelings must come out. Often, they surface with the next pregnancy.*

PAM: In retrospect I feel if I had really been more aware I would never have agreed to go along with the system and have a cesarean. I believe that having a first baby is such a learning experience. Boy, was I naive! I'm no longer angry about what happened. I truly believe it has changed the way I see and do things. I now realize that I am the one who makes things happen in my life.

The Birth of Sean

PAM: I first heard about VBAC at a lecture given by my gynecologist at a local mother's center. Knowing that VBAC was possible was the deciding factor in having a second child and going through a second pregnancy. At least there was hope of having a vaginal delivery!

But becoming pregnant brought out all of my buried feelings of inadequacy surrounding my daughter's birth. Somehow I had to do better this time, but how? I contacted my birth instructor from our first experience, who put us in touch with Lynn.

COMMENTS: *Pam and Keith joined my VBAC class.*

PAM: At first I felt uncomfortable being with this new group of people at Lynn's house. But when we heard what they had been through, and we realized that they listened to us without condemning us, we were making progress. Before I could successfully have this baby vaginally and guilt-free I had to work through many emotions. This healing process took many months, and much help, effort, and support.

The pregnancy went too fast in terms of going over the previous pregnancy and working things through emotionally. Any woman who has had a cesarean should receive (and seek it out if it's not readily available) emotional support instead of burying all those feelings. They go too deep.

COMMENTS: *Pam and I worked individually as well as in the class on helping her to feel confident that she would not have another outbreak of herpes. We discussed diet and supplements that would help to avert a herpes outbreak. And we worked on the emotions that are often connected with herpes—guilt, anger, frustration, and fear for the baby.*

We discussed the use and misuse of the herpes cultures which empowered her to make her own decisions about whether or not to have the prophylactic cultures done on the usual schedule of once a week from 36 weeks to onset of labor. She decided to have one culture done. But the wrong test was done. The doctors wanted her to come in to have a retest, but she refused. Pam had begun to trust her own body's signals.

As she began to feel more comfortable with herself, with or without herpes, she began to feel her own power.

PAM: At first I thought my greatest fear was rupture of my incision. But it really wasn't—it was being able to let go, and at the same time not let someone else step in and take over my responsibilities. My body is mine, yet I have been raised to look up to the medical profession—to listen and do as told. This was going to be different. I was going to have our baby, I was going to hold our baby and nurse him immediately — no one was going to separate us.

We continued to use our previous doctor for this pregnancy. He now had a new partner. Dr. G was supportive of VBAC's but his partner, Dr. O, was another story. "Against VBAC's" should have been his name. When confronted with our list of requests his back went right up against the wall. When I went into labor he wanted me "in the hospital immediately because anything could happen." He told us all kinds of things to try to change our minds. So, instead of feeling that we had no choices, with Lynn's support, we arranged with another doctor who practiced further from our house to act as a backup in case Doctor O was on call when I went into labor.

COMMENTS: *When Pam related Dr. O's attitudes about VBAC to me, I advised her to find another doctor. But she felt so good about Dr. G, that she did not want to leave his practice. So, I suggested that she talk to Dr. G, to ask him to be on-call for her rather than taking her chances with the luck of the draw. In addition, I suggested she contact another doctor, Dr. L, whom I knew to be supportive of VBAC, to ask him to act as backup in case Dr. G didn't come through for her. Much to my surprise, Dr. G promised Pam that he would be there for her, that she could count on him attending the birth no matter who was on-call when she went into labor. In addition, Dr. L agreed to act as backup. Pam would not be stuck with the luck of the draw!*

PAM: My "due date" was November 17. Keith and I walked everywhere. I thought I'd walk this baby out. I had strong Braxton Hicks (pre-labor) contractions daily, and was this baby low!

Well, the 17th came and went. So did the 18th, 19th, and 20th. Finally, on the 21st when it was time for bed I started having contractions every 20 minutes. Mild, but strong enough to have to breath deeply through them. I spent the night on the couch. I knew I was in labor but I stayed very calm. Because this was my first real labor I knew it would probably be a long one. A few times I got up and went to the bathroom. Loose bowel movements and steady contractions. Keith was asleep and I tried sleeping in between contractions.

About 5:00 in the morning I knew things were changing—the contractions were coming closer and I could use some support. I called my midwife, Lynn, to tell her I was actually in labor. She and her assistant arrived at my home. I was pretty proud of myself for having gone through the night alone. But now I knew I needed support and was glad to have it. We all had tea and toast, and talked as I walked around beginning to feel more uncomfortable.

COMMENTS: *Pam made wonderful progress. At 8:00 A.M. though the head was still a bit high, approximately −2 station, Pam's cervix was 4 to 5 centimeters dilated and 75 percent effaced (thinned). An hour later she was 7 centimeters dilated and station 0.*

PAM: Keith called the office and Dr. O was on call. He told Keith to get me right in! I was doing wonderfully, no way was I going in! My plan was to get to 9 centimeters, and then go in. No sooner. When I found out Dr. G wasn't on-call I was mad, especially because he had promised me he would be there for me.

The phone call really set me back. I tensed up, holding my baby in. I could feel that the baby had moved back up again.

COMMENTS: *The moment Pam got on the phone to talk to the doctor, her energy changed. After all these hours of smooth labor, she suddenly began to have difficulty coping with her contractions. When she got off the phone, I suggested to Pam that we could transport to Dr. L, who had agreed to act as backup. But she did not want to have to travel such a great distance in labor (about an hour).*

PAM: I decided to try to have the baby at home, so Lynn set up for a home birth. But hours went by, walking and contracting. I made progress but if we hadn't called the doctor I know I would have done better.

COMMENTS: *Instead of Pam's contractions growing stronger and closer, her contractions spaced out. She was still making progress, but the rate of progress had slowed down significantly. At 11:30 she was 8 centimeters, fully effaced, and the baby's head was back down to station 0, which was certainly heartening. At 12:30 she was 9 centimeters, and was feeling a bit pushy.*

PAM: It was a very warm day for late November. The sun was strong and the sky was a bright blue. I wanted to see my baby and hold him. I had to pull myself together.

Whoever thinks having a baby is easy is crazy. It's hard work. It's a test of endurance and it hurts! Thank God I had the support I had. I thank God I stayed home for as long as I did. I was not going to a hospital to have tubes in my arms, drugs pumped in, and have another cesarean.

COMMENTS: *At 1:30, Pam still had a cervical lip (she was fully dilated except for a "lip" which was still in front of the baby's head). The lip was slightly edematous (swollen). I massaged her cervix, and during contractions when the head would move down, I could push the lip up behind the head. However, between contractions the baby's head would slide back up, the cervical lip would come back down, and we were back to square one.*

We asked her to try to urinate to give the baby more room to come down, but she was unable to do so. So we catheterized her. However, this made no difference whatsoever in the station of the baby.

Judging from the initial fast progress of the labor and the ease of the initial descent of the baby, it appeared to me that something besides a mechanical process was holding up the birth of this baby. It was then that I asked Pam if she really would prefer to have her baby in the hospital, if she would feel safer there.

PAM: Everyone could tell, myself included, that I was holding back. I was afraid to have this baby at home.

COMMENTS: *A woman's emotional state, how safe she feels, has an immeasurable effect upon the course and outcome of her labor. When a woman feels safe, she lets go easily. When she is in conflict, she holds her muscles tight, holding the baby up, and at times may even reverse the progress of labor. Whenever a woman's progress appears to be impeded, especially if she has gone backwards in labor, we must assess the psychological environment. Regardless of whether the birth is planned for home or hospital, the environment can be a significant factor in the outcome of the birth. We must always be ready to change our plans in order to find a safe place to give birth.*

PAM: We called the doctor's office again, and this time Dr. G was on call. He would meet us at Stony Brook. From that point on my contractions became controllable to me again. They still hurt like hell, but I felt at ease somehow. We got to the hospital at 4:10 P.M.

COMMENTS: *Upon examination by the doctor, Pam was 9 centimeters dilated, and the head was "high," no further definition being given. She had arrived at the hospital at just the dilatation she had originally envisioned.*

However, although she had made arrangements with the doctor in advance to be able to have both her husband and another labor coach with her, when we arrived, the nurses refused to allow her more than one labor support person. So I left the hospital, waiting to hear the news of Pam's birth from afar.

PAM: I gave birth to my son at 6:10 p.m., November 22. All 22 1/2 inches and 8 lbs. 10 oz. of him—without an IV or any other interventions.

My emotions were so mixed—I was tired, my bottom was sore and swollen. But I was drug-free, awake, and I had done it! I was so proud of myself! What a thrill to hold my Sean and nurse him right after he was born. I cried, I laughed, I did it!!

Later that night Dr. O. came into the room and said, "Congratulations, I want to know you're the talk of the hospital."

"Ha," I thought to myself, "not if you'd been here."

Even though I hope that if I were to have another child I could have that baby at home, I felt I made the right choices for Sean's birth. I'm glad that Lynn fully supported my decision to go to the hospital when I did. Perhaps that small fear of the unknown, not knowing if I could actually do it, held me back from a home birth.

It was so wonderful to tell everyone I had a VBAC. Even now two years later so many people I meet still believe, "Once a section, always a section." Thank God there are women that know in their hearts that their bodies are theirs, and to trust in themselves. If we don't, we are being robbed of the best experiences in our lives. I only pray that more women start questioning their experiences, and know that there is so much more out there.

My son's birth has been a changing point in my life, a very rewarding growing experience.

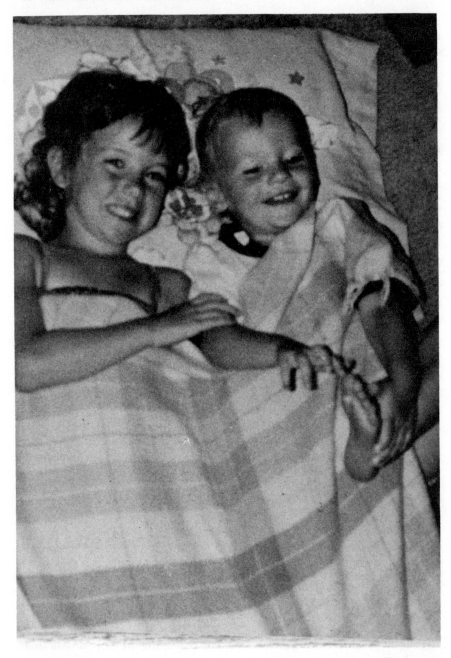

Erin (4½) and Sean (1½) Morrison

10

Laying the Bugaboo of Uterine Rupture to Rest: VBAC After Four Cesareans

MARY JO CAMILLUS

The Birth of Sheila

MARY JO: My husband and I attended "natural childbirth" classes during our first pregnancy and felt that we had prepared ourselves as well as possible for the birth. The class consisted of factual information, relaxation, and breathing, but there was certainly no attempt at educating us for cesarean prevention. Because I was in fine health and the pregnancy was completely uncomplicated, we hardly gave that possibility a second thought.

Our baby's due date was December 15, 1972. When I went into labor, it was December 28. My contractions were about 5 minutes apart when we set out for the hospital, 35 minutes or so away. By the time I arrived at the hospital, the contractions had slowed down. When the doctor did an internal exam and discovered that I had not begun to dilate, the immediately ordered pitocin and broke my waters. I was on my back with an external fetal monitor.

Suddenly I had a sustained and very painful contraction, unlike any other I had had. The fetal monitor showed a sudden drop in the baby's heart rate. The doctor decided the placenta must be in the process of detaching, and he immediately ordered the nurse to "prep" me for a cesarean, to "save the baby."

COMMENTS: *Although it may appear that the doctor was a hero because he did a cesarean to save the baby, the very emergency which threatened the baby's life may have been caused by the doctor's mismanagement of the labor.*

Artificial rupture of membranes (ruptured intentionally by the practitioner) can potentially cause fetal distress because the baby is no longer protected from the force of the contractions. Imagine yourself squeezing a water balloon as hard as you can with an egg inside of it. The egg is protected from the force by the water balloon, and is very difficult to break. Now, imagine breaking the water balloon, and exerting the same amount of force directly on the egg. The egg would shatter. Clearly, then, the longer the membranes remain intact, the less stressful labor will be for the baby. Therefore, artificial rupture of membranes increases the risk of fetal distress to the baby, and should be used to stimulate labor only after all other less risky methods have been attempted first.

The supine position (lying flat on your back) increases the risk of fetal distress because the weight of the pregnant uterus presses on the vena cava, thus preventing adequate blood flow return, and causing poor oxygenation to the fetus.

It has been known since the 1940s that the dangers of pitocin include abruption (the placenta tearing away from the wall of the uterus before the baby is born), fetal distress, and even uterine rupture. It is precisely for these reasons that the monitor is used routinely with a pitocin stimulation of labor.

However, practitioners rarely discuss these risks with mothers. In some states in the country, it is now requied by law that physicians and hospitals enumerate the risks (as well as the benefits) of any medication or procedure they plan to use for a woman in labor. If a woman has had a pitocin induction without being informed of the potential risks, she may be in a position to bring suit again the practitioner and the hospital. If more women would have the courage to bring suit for an unnecessary *cesarean (especially when uninformed consent is an issue), then practitioners would become influenced not only by a fear of malpractice suits for* not doing a cesarean, *but fear of suits for performing* unnecessary *cesareans as well!*

MARY JO: My husband, who had planned on being with me throughout the birth, was whisked away. He was told that they were working quickly, not only to save the baby, but to prevent me from rupturing and being in danger. So, while my fears were focused on the baby's well-being, he was left out "in the dark" with mortal fears for both me and the baby.

I was offered the "reassurance" that I would have a spinal, rather than general anesthesia, and would thus be awake to "see the whole thing."

COMMENTS: *Usually if a cesarean is a "true emergency" (the life of the mother or the baby is* at risk now*) spinal anesthesia is contraindicated. Spinal anesthesia takes much longer to administer than does general anesthesia (which means it will take much longer for the baby to be born). In addition, if the "emergency" is related to blood loss (as it certainly is with a placental abruption), spinal anesthesia is most certainly contraindicated. Spinal anesthesia almost always lowers the blood pressure to some degree. If the blood pressure is already low because of blood loss, the spinal could create dangerously low blood pressure, thus possibly causing a maternal death.*

It seems doubtful to me that the "emergency" that the doctor depicted to Mary Jo was indeed so emergent. Had it been a "true emergency" I feel quite certain Mary Jo would have received general, not spinal, anesthesia.

MARY JO: A classical incision was made in my uterus, and our daughter was born very quickly. She was—thank God—*alive,* and so perfectly beautiful. Everyone seemed so busy that I had to ask at least 3 times, with mounting insistence, that someone go out and tell my husband. I remember assuring myself that not only did the baby seem fine, she must be, or the doctors wouldn't be talking about football scores as they stitched me up!

Although my husband and I both saw our baby in the corridor, neither of us were permitted to hold our daughter. I assumed Sheila would be brought to me at the regular nursery feeding hours. But she was not. I was desperate! Finally, seven tearful hours later, I held and nursed my baby.

The cesarean was certainly a major disappointment— especially because I was told to expect that all future births would also have to be sections.

The Birth of Johnny

When I became pregnant for the second time, I was still with the same doctor. I had no notion that I could question his assumption that the delivery would have to be by cesarean. My main concern was to have the baby with me much sooner after birth. I contacted the pediatrician in advance at the hospital and got a promise that he would waive the 24-hour observation in the special care nursery that was still routine for cesarean babies. Unless there was some specific contraindication, I could have the baby with me as soon as the usual nursery rituals (eyedrops, weighing and measuring, etc.) were complete.

The baby's due date had been set at September 30, 1975, so the cesarean was scheduled for one week before that date. However, early in the morning of September 16, my waters broke, and the doctor delivered our Johnny a few hours later.

Emotionally, this birth experience was easier than the first, because it didn't have the "emergency" character and aura of fear around it. Besides, I did get to have Johnny with me within a few hours. Physically, however, my recovery period was the hardest of my four cesarean experiences. It was hot in the hospital; I was feverish when my milk came in; I had the usual stomach-gas problems after surgery. I missed Sheila terribly. We had some teary phone calls. I didn't see her from Tuesday (when John was born) until Saturday, when—against hospital policy— my husband Joe smuggled her in to see me. By the next day, I had convinced the doctor to let me go home.

My mother was able to come from out of town to help me this time. Her presence, from the day after John's birth until almost three weeks later, was a tremendous blessing in terms of my recovery.

The Birth of Tina

By the time of our third pregnancy, two years later, my husband and I had read a newspaper article about the new cesarean support group, C/SEC, and we went to one of its meetings.

With C/SEC's help, we were able to find a hospital in Boston where my husband could be present for a cesarean birth, where the baby could be with us in the recovery room, and where the older children could visit daily. We also found a doctor on its staff who would permit my husband to give the baby a Leboyer bath right in the OR. This doctor was recommended to us by C/SEC as one of the more likely doctors to consider a vaginal delivery, because by this time we had heard of some exceptions to the "once a cesarean, always . . ." rule. On inquiry, he said he would have considered it after one cesarean, but that he knew of no one, himself included, who would allow it after two. At my request, he did agree to deliver the baby only after I went into labor instead of scheduling the birth. This request was made, not so much out of any great respect for mother nature's sense of timing, as out of my husband's and my flicker of hope that if the labor progressed fast enough, we might finagle our way into a natural birth after all.

On the morning of September 21, 1977, when this baby was already a few days overdue, I began having occasional contractions. We stayed home until shortly after midnight, when the contractions were coming at about 5-minute intervals. When we got to the hospital, the doctor arrived shortly, ready to operate. When I asked for an internal exam, he did one, but dashed our hopes with the announcement that I was less than 1 centimeter dilated and we would certainly have to go ahead with the cesarean.

Having Joe there for the birth made so much difference—the miracle of watching together as that new life emerges! I still had the screen between me and the surgery, but he stood up and looked around it, giving me the "play-by-play account" as our little Christina was taken out of my uterus. I really can't say who enjoyed the Leboyer bath more—father or daughter! It was just bliss for both! We had Tina with us for well over an hour in the recovery room and I was able to nurse her for most of that time.

After the first two births, I had remained catheterized for a day or two and on IVs for even longer. This time, the doctor removed the catheter before leaving the OR and allowed me to drink liquids in the recovery room. By the next mealtime I was eating real food! What a morale booster that was!

After Tina's birth, I had much less discomfort of any kind and gained strength much faster than after the first two. I feel my faster recovery can be attributed to the differences in procedures after the operation, and that I had a different kind of incision. Although this doctor entered through the same vertical incision externally, he did not use the classical uterine incision (an incision which runs vertically from the top of the uterus down to the cervix) that I'd had the first two times. He did a low cervical uterine incision (a transverse incision just above cervix). I was able to walk without clutching my abdomen by the time I left the hospital! I hadn't been able to do that for weeks after the other two!

The Birth of Rebecca

If a vaginal delivery was out of the question after TWO cesareans, there was certainly no hope for it in our minds after three. So Rebecca was born March 10, 1980, in a C-section scheduled a few days before her due date. Joe was again able to be there and to give her the Leboyer bath. In many ways, the details of her birth and my recovery were similar to those of Tina's birth.

The Birth of David

How did we get from there to a VBAC for baby number five? By an odd route indeed!

Joe's mother lives in India, where cesareans are considered to be high-risk procedures, and tubal ligations are always done with the delivery of a second cesarean baby. She had already spent 18 months "on her knees" through the last two pregnancies, and the news of this one — as delightful as it was for us — was liable to cause her heart failure! So I pulled out an old list of C/SEC phone numbers to try to gather reassuring statistics on the safety of cesarean births to send to her.

However, the person I happened to connect with was Nancy Cohen, who was hard at work on a book about VBAC and cesarean prevention, *Silent Knife*. I was apprehensive, but intrigued. We talked at length. Nancy gave me the names of four doctors whom she thought might consider doing a VBAC in my, admittedly unusual, case. Joe and I had had a lot of fear (particularly of uterine "rupture") instilled in us along the way. So a VBAC after four cesareans—particularly with a classical incision—sounded to us like a pretty awesome undertaking. On the other hand, we hoped for more children after this one and did NOT relish the thought of more and more surgery. So, we decided to make an appointment to talk with Dr. Richard McDowell.

We had thought that upon hearing a history of four classical C-sections, any doctor might climb the walls at the suggestion of a vaginal delivery. But, in his own low-key way, Dr. McDowell received the request thoughtfully. In our presence, he phoned a colleague who had also had a great deal of experience with VBACs, and conferred with him about it. In the end, his conclusion was that, if all went well with the pregnancy, and if there should prove to be no contraindications in my medical records when he received them, he would be glad to help us give it a try. He would want to take certain precautions, such as having cross-matched blood available and a heparin lock in place on my wrist (to allow quick insertion of an IV if necessary).

Dr. McDowell felt strongly that we should attend a VBAC class. We found it incredibly helpful. We started the class with some serious misgivings about the wisdom of a VBAC for us, and ended it fairly bursting with confidence and optimism. In the meantime, Dr. McDowell had put us in touch with a midwife, Kim Brodie, whom he recommended as a labor support person.

COMMENTS: *The creation of the birth team—the childbirth educator, the midwife, the doctor, the mother, and the father—all knowing, trusting, and supporting one another is a tremendous asset in preparing for a positive birth experience. Unfortunately, many doctors feel threatened by the presence of a midwife/labor coach at the birth, and do not understand that the midwife is not there to usurp the power of the doctor. However, Dr. McDowell clearly did not harbor those fears. His recommendation to Mary Jo to not only take classes, but specifically to take VBAC classes, and his recommendation of a midwife/labor support person demonstrated his true support of Mary Jo's VBAC. His efforts created the cohesiveness of the team. When a VBAC mother knows that she has an entire team surrounding her to support her in her efforts to give birth vaginally, she feels much more strength and faith in her own abilities to birth her baby.*

MARY JO: The baby was due March 30. Time crept by until just before midnight, April 12, when I felt fairly sure my waters had broken while I was on the toilet. I began to have some contractions, but at wide enough intervals that we decided to go to sleep until the pace quickened. By about 6:00 A.M., they were coming at 5-6 minute intervals and we decided to head for the hospital. We arrived at the hospital at 7:30 A.M. Labor and delivery was extraordinarily busy, and Dr. McDowell was having a busy morning himself. So we were doubly glad to have Kim, our labor support person, with us the whole time.

COMMENTS: *Though many women presume that their doctor will be with them during most of their labor, rarely is that the case. Even, with a doctor like Dr. McDowell who has a reputation for giving lots of labor support, the support of a midwife or other knowledgeable professional labor support person is quite often of the utmost importance. Having a skilled support person with the mother during labor encourages relaxation and flowing with the course of the labor. The mother feels "mothered" by another mother—woman to woman.*

MARY JO: At times, during their intermittent checks with the external fetal monitor, the labor room nurses had difficulty picking up the baby's heartbeat. But Kim was usually able to track the heartbeat down with her stethoscope.

COMMENTS: *Though the hospital staff usually feels dependent upon the fetal monitor for monitoring the baby's heartbeat, a skillful attendant can monitor with a fetascope or stethoscope. Since electronic equipment can fail, it is much to the laboring woman's advantage to have an attendant skilled at auscultation of fetal heart tones.*

MARY JO: I got up to walk around a couple of times during labor, but that seemed to stop my contractions rather than to strengthen them. In the end, I seemed to labor best and most comfortably lying on my left side.

COMMENTS: *Walking or moving about usually enhances the power of the labor. However, sometimes the activities of the woman's surroundings may be extremely distracting from the inner process of her labor. She may need absolute peace and quiet, perhaps even isolation, in order to feel able to give her labor her complete inner focus and permission to relax into her labor, to let it happen.*

MARY JO: Early in the afternoon, the contractions were getting closer and harder. I was laboring pretty quietly, and I think the labor room nurses might not have realized how close to delivering I was if Kim had not alerted them.

At about 3:00 P.M., the urge to push seemed to come on very suddenly. I was fully dilated. "Go ahead and push." The doctor arrived. The nurses tried unsuccessfully to pick up the baby's heartbeat. I was rushed to the delivery room. Because of the staff's concern for the baby, I was urged to push hard, even between contractions. At Dr. McDowell's request, a padded, desk- type chair was brought in and draped. I knelt on the seat of it, leaning over the back, and pushed for all I was worth. Our son David seemed to be born very quickly (at 3:36 P.M.) and was also quickly determined to be fine.

COMMENTS: *Mary Jo's first and last labors were very similar. Although the first labor ended with a cesarean, and the last ended with a vaginal birth, in both of these labors the possibility of fetal distress created an emergency aura around the birth.*

Often, the blocks which "caused" a woman to have a cesarean, reappear in her VBAC labor as hurdles that must be vaulted in order to deliver vaginally. Mary Jo's hurdle was fetal distress, which she most certainly vaulted.

Mary Jo might have been so frightened by the pressure to perform—to push even when her body was not calling her to push— that she might not have been able to push her baby out. A cesarean would then have been necessary. However, when the pressure was on, Mary Jo pulled through for her baby. Though the birth was far from ideal, she did what she needed to do to give birth to her own baby. She had a successful VBAC.

Each birth subsequent to Mary Jo's primary cesarean was a step along the way to her VBAC. With each birth she saw to it that more and more of her needs were fulfilled. With each birth she needed to sacrifice less of her own needs in order to assure herself the safety of her baby. As she "pushed through" the emergency and the fear of fetal distress, perhaps she "pushed through" not only the issue of self-sacrifice in birth, but also self-sacrifice in life. We all deserve to and can get our needs fulfilled without hurting those we love. Perhaps this birth may be the key to fulfilling Mary Jo's goal of a peaceful birth with her future pregnancies.

MARY JO: I was in great pain while I pushed, and was bleeding profusely. Although my uterus had "done fine" and the VBAC was a success, I had suffered deep tears in my vagina which required immediate, painstaking, extensive suturing.

COMMENTS: *Whenever the second stage is forceful, the possibility of severe tearing increases. With the emergency nature of Mary Jo's second stage, she pushed even between contractions. Her vagina did not have time to slowly stretch to accommodate her baby without tearing. If she had another baby with the same size head, and the second stage were taken at the pace her own body were dictating, she definitely would not experience such a severe tear as she had with David's birth. Chances are she might not tear at all.*

MARY JO: Once I was able to go to the recovery room, I held and nursed my baby. Despite all my blood loss after the delivery, I found my recovery at home to be significantly easier than with any of the cesarean births.

Obviously, our VBAC was a mixed experience for us. We felt tremendously pleased that a vaginal birth had been possible. For us, this laid to rest the bugaboo of uterine rupture once and for all. Besides, my recovery was immeasurably easier than after the cesareans, even in spite of the complications and blood loss from the vaginal tearing.

On the other hand, we certainly did not have a birth experience that would be anybody's ideal. The tears and their repair were painful and frightening, and our hopes for a calm, pleasant welcoming of the baby were side-tracked by that emergency. Even if we could have known in advance how the birth would go, I think we would still have opted for a vaginal delivery, in spite of the extraneous complications we met.

COMMENTS: *Although Mary Jo did not have an "ideal" birth, a "pure" birth, or a "perfect" birth, she did have a VBAC. She had a VBAC which was perfect for her. Through it she faced her fears and vaulted the hurdles. She grew. Her lessons were not simply about birth, but about life.*

To seek a "pure" birth may be a path through which we learn to recognize our own needs. But to require a "pure" birth is only a set-up for failure. Life is not ideal, nor is it pure. Birth is but a small moment in life. Although some births appear to be more ideal, more pure, I have rarely known women who actually had a "pure" birth—a birth that measured up completely to their ideals. Yet, every birth is perfect. Every birth teaches us the perfect lesson, through which we become more beautiful and courageous.

The Birth of Katie

MARY JO: On August 21, 1985, our sixth baby, Katie, was born. Once again there were symptoms of possible fetal distress on the monitor. But our fears were allayed as the results of the scalp sample were good and did not indicate that the baby was in distress. This time Dr. McDowell did not ask me to push between contractions. I pushed only during contractions, and without the emergency aura which had been present at David's birth. Katie was born pink and healthy, and I had only a small skin tear. But most importantly, both my husband and I were fully present to welcome her into the world.

In retrospect, I wish that we could have refused all the technology. I wish that we could have trusted ourselves, our feelings that the baby would be healthy. But when I felt that the baby's life could be on the line, it wasn't something I could fool around with.

COMMENTS: *Trusting our intuition in a technological era is profoundly difficult. Before the technology was available, we had only our skills and intuition upon which to base our decisions. We had only God and our own conscience to answer to if the outcome was less than perfect. Through spiritual growth we accepted death as part of life.*

With the miracles of technology, we sought to avoid death. Although the motivation is admirable, the technology is often no more accurate than the skills and intuition of a good practitioner. However, today we are accountable not only to ourselves and God, but to a legal system which seeks "proof that everything which could have been done had been done."

Practitioners and parents often feel they are a rope in a tug-of-war between their inner-most voices and the power of technology. The struggle between the spiritual God and the god of technology is the modern dilemma which is epitomized and reflected in the way Americans are giving birth.

Those of us whose consciousnesses are becoming aware of this dilemma have a responsibility to ourselves and our children to find the balance between these forces for ourselves, and to help society to realize the need for the balance as well. If we sit idly by, soon the power will be given totally and completely to technology, and we will have lost perhaps the most vital piece of life.

MARY JO: We certainly ought to be a "landmark case." Our message to VBAC "candidates" would be: "Don't let anyone frighten you into a routine repeat cesarean. If a uterus with two classical incisions and two low cervical incisions can do the job, why shouldn't yours, too?!"

11

VBAC Triplets

MEG WESTON

MEG: Ten days after the due date for my first baby, my water broke and contractions began immediately. My husband and I went to the hospital at 9 A.M. By evening, our obstetrician (who had not exactly been around all day), appeared to tell us that he was leaving the hospital because he had tickets to a Bruins hockey game. I remember saying, "If I weren't such a rabid hockey fan, I wouldn't let you get away with this." His associate would take over, he said. His associate turned out to be the same doctor who had done a D and C when I miscarried our first baby. We did not hold that against him, but we felt a sense of foreboding.

COMMENTS: *A "D and C" is an abbreviation for "Dilatation and Curettage," a procedure done almost routinely to complete a miscarriage, and is most certainly indicated if the woman's life is threatened due to excessive blood loss. Under anesthesia, the woman's cervix is dilated. Then, using an instrument called a "curet," the wall of the uterus is scraped to remove all the products of conception and/or any other source of bleeding. At times, now, a vacuum aspirator is used instead of the curet to remove the contents of the uterus.*

The procedure can be very frightening, especially if it has been preceded by the loss of a much-wanted pregnancy and/or heavy bleeding. Though we do not consciously choose to repeat patterns in our lives, such patterns are often unconsciously repeated. The forboding feeling Meg experienced was the fear of a repeating pattern in her life—a repeat either physically or symbolically of her miscarriage and the surgery that followed.

MEG: This same doctor came in later in the day with his crochet hook. Unable to believe that the amniotic sac had ruptured at home, he attempted to rupture it artificially. Why wouldn't he take my word for it?

My labor was all back labor, and my husband helped by pushing against my back during contractions. Around 10:00, the nurse came in and recommended demerol—"Because you've been working so hard." We were at 9 centimeters, and the nurse implied that relaxation would get us that last centimeter we needed. We negotiated on the dosage (cut in half), but we never should have accepted it. After I had the demerol everything came to a halt. Nothing progressed. Everyone went to sleep, including the baby.

The next thing I remember is the doctor arriving with the pitocin drip apparatus. He said that the baby was "turned" and that I should push while he tried to rearrange him. He was not successful, however, and I remember thinking afterward that maybe I just hadn't pushed hard enough or breathed right.

He motioned to the nurse to take away the pitocin. It would not be possible, he said, to deliver this baby other than by cesarean because, although the baby was vertex (head down), he was face sideways. He was very far down because, of course, we had been in labor for sixteen hours, and we hadn't seen the doctor all evening. We couldn't help thinking that if the doctor had shown up sooner, the baby would have been easier to manipulate.

COMMENTS: *Technically speaking, a baby that is stuck deep within the pelvis but is facing "sideways" is said to be in "transverse arrest". A persistently transverse head cannot negotiate the pelvis because of the shape of the normal pelvis. Therefore, the baby must be rotated in order to be born. This rotation can be accomplished by maternal position and/or manual rotation by the practitioner, and should be done as early in labor as possible.*

MEG: Then came the worst part of the whole experience. Jim, my husband, faithful to the end, suited up and with three cameras loaded (instant, SLR and sound movie), was told that he would not be permitted in the operating room because they would be administering general anaesthesia. It was devastating. Jim had *been there* for me throughout the labor. The doctors had not.

I was very frightened in the operating room. It reminded me of my miscarriage. I was having surgery at night with the same doctor. I feared that all I would have to show for it was another dead fetus. They brought me out of the anesthesia just long enough to tell me that I had a boy. I woke up alone in the recovery room. My husband had been barred from recovery also. They told me he had gone with the baby to the nursery. Was the baby okay? Yes, they said. Would his father be able to hold him? Yes, they said.

Well, they wouldn't let my husband hold the baby. They put the child in an isolette to control his temperature. His apgars had been 9 and 10. He weighed 7lbs. 13oz., and his feet and hands were peeling from postmaturity. He was born at 3:15 A.M., after 18 hours of labor.

At around 5:00 A.M., they brought me back upstairs to see the baby. My husband was sitting all alone in a dark lounge.

The recovery was very slow. I was drained by the effort, physically and psychologically. I felt I had failed. I felt the doctors had failed us. I felt the hospital had failed us. I was nervous about nursing. Would I fail at that, too? Why couldn't this baby learn to latch on? I was despondent, and monosyllabic when the doctor removed my stitches weeks after the birth. It took about four months (spring came) before I felt like a human being again.

I never really trusted the doctors in the group after that. With our next pregnancy we changed doctors. We deliberately changed to someone who was sympathetic to VBAC. Our VBAC baby, we thought, would be born and "show everybody" that we could "do it." Wrong attitude, but there it was.

We went for ultrasound at 12 weeks, fully expecting to be told we had twins. My maternal grandmother had had two sets of twins: one set of boys too small to survive, and a boy and a girl set, who lived. Then the ultrasound technician said, "Wait a minute. I think I see a third one." Gulp. I was glad I was lying down. My husband was sorry he was standing up. He remained upright, but we'll never know how. Afterwards we whispered in the hall, panic-stricken. "We'll have to put an addition on the house. Holy mackerel! Three of 'em. What'll our son say?"

Then it hit us. Who would deliver triplets vaginally at all, let alone VBAC? Nobody. Nobody in his/her right mind . . .

We went home and that very day began to draft questions, to read and take notes. We decided to interview our new obstetrician first. She recommended another cesarean. She even arranged guest privileges at a large city hospital, because we were beginning to balk at having the babies away from a neonatal intensive care unit.

We couldn't accept the decree of an automatic cesarean. We decided to seek another physician who might give us a chance at an attempted VBAC. After all, we thought, the Dionne quintuplets were born at home in 1934. There was no cesarean. They had two more babies than we had, and we were having two more babies than most people have at one time.

I spent what seemed like hours on the phone with friends, friends of friends, nurses, birth counseling agencies, anybody who would listen. Our interviews with doctors ranged from , "I think you're nuts," to "You should gain no more than thirty pounds." Finally we located a physician who had delivered a friend's twins. He seemed very sensible and down-to-earth. We liked him. I saw him once after we interviewed him, then left for a week in New Hampshire with his blessing. I was 22 weeks along.

Upon our return, we found a registered letter stating that as of the date of the letter, I was no longer officially in his care. My due date coincided with a meeting he had agreed to chair, the date of which had been moved. All during our vacation, there had been nothing binding him to us in terms of care. We felt that the manner in which the relationship was severed was a bit cold. When we telephoned, he gave us the names of two other doctors, both of whom, we knew (and he did too), were vehemently opposed to VBACS.

Twenty-three weeks, and back on the phone. Interviews with the two recommended doctors had revealed their aversion to VBACs. We sought other referrals and got lucky. We turned up three excellent doctors who were willing to give it a try. One, however, was going on vacation for the next three weeks. We arranged interviews with the other two, and were charmed by both of them. The determining factor was that the other doctors in the respective groups had differing views on our case. One doctor, with whom we had an almost instant rapport, told us frankly that his associates had said things about possible malpractice suits, and one had said, "What's the matter, David? Your mother didn't love you enough? What do you need this for?"   So we settled on the doctors whose associates (his juniors) were willing to consider the case on our terms. We never insisted that we had to have a VBAC, just that we wanted to try.

COMMENTS: *In the struggle to find a doctor supportive of VBAC (especially in special circumstances such as twins, triplets, or breech) we are often so happy to find someone, anyone, who will agree to our wishes, that we often neglect to investigate the attitudes of the partners or associates of the doctor we like. Meg was indeed wise to investigate this further, and to make decisions that followed her instincts about the ability of those doctors to give her the support she needed to have a VBAC with triplets.*

MEG: All summer long I had been working with a psychiatric nurse, actively recalling my first cesarean and working on my feelings of rage and disappointment. She had access to medical journals, and and we dug up articles on VBAC, anesthesia, triplets. Then I went to a weekend VBAC workshop with Nancy Wainer Cohen.

After our initial consultation, I saw the doctor only one more time before I went into labor. It was a Monday night of the long Columbus Day weekend. I had not expected to go into labor so soon, but statistics had indicated that it could happen. The average date for delivery of triplets is 33 weeks. We were, we thought, at 31, though the hospital pegged the babies at 32.

At any rate, there it was again, another ruptured amniotic sac and fluid all over the place. Was it one sac? Two? All three? It was 10:30

P.M. We telephoned the doctor and said we were coming in. There would be some attempt to stop the labor so that the babies could be given betamethasone to help mature their lungs.

COMMENTS: *Betamethasone is a corticosteriod which has been found to be somewhat effective in assisting the maturation of the fetal lungs, when given to the mother at least 12 hours prior to the birth of the premature fetus.*

Prior to the use of corticosteroid for this purpose, observant practitioners have noted that early rupture of membranes also appeared to be a significant factor in maturation of fetal lungs. The longer the membranes had been ruptured prior to the birth, the more likely were the lungs to have matured adequately to support extrauterine life.

MEG: The resident began to speak about our IV, our surgery, our cesarean. We spoke about not having anything like that. He began to think we were cuckoo. We asked him how far dilated I was, thinking I was at 3 or 4 centimeters, like the last time. He said, "Quite a bit." We said, "How much is 'quite a bit'?" He said, "All the way." We knew then that they would not be able to stop the labor. Our babies, if they survived the birth, would be conveyed almost instantly to the best neonatal intensive care unit around.

We were grateful that our doctor lived nearby. He appeared sooner than we thought he could, and informed the resident that since the first baby was head down, he would deliver her "from below." Down we rolled to the delivery room, so full of attendants (for me and for each one of the babies) that one baby bed had to be kept in the hall.

The psychiatric nurse who had counseled me through this pregnancy and the labor coach we had hired arrived, breathless. They had been speeding into the city, hoping for the police to stop them so they could get there even faster with an escort. However, they were not permitted in the delivery room because there were so many people in the room.

At 12:45 A.M., our daughter Kate was born, as I squeaked delightedly, "There's a baby coming out!"

Our second baby, however, was not vertex anymore. Ultrasounds had shown all three babies head down in September. Perhaps when his sister left their cozy womb, there was more room and he flipped to a breech position. The doctor said that he was clearing the room for an emergency cesarean (maybe classical incision) because of the breech presentation. As he said that, the baby came down of his own accord, and they had to deliver him vaginally. My husband was bouncing up and down on his stool, saying, "They're gonna do it! There're gonna do it!" I could hardly believe that we had escaped a second cesarean. Even now that baby is absolutely fearless—that's his style.

Our third baby was vertex but up high and still intact in his amniotic sac, so I was given halothane (an inhalation anesthetic) while the doctor manipulated him into position. While our second baby, a boy, was born 10 minutes after his sister, our third baby took 55 minutes before he appeared on the scene. He looked the most "preemie" so we assumed that he just wasn't ready to be born yet. Since then, he has reached each developmental milestone ahead of his siblings. It had all taken 3 hours and 25 minutes.

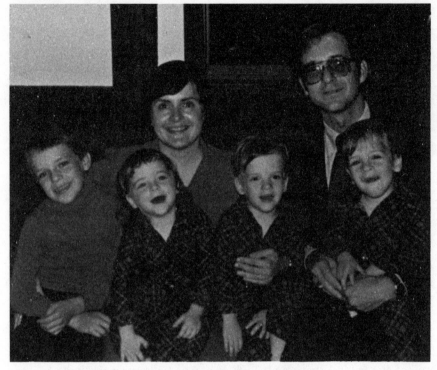

Meg and John Weston, with Adam, Kate, David, and Mark.

I woke up in the recovery room on my stomach with an oxygen mask on. I knew it must be over because I was on my stomach! My labor coach said, "You did it, Meggie."

My husband told me all about the babies and how well they were doing in intensive care. I was particularly concerned about the third one's exposure to anesthesia, but our obstetrician said his heartbeat had remained strong throughout. I wanted to see them up close, not from out in the hall. So the nurses went out of their way to find a gurney narrow enough to be rolled into the nursery next to the babies' isolettes.

My recovery was excellent. While I was in the hospital myself, I negotiated several trips a day down long halls with ease, in order to see all my babies. I remember one poor soul "doing the cesarean shuffle" with her IV pole. Less than a week after they were born, I was walking quickly and confidently into the hospital to visit the babies.

The babies spent about three weeks at the hospital where they were born and about one week at our local hospital before they came home, four weeks before their original due date. We began to work very hard at taking care of them and of our oldest son, (who was then almost four), and we've been working very hard ever since!

12

Home Alone for Four Days of Labor

DIANE WIRKKALA

My first baby was a little girl. She was born vaginally after 3 days of leaking membranes, 14 hours of labor, and only 15 minutes of pushing. She weighed 8 lbs. 7-1/2 oz., and was born at full term. I was given a drug for pain, which made me drowsy, but I considered it a good birthing experience.

For some reason during my second pregnancy, I felt there was something wrong. But when I talked to my doctor, he was no comfort. When I was about 7 months pregnant I was told that my expected due date did not correspond with my uterine size. So I had a sonagram. The only information that I was given about the results of the sonagram was that there was only one fetus present. As my delivery date grew closer, I grew more concerned. Still my doctor acted as if I were stupid, and said that everything was fine.

I went 3 weeks past my due date, and had my 10 lb. 6 oz. son by cesarean. It was a nightmare. I had only labored for 4 hours when I was examined and told my baby was breech, and that a cesarean would have to be done.

I had no idea what to expect. I begged for my husband to be with me, but was told that that was not possible. I saw my son at birth, but was not allowed to hold him. I imagine you know how the rest of it went. I was so sore, angry, and frustrated afterwards that I just could not handle my baby. My arms felt like lead . My tummy felt like I had been beaten with a bat. I could not urinate and my bladder felt as if it were about to burst. I did not see my son for 14 hours.

I went through a guilt trip for several months afterward. I felt I had not given "real birth," and I blamed my doctor for my feelings. I could not get enough rest, so I was tired and grouchy. I did not get proper support—everyone, including myself, thought that I should bounce back after surgery. We just didn't know how long recuperation after a cesarean could take.

Almost four years later, during my third pregnancy, I knew I did not want to have another cesarean. We changed our residence and I changed doctors. It's worth it financially to shop around for an empathetic and understanding doctor.

I sent for my medical records. When I read them I realized that my doctor knew from the sonagram results at least two months ahead of my due date that my son was breech! Not a word was ever said to me about it—*nothing!*

COMMENTS: *Medical training does not encourage sharing information with patients. Perhaps he thought that he would "protect her pretty little head" from worry. However, she was already worrying. Her intuition told her something was different, and had asked the doctor if something was wrong. In all likelihood, the doctor chose to keep the breech lie a secret in order to maintain his own power over his patient. He protected himself, not his patient.*

DIANE: At the beginning of my third pregnancy, I had very little knowledge about VBAC. I began to send for materials, and some of them took months to reach me. I was very impatient. I was getting bigger every day. There were no support groups and I knew no one who had had a VBAC. The only person who really understood was my husband, Jerry. He stood beside me all the way. We had learned from our cesarean how much a mother needs the support of her husband.

The doctor I chose was the only one I could find within 500 miles who was willing to try VBAC. I was a little skeptical, however. Doctor Lovett was new to the area and fresh out of residency. It was a small hospital with no on-call in-house anesthesiologists. Everything I had read about criteria for VBAC included having the anesthesiologist standing by at the hospital.

COMMENTS: *Most community hospitals (where low-risk births are done) are not adequately staffed to provide 24-hour, on-call, in-house anesthesia. This arbitrary limit set by ACOG (American College of Obstetricians and Gynecologists) only serves to feed VBAC women into tertiary care centers. There, they will not only have an on-call anesthesiologist, but will be treated as high-risk consistently—throughout their pregnancies, labors, and births. Having a VBAC in a high-risk center makes VBAC women more high risk for having more iatrogenic (practitioner-caused) complications and more iatrogenic cesareans. Luckily, the only physician willing to try a VBAC for Diane was not in a tertiary care center, and was not a high-risk physician.*

DIANE: When I was about a week from my due date, my doctor informed me that a cesarean would be necessary if I went two weeks past my due date. I panicked, started going through all my books and pamphlets, and found Lynn's phone number.

COMMENTS: *As Diane's pregnancy progressed, her physician came upon further conflicts with ACOG's VBAC guidelines. Her fetus was clearly over the 8 lb. 8 oz. weight-limit, and her time limit was nearly up (42 weeks gestation). His courage to throw all three of these guidelines to the wind was waning.*

DIANE: I asked her how to start labor. She told me I should talk this over with my baby to make sure the baby was ready to be born. She suggested warm baths, making love, exercise, and a castor oil-booze-and-orange juice recipe for at-home induction of labor.

I enjoyed our talk—felt better, relieved—and I wrote down her advice in case I needed it. But most importantly, I had found someone who had a VBAC, and at home to boot! What surprised me most was that she said I didn't have to sign a release for a cesarean. It had never occurred to me to disagree with my doctor. After all, his reason that I was a high risk (previous cesarean, overweight, brief period of high blood pressure, history of large babies) seemed sound. But when I talked with Lynn, I became inspired and determined—rejuvenated. Yet, I still hoped I would not have a big confrontation with my doctor. I was scared to disagree with him. After all, who was I to argue? He was the doctor. Until I spoke with Lynn, I did not realize that it was his job to give me advice, but it was up to me to decide whether or not I would follow his advice.

On my next visit (with my husband, Jerry, for moral support,) I told my doctor I would not sign papers for a cesarean just because I was overdue. He turned beet-red, and I was afraid that he might refuse me care as a patient.

This confrontation upset me more than I allowed to be apparent to the doctor. I needed more support, so I called Lynn again. She gave me phone numbers of doctors and midwives in California who attended VBACs. I called them in hopes that they might consider me as a patient. Through them I got names of midwives in Nevada. But no one would accept me. Boy! Was I frustrated! I gave up.

I returned to my doctor for my last visit. Filled with contradictions— I was determined, yet a little unsure. I kept quiet in fear of another confrontation. I could tell he figured I'd go for a cesarean, if it came down to it. And I just figured I'd let him think so, even though I was determined to have a VBAC.

I tried *all* Lynn's suggestions for starting labor. They must have worked, as labor started two days later. I called her one last time. I was in the 2nd day of my labor by then, and 6 days past my due date. I had seen my doctor that day. He checked the baby's heart beat, asked how I was, and said to come in the hospital when my labor pains were 5 minutes apart and consistent. I felt, as Lynn had suggested, that the longer I stayed away from the hospital, the better. I felt the hospital environment would not be the best atmosphere for labor, especially when they would start running IVs, and tests, etc., so I packed Lynn's phone number in case I'd need it at the hospital.

The first 4 days of labor were really different than my labors with my other two children. The labors with the other two did not last as long. With this labor, at night my pains would be from five to twenty minutes apart, and then stop. I'd wake my husband several times and have him time the contractions, but they just weren't consistent. By morning they would become very strong. I would think, "Today is it!" and Jerry would stay home from work. I walked around the house, cleaned a little, cooked meals, and washed dishes. Mostly, I took care of my other two children. My contractions during the rest of the daytime were very light, and all in my stomach area. I could not believe they were so light! During my other two labors, my contractions had been really strong, in my back, and hurt! These were so light they were almost "tolerable"! My "plug" had begun to fall out a little at a time on the first day of labor, and continued every day of labor. I knew I was getting close, but when?

COMMENTS: *Technically, this kind of stop and start labor is called "prodromal labor", prelude to "real" active labor. This type of labor can be very confusing and disheartening. Fortunately, Diane was intuitive about this phase of her labor, and did not feel threatened by its inconsistency, an attitude which was essential for her to continue to have a progressive (albeit slowly progressive) home labor.*

DIANE: Throughout the 4 days of easy labor, I didn't worry *too much.* My Mom kept stressing that I was going to wait until it was too late, but I felt I knew what I was doing. On the 4th night I had labor pains all night, and woke up knowing they were different this time. They got stronger all day the next day, but they never were consistent.

COMMENTS: *This change in gears was active labor.*

DIANE: At 3:30 that afternoon I sent my husband to the store and regretted it immediately. We lived about 4 miles out of town and it took him about a half hour to shop and get back. When he was gone, I realized that the sensation I had been having that afternoon was the baby moving down. Now, I was pushing! I was surprised because again it was so different and light compared to my first vaginal delivery.

Jerry was gone! Mom was extremely nervous and wanted to leave for the hospital before Jerry returned, but I wouldn't go without him. By the time Jerry got back, my labor was really strong, and I began to worry that maybe I waited too long. We rushed to the hospital. I was examined, and the nurse said I was fully dilated. She called for my doctor .

In the delivery room I was surprised again. This was hard work— it did not feel good to push. With my first vaginal delivery, I wanted to push. It felt good to relieve the pressure. Not so with this delivery!

COMMENTS: *Some women have a strong urge to push. Some women never have an urge to push. Some need to push and push hard in order for the baby to be born. Others only need to breathe and let the uterus do the pushing.*

Usually, in a hospital delivery, however, very little space, (if any) is given to a woman whose body seems to be indicating that she should simply breathe her baby out. If the rest of her labor had been quietly slowly progressive, it stands to reason that the "pushing" phase of her labor would follow suit. Had she been permitted to assume a vertical active position (such as squatting, standing, or hands and knees), and to follow the cues of her body (how, when, and how much to push) her baby might have been born just as "painlessly" as the rest of the labor had been.

DIANE: After a half hour of pushing, Dr. Lovett said, "Come on, Diane, push! This baby is ready to be born." I tried, but made little headway. Then he said, after another fifteen minutes, that he would have to use the forceps if the baby wasn't out soon. I didn't want the forceps used!

Jerry really helped. He coached and talked to me. I think I would have cried if not for him. He kept saying, "You can do it. It's all right." I felt the doctor was talking too rough to me.

After a few more pushes, David's head was out. Dr. Lovett then told his assistant to grab the baby's shoulders and pull.

COMMENTS: *Whenever the head has been born, but the shoulders do not slip out easily, assistance may be needed to complete the birth. Technically, this situation is called "shoulder dystocia," which means that the shoulders don't fit. Actually the shoulders do fit, but they need some assistance in making the maneuver under the pubic bone. Although sometimes this situation can be life-threatening to the baby, usually it can be resolved relatively quickly. This situation is more common with big babies; however, it is possible for even a small baby to have shoulder dystocia.*

DIANE: My 10 lb. 3 oz. boy was born after 55 minutes of pushing! All this, with no mirrors—I couldn't see much! Not exactly an ideal birth!

DIANE: As soon as they brought David to me, I nursed him right away, even though the nurse was against it. She said the baby had too much mucous to nurse.

COMMENTS: *It has been my experience with babies whose births I have attended that early and frequent nursing helps babies to rid themselves of mucous. Sometimes it's handy to have a bulb syringe to assist the baby in this process. If the baby sounds mucousy or gags, quickly suction, and return the baby to the breast.*

DIANE: I felt my triumph! It was just like a battle had been won. I was victorious!

My husband didn't say much. He was beaming with pride— smiling all the time. This was the first child he had seen delivered! He said he was impressed with my efforts and could appreciate what mothers went through to give birth. He was tickled pink with me and the baby.

The next day I was pretty exhausted. My arms and legs ached and trembled. One nurse made the comment, "Natural childbirth is not all it's cracked up to be, is it?" I said, "Maybe not, but it sure beats the hell out of another cesarean."

13

Turning Around More Than 180 Degrees

ED AND MARIA ANDERSON

ED: We were married about 4 or 5 years when we decided to have our first child. We went through the usual routine. We went to see the obstetrician and he verified the pregnancy, which of course Maria knew anyway. He gave us an estimated birth date. One of the running jokes throughout the pregnancy was that he told us when the conception occurred and we told him when it happened. We were there, he wasn't. As it turned out, the actual date that Christine was born was much closer to our calculations than his.

COMMENTS: *Health practitioners are taught that they have a "method of calculation" to determine the date of conception and the due date which is accurate. Regardless of whether or not the dates the practitioner calculates are in conjunction with the experiences of the woman, the practitioner will trust his/her own calculations over and above the observations or experiences of the woman/couple. Practitioners are taught that they cannot presume that the patient accurately knows her own body, her own experiences, or has any understanding whatsoever about how conception occurs. They are taught to presume that the patient knows nothing.*

If the practice of obstetrics is to change in this country, the presumptions of training need to be changed. We need to train practitioners to presume that:

1. Women/couples have the innate ability to learn about their own bodies, to understand the normal process of pregnancy, labor, and birth; to understand the possible deviations from normal, and the use of interventions in that process; and, to learn skills and make decisions involved with these processes.
2. Women/couples have the innate intuition about themselves and their babies, which, along with the intuition of the practitioner, can and needs to be trusted.

ED: We had Lamaze training, the usual kind. When Maria went into labor, I was working in the city at the office. I left immediately for home, but by the time I got back to Syosset, she was already in the hospital. She had called the doctor, told him she was in labor, and he immediately sent her to the hospital. He broke her water as soon as she got there, which kind of placed her permanently there.

MARIA: I told the nurse that I wasn't staying, and the doctor told the nurse, "Yes, she is."

ED: By the time I got to the hospital, she had been there 5 hours, by herself. I came in not really knowing what to expect. Maria was very upset and uncomfortable and she appeared to be pleased to see me. So, I just stayed with her. There wasn't much for me to do until the labor started to become much stronger.

Maria's labor progressed and everything seemed to be fine, except the baby was posterior. Then Maria became fully dilated. She pushed for three hours, and the baby still wasn't crowning. It was just about 22 hours into the labor, when the doctor took me outside.

COMMENTS: *When the doctor takes the husband outside to talk "man to man", the husband then becomes "one of the boys". The doctor plays on the father's natural instinct to want to "do something" to help his wife. And the obvious*

"something" is a cesarean. The doctor and the husband then become "comrades"
in the battle to convince the "little woman" to be rescued by a cesarean.

ED: There he told me that he thought that inevitably a section was going to be necessary. At this point, I agreed with him. To a large extent I was relieved, for myself and for Maria.

So they did the section. I was in the room with her. And after it was all over, I remember Maria telling me she felt like a cold pork chop. She couldn't feel anything. But for me, (except for the discomfort she had after the surgery which was expected) I had a healthy wife, and a beautiful child. The major difference between what we had expected with Lamaze training and what we actually got was that Maria had to spend a few extra days in the hospital.

MARIA: Being a surgical patient is not the same as being a new mother. At the time I wasn't distressed about the cesarean. My roommate had more problems than I did, was in the hospital longer than I was, and she had delivered "normally." So from my perspective, at that time, the cesarean wasn't all that bad.

It wasn't until it came time to have another baby that I started to look back and say, "No, it wasn't right, it didn't go well."

COMMENTS: *Maria and Ed's response to her cesarean—feeling happy she and the baby were healthy, and accepting it as "not all that bad" is perhaps the most common initial response of all cesarean parents. For many of us birth is easily seen as only a means to an end—a healthy mother and baby. And while no one would ever quibble about the outcome (a healthy mother and baby), it is often not until the subsequent pregnancy(ies) that the mother begins to realize that the birth process itself is really important to her.*

This common process of first denying the negative feelings, and then identifying them, exploring them, and resolving them is the same process that we go through when a relative or friend dies—grieving and healing.

ED: Maria became pregnant with Julie 12–14 months after our first child was born. We went back to the same doctor to verify the pregnancy and go through the routine.

MARIA: When I used to go to the appointments alone, I got a certain degree of cooperation from the doctor. However, if I really wanted questions answered, I would make Ed put his suit on, bring his briefcase, and sit. We'd have the first appointment in the morning, and I'd make him sit so that as the doctor walked in the door of his waiting room, the first thing that he would see would be my husband, sitting there all set to do business. It would absolutely unnerve the doctor. He would answer any question I wanted. Usually I would give Ed the handwritten list, and he would ask my questions, because I couldn't get the doctor to answer all of them when I was doing the asking.

COMMENTS: *Doctors often treat women differently when they are accompanied by their partners. If they are accustomed to treating their patients like little girls, it is far more difficult to be as condescending to their male partners. If your doctor treats you like a "nice little girl," it may be time to consider: 1. Using Maria and Ed's technique; 2. Writing an "Optimum Birth Letter" (a letter of requests for your birth), and demanding that the doctor respond to you in writing; 3. CHANGING DOCTORS!*

ED: Maria had been doing some reading on vaginal birth after cesarean. We decided to discuss VBAC with the doctor.

He gave us every excuse in the world. It would be expensive. We would have to pay to have an anesthesiologist on-call (which, of course, we had done the first time anyway). All of his excuses were economic. None were medical. Then he looked at Maria and said, "Besides, you wouldn't want to have to go through labor again, would you?" which infuriated Maria.

He told us there were some doctors who, in order to attract business, were starting to talk up vaginal birth after cesarean. But he wasn't really in favor of it. However, if we really insisted, he would try to go along with it. Neither one of us really believed that he was sincere.

MARIA: I continued to see him for another three or four months. It seemed that once we had agreed to work with this doctor, (as long as he agreed to let us have a trial of labor) he presumed that we would be having another cesarean. He was setting up with sonograms, and scheduled surgical dates, and everything else. He was setting me up for a second cesarean! With all the reading I had been doing, I was hysterical about having to go through surgery again. So, I said to myself, this man's not even going to give me a chance. Breaking away from him to go to another doctor was very difficult, but with my mental state at that point, it was necessary.

I found another doctor who said, "Of course, why would you want to skip labor? You should go through labor. There's no reason to go directly into cesarean, unless it is a last minute emergency." This really made me feel positive. Unfortunately, his partners weren't so positive.

By this time, I had done a lot of reading, and had already concluded that most of what had happened during my last labor was caused by interference on the doctor's part. Ed skimmed over the reading, or I would read him a few lines here and there out of books. He would say, "Yeah, okay . . . all right . . . if you say so." But I always felt as if he were only pacifying me.

ED: I felt I was not pacifying Maria. Maria *had* done a lot of reading, and a lot of this was happening to *her*. It was her body that was going to go through labor or having a cesarean. It wasn't mine. I was going to be able to watch it, but I wasn't actually going to do it. I would have gone along with whatever Maria wanted to do. I wouldn't have stopped her from it. But what Maria didn't like was that I was not committed to supporting her, "tooth and nail," for having the VBAC.

COMMENTS: *Opposing attitudes between the mother and the father may create intense conflict. In order to find a peaceful resolution, both the man and the woman may need to take direct action by giving their own and one another's feelings focus and understanding.*

MARIA: Ed knew I was upset, but until we went to the La Leche League conference, where Lynn and Barbara gave a VBAC workshop, he really didn't understand very much about it.

ED: Lynn described some of the interventions that can lead to an unnecessary cesarean. As she described the posterior presentation, the breaking of the water, and why this aggravates rather than resolves the problem, I said to myself, "This woman is recounting the entire process that lead up to our cesarean section."

Up until this point, I was relatively closed-minded to the idea that the doctor and I, in fact, had aggravated the situation. But, when I heard her words, for me, a light went on.

We signed up for Lynn's VBAC class. After the first class we got into a very very big knock-down-drag-out fight on the way home. Maria accused me of everything but cutting her myself—conspiring with the doctor, holding the baby in so that she couldn't deliver it. I mean, she accused me of everything. I had been totally unaware of the anger, the frustration, the pain, and the hurt that came out that night. I could see it was there, but I couldn't understand it. Even to this day, I don't really fully understand it.

MARIA: Every pent up suspicion or black thought that ever had arisen in the back of my mind came out that night. The flood gates opened. It all came out, and Ed got it, but good.

ED: I think we left Lynn's house at 10:30, and walked into our house still angry with each other at about 2:00. And it's only a 30-minute drive. We just kept driving.

MARIA: Then we sat in the house until about 4:00, just discussing and discussing.

ED: As we went through the classes, it was my idea that we would learn, we could become knowledgeable, we would stay home much longer, but that we were going to have another hospital birth. And, if everything went well, that it would be a vaginal birth. The idea of a home birth never really seemed real to me. The other people in the class were so committed to this whole birth idea. I said to myself, "That's fine for them. I wish them a lot of luck and every good fortune," but I didn't see it happening to us.

MARIA: I was sitting in class saying to myself, "I want to deliver this baby without going through surgery. Whatever I have to do to do it, I'm going to do it." And if it made Ed happy that we were going to the hospital, fine, we were going to the hospital. But he wasn't going to get me there to sit alone in a room with no doctor, no nurses, no husband, for five hours in labor again.

ED: As we went through the classes I became interested. I have to describe myself for the record, as being what I consider to be a scientific person, an analytical person. I try to reason things out with logic, and sometimes seem a little cold. I still didn't see anything wrong with doctors and hospitals.

I started reading more. I started understanding more of what Lynn was trying to teach us, not only the factual items, (which I went after very hard), but the psychological situations for the mother and father as well.

It's a frightening thing for a man to see his wife in such pain, and not understand what's going on. Men are in the protect mode—defend and support. When a man sees his wife in pain, his impulse is to either do something about it himself or find someone else who can stop the pain. But once a man understands that the pain is not dangerous pain, then he can let the pain go on without trying to stop it. Once I learned that pain was not necessarily a bad thing all the time—that sometimes pain is part of the act—then I wasn't afraid of pain anymore.

COMMENTS: *It is often forgotten that men go through their own kind of pain in childbirth. The pain is not physical pain for themselves. The pain is psychological. The pain is wanting to take control of something that is out of their control. Once the man's pain is acknowledged and addressed as "real," then he can begin to deal with his fears of his wife's pain. Only then can he be of real support to her in labor.*

ED: I became more and more committed that we, not the doctor, would direct this birth; that he was there to help us, we were not there to help him.

I still remember asking Dr. Levine some questions. He looked at me, and said, "Are you a doctor? Did you study medicine or something like that?"

MARIA: Then he said, "You better be careful or you'll know more than I do." We had a lot of information at that point and we were asking him a lot of questions.

ED: I was beginning to feel uneasy about not knowing which doctor would actually be there for the delivery. Before the classes it had simply never occurred to me that there would be any question about who would deliver the baby. I was under the presumption that if you go to see a particular doctor prenatally, even if he has three associates, this doctor does the delivery. So, I was quite unnerved by the idea that you develop this whole rapport with someone who might not be there anyway. You could still end up having a stranger at your birth!

In addition, if I had read the stories of the births of the other people in our class, I would have said, "Hogwash! These stories aren't real!" But I sat with these people. I became friendly with these people. The more I heard from their horrifying experiences, the less acceptable the hospital was as a solution for us. I would not say that the hospital was *unacceptable,* but just less acceptable.

COMMENTS: *Ed and Maria's attitude—the hospital as less acceptable, not unacceptable was a key to their success in having a simple, straightforward VBAC. To allow a home or a hospital birth to be acceptable gives permission to let go.*

ED: Until about two months before the birth, we were still going to have a hospital birth. We had asked Lynn to be our labor coach, so that we could comfortably and with confidence stay home as long as possible. But we were still going to the hospital.

COMMENTS: *I remember Ed saying, "We're planning a hospital birth, and if everything goes perfectly, we'll stay home."*

ED: I was beginning to go through a change.

MARIA: Each class would dig out something else in Ed. He would come home annoyed about something new every time.

ED: Lynn is very good at spotting and attacking weak points, and hidden points. It seemed that any time that I would vacillate on a point, or sort of approach it with a soft or casual attitude, she would nail me on it. And being a relatively argumentative person, we got into some very interesting discussions in the class. But every time we walked away from there, I felt more and more uneasy about stepping into the hands of a hospital, and a doctor, and saying, "Here are our bodies. They're yours now. Do with them as you will." No longer was it my wife's body. She had lost a piece of the ownership because now I was in it. I really felt committed and part of this, which I had never felt before.

The more I fully understood the process, the more I fully understood the psychology. Lynn spent a great deal of time on the psychology of birth. With understanding came ownership. I was beginning to feel that fear and anticipation of labor myself.

If we had had another cesarean section, I would have felt no failure. We would have done our best, and as long as mother and child were healthy, I would have felt the mission had been accomplished. But it would not have been the way we wanted it. More and more, I wanted it to be our way.

I was learning more, I was understanding more. Learning how to palpate (to feel the lie and position of the baby with my own hands) was crucial in building my confidence. I think the first time I actually found the baby, felt the baby, knew where the parts were—that was probably the turning point. Now I knew something that even that damned doctor didn't know. He needed $25,000 worth of equipment (a sonagram) to tell what I could tell with my hands. And I said to myself, if I could do this, then there's no reason why I can't help my wife in labor.

MARIA: At one visit, I said to the doctor, "Is the baby still in an anterior position?" And the doctor did a doubletake. The doctor said, "How did you know that?" I said, "My husband and I are learning how to palpate for the baby's position." And the doctor said, "Hmmm." I swear he was making a mental note to put on my chart, "Be careful with this one. They know too much."

ED: We had started checking the baby's heart and position every two days. I still have the sheet with all the readings on it. At one point Maria felt that the baby had flipped over into a posterior position. I checked, and she was right. We were both a bit concerned because the posterior position had been a problem with the last delivery. But we knew from the training that we received that it was normal for the baby to flip, and that it could just as easily flip right back over, which the baby did three days later.

Knowing what the baby's normal heart rate was, knowing the baby's position, gave me such a feeling of confidence. I could feel, I could touch, I could sense, I knew exactly what was going on. Knowledge is power, and once you know what you're doing, you can do anything. I was beginning to feel confident in myself as a person who could be competent to understand my wife's needs, to look after her needs and to recognize danger signs. Once I started feeling comfortable within that, I began to feel more confident in our ability to do it ourselves.

I came to realize that the doctors were treating pregnancy as an illness. It wasn't an illness. I didn't really need to know a lot of illness skills, because we weren't ill. But if we became ill, then we would go to the doctor.

I knew in my heart that once we walked through that hospital door, I would have turned it over to the doctor and the staff. Try as I might to fight with it, I wouldn't have. The only reason we would be in the hospital at that point would have been that it was beyond my ability to deal with it—not Maria's ability, my ability. I knew that once I would have made the decision to go to the hospital, there would have been no turning back on it. I would have already done everything I could do, and now it would be their show.

About two or three weeks before the labor, I think it was the most critical point because Maria had bought the clamps. I was reminding her, "Did you get the sheets, the plastics for the mattress? Do we have the drop cloth, just in case?" I was making sure that the van was in good operating condition so that if we needed to transport quickly, we could. We had called a pediatrician, and spoke to the pediatrician together. We said, "Should, by some wild happenstance, this baby be born at home, suddenly without expectation, would you come to the house to see the baby?" And he said to us, "If the baby needs me, I will come." Again, now I had another support source.

One afternoon about 2:00 Maria called me at the office, saying, "I don't know for sure if anything's really going on, but why don't you come on home." I caught a 3:00 train, and was home at 4:00. When I arrived, Maria was in a case of the screaming labors. She had just called Lynn.

MARIA: I had been in Manhasset for an appointment with Lynn, but we miscommunicated and she wasn't there for the appointment. On my way home, I was having to stop the car for my contractions. I had had fried chicken for lunch, and I had thought, "Boy, I'm never going to eat that fried chicken again." I really thought that it was gas from the fried chicken and the cole slaw. I had been uncomfortable for about a day and a half, and I now understand that that was my pattern from both labors—mild discomfort for about a day and a half, and then all of a sudden I was in labor, *wham.*

ED: The only place that Maria was comfortable was sitting on the toilet. It was now about 4:15. Christine, our two year old, was in the living room talking to Anne, our neighbor. Maria let out one good yell, and Christine said, "Mommy's having a baby." And then she went back to her play as if she knew everything was fine. Christine was here for the whole delivery.

COMMENTS: *Though often parents are hesitant to have little children present for the labor and birth, when children have been well-educated most often the children accept the sights, sounds, and smells of the process more easily than adults as simply a part of life. The labor happens, the birth happens, and their life goes on as usual.*

ED: At 4:30 Lynn was not here yet, and Maria was screaming bloody murder. I was in the bathroom washing my hands, because it looked as if I was going to deliver this baby. Now, I'm the kind of guy that likes to try something new. But not that new! I was all prepared to do it if I had to. I wasn't hesitant in any way. The only problem was that the only position that Maria even wanted to talk about having this baby in was either sitting on the toilet or standing at the foot of the bed—the only two positions that I really couldn't deal with. Now I understand why the doctors want women to lie on their backs on a nice, flat table.

MARIA: All during labor, I could *not* sit down! About two hours before the birth I was going to sit down in my rocking chair to try to talk to my neighbor. This had been the only chair that I could be comfortable in for the last few months of my pregnancy. But each time I would go to sit down in labor (even in my "comfortable chair"), I would get within three inches of the pad and say, "Oh, well, Anne, I guess I'm going to walk around." I could not sit. I could not even get on hands and knees. I could not lie down. Sitting was terrible. Lying was the pits. There was no position I could be in comfortably. At least, if I sat on a toilet seat I could rest for a few seconds.

COMMENTS: *The toilet is one of the best places to labor, especially in the later stages. It is the place we associate with release. It is basically a supported squat position. It opens the pelvis, and opens the mind simultaneously. It is often used by midwives to enhance a slow-to-progress labor (referred to as "toilet-torture"). Maria simply followed her own natural instincts in finding the position that assisted the descent of her baby the most. Unfortunately, however, though toilet labors are marvelous for the woman, toilet births are not particularly relaxing for the birth attendant, no matter how experienced. One midwife who attended one such toilet birth described the outcome as, "The baby's apgar was 10; the midwife's apgar—0!" So, both Maria and Ed were in good company!*

ED: It was now about a quarter to five. I had decided that this baby was coming, and it was me that was going to catch it. I was trying to maneuver

Maria into any position that I could deal with. She wasn't going to sit, she was not going to lie. I tried to get her on her hands and knees. But the only place she would sit was on the toilet, and I was really afraid that she was going to drop the baby in the pot. For the last five minutes before Lynn arrived, Maria kept saying, "Lynn, where are you? I want Lynn. Go get her. Go call her again. Go find Lynn. She's lost." It was easy to see that Maria had taken scotch tape to hold this baby in until Lynn got there. So, Lynn walked in through the door, and Maria screamed a sigh of relief.

COMMENTS: *When I received the phone call from Maria that she was in labor, the labor seemed mild. I fully expected that the labor might take the better part of the night. One thing I knew for certain was that she wanted Ed to be there with her. She did not want to feel abandoned again in labor. I knew she would wait til he was with her to let the labor get stronger. But I NEVER suspected that as soon as he was there she would be ready to give birth!*

When I walked up the path to their house, Anne was screaming to me from the door, "Hurry! The baby's coming!" Half in disbelief, I quickened my pace considerably.

I found Maria sitting on the toilet, telling me not to bother checking the baby, because it was already here. Ed asked me where she could have this baby. I said, "Anywhere but here!" (on the toilet).

ED: So, Maria took a stand at the foot of our bed, which is a cannonball bed with a big rail in the front of it. Lynn played catcher, and Maria just let her breath out and the baby dropped. Then I saw something which I never had seen before, and will probably never see again—such a look of exhilaration on Maria's face! I think at that point she could have done anything. She said, "We did it," which meant a lot to me, because I knew she meant her and me.

And there was the baby—a little ugly, ratty-looking thing. I'm glad Lynn was here for the delivery, because there was more blood than I expected. I would have become frightened. We probably would have run to the hospital for nothing. In any case, the baby was fine. Maria delivered the placenta fine. Lynn was terrific in both what she did and what she didn't do. She could have very easily just totally taken over the situation, and been just like the doctor. But she didn't.

I was snapping pictures, because it was the only thing I could do at the moment. Lynn told me to put the camera down, cut the cord, and hold the baby—things that I should be doing, which I had forgotten.

A little while later, Maria was in the bathtub, getting cleaned up. Lynn looked at Maria, saying, "I'm teaching a class tonight at 8:30. Do you need me here? Should I cancel class? What do you want me to do?" And Maria said, "Why don't you have the class here?" I was absolutely floored! What a great idea!

We had the most wonderful birthday party right after the birth, which is the most appropriate time to have a birthday party. Everybody brought cake and ice cream and cookies, and we took pictures.

COMMENTS: *Though many families have birthday parties after their home births, this party was very special. All the couples who had given Maria and Ed the impetus to have their baby at home were invited to the party. These same people were all still awaiting the births of their VBAC babies, and since their previous births had been by cesarean, they had never seen or held a baby who was only hours old—not even their own babies!*

ED: After everybody left, Maria and I went into the bedroom, and lay down in bed with the baby between us. I remember leaning over and looking at Maria, saying, "This is the way it's supposed to be. This is the way you're supposed to have babies." That moment was probably one of the most fulfilling moments that I can remember, because we did something that I had previously thought we couldn't do. I hadn't been afraid that Maria wasn't going to be up to it. I had been afraid I wasn't going to be able to deal with it. I had had a lot of fear. We overcame that fear. We did it!

I made a big turn-around. It was easily 180 degrees. If you could go more than 180 degrees in a more opposite direction, then that would describe the changes I made. If I could make that turn-around, then a lot of people could make that turn-around. But it takes a lot of work. It's not something you enter into lightly. I guess it's like marriage in that respect. You have to spend a lot of time and a lot of effort. It's an experience I would recommend for anyone who has the nerve for it, who has the guts for it. It's not an easy thing to do. But if anyone has any doubts about whether children can be born at home healthy and happy, tell him to come and see us.

14

What a Difference Support Can Make

GINA AND RICHARD BERQUIST

G INA: At 23 years of age, more than eleven years ago, I became pregnant with my daughter, Lia. I was very excited about the pregnancy and the baby.

When I had a prenatal with a doctor he checked my pelvis and told me that everything was fine. But my sister had had a cesarean about a month before I got pregnant, so I wondered if there would be anything wrong with my pelvis.

COMMENTS: *Cesarean seeds had unintentionally been planted for Gina by her sister's recent cesarean. Such seeds are quite powerful and need to be dealt with creatively in order to release and diffuse their power.*

GINA: We lived in Colorado in a small mining town of about 600 people. There were no childbirth classes. I just left my labor and birth up to mother nature. I had a good attitude about birth because my mother always had a very good attitude about birth.

During my pregnancy, I was pretty content. Richard never got too involved. Although I really wanted to have a baby, he was not really into it. So it was therefore considered my pregnancy and my baby. I went through my pregnancy with very little support. A friend of mine gave me a Lamaze book which I read from cover to cover over and over during my pregnancy. I asked Richard to read his section for fathers, but he said he wasn't interested. I felt hurt.

COMMENTS: *Although many women whose husbands do not wish to participate in their pregnancies or births feel hurt and unloved, nonparticipation by fathers in birth is not necessarily negative. In most primitive cultures fathers never participated in the actual birth process, although they certainly did participate in their own rite of passage into fatherhood. Only recently have fathers been expected to be involved in the birth process. However, although women do not always need to have their husbands present at the birth of their babies, pregnant and birthing women need to know that their husbands support them deeply and powerfully. Support is loving communication about needs and desires—physically, emotionally, and spiritually. The choice about when, how, and where this support is given is a choice which must be made individually by each couple.*

RICHARD: I knew Gina wanted me to be there by her side for the birth. Although I was very confident that labor was a very natural happening, and that everything was going to work out fine, it still scared me to be involved. I was reluctant and kind of frightened at the prospect of being involved with an operation. Even though I wasn't anticipating a cesarean, I saw it as an operation. I had seen a natural childbirth movie while I was taking an EMT (Emergency Medical Technician) course. The movie was very scary, and left me thinking that I wouldn't want to have to be too involved in a birth.

COMMENTS: *Seeds had also been planted for Richard—seeds of fear by his EMT training. Both Gina and Richard entered the birth of their first child with conflict between their conscious and unconscious beliefs. Consciously, they each believed in the natural process, but unconsciously perhaps they each anticipated an operation.*

GINA: When I was about two weeks overdue I called my doctor, who was about 50 miles away, and said, "Oh, please, I'm so uncomfortable. Isn't there some way I can get this going?" And he said, " Come in for your next check tomorrow, and we'll see how you are." After he determined that I was far enough along, he gave me some castor oil. My husband and I checked into a nearby motel. I hardly took any of the oil, but it was enough to get my labor started.

COMMENTS: *Being overdue is difficult because of pressures from within ourselves. Because we are so conditioned to have everything in our lives under our control, we often find it difficult to allow nature its own timing with regard to the onset of labor. We want to know when labor will begin, how long it will last, how painful it will be, and what will be its outcome.*

Our very desire for guaranteed answers to these questions has in many ways created the medical interventions which we now fear and disdain. If we are ever to reverse the trend of greater and greater intervention in the birth process, we must first be willing to reverse our desire as mothers to control a process which is innately uncontrollable—the process of labor. In order to release our desire to control we must be willing to accept that we will not know when labor will begin, how long it will last, or how painful it will be. We cannot be guaranteed anything—not even a healthy baby. When we are willing to accept nature's timing, her process, and her outcome, then we will be ready to have a truly natural birth.

GINA: When I went into labor, I had incredible back labor, which I later discovered was due to my baby's posterior position. I was lying on my side and on my back throughout my whole labor. I had very little support and felt very alone during my labor. At one point a nurse rubbed my back, which felt very soothing and comforting. But her shift changed, and she was gone.

I was in labor for about 36 hours. I was thirsty throughout it, and never got anything to drink. My husband just hung on the side of the bed, exhausted, not knowing how to help me or what to do for me. I knew it was causing him a lot of emotional pain for me to lay there that long in labor. But he didn't know how to do anything for me. I became angry during my labor, feeling that he could have helped me, if only he had taken more interest during my pregnancy.

RICHARD: I was totally unprepared for the birth of our baby. I thought labor would be painful and would take time. However, I had no idea what it would be like. I had no instinctual knowledge. I was totally dependent on my own wife's instincts and upon the doctor. He was God as far as I was concerned. Whatever he said, I was going to have my wife do.

I didn't see myself as having a role, other than trying to encourage and support my wife in whatever way I recognized. Unfortunately, I didn't recognize much. I felt like I had very little to do except hold her hand. I couldn't share her pains. I couldn't share anything with her really because I didn't understand much.

I felt helpless because I knew and understood so little about what was happening. Nobody attempted to explain anything to me. I was told to go away whenever any kind of checking procedures were done (like checking her cervix). I was kept very much in the dark. The atmosphere wasn't very friendly or warm—just very technical.

COMMENTS: *Since birth has been removed from the home and family, techno-birth has removed all "unqualified persons" (including the mother and father) from the richness of birthing. Techno-birth PERMITS only a token amount of involvement for all unqualified persons. Techno-birth encourages all unqualified persons to remain unqualified, uninformed, and uninvolved—turning over their responsibilities to those who are considered to be qualified. Richard's experience clearly demonstrates that whenever we choose techno-birth—to see ourselves as unqualified, uninformed, and uninvolved—we place ourselves in a position of powerlessness and helplessness.*

GINA: The doctor finally came and told me that he felt that I wasn't making any progress. I had dilated to only 5 centimeters. He said my pelvis was too small for her and that I had uterine inertia. He told me that my baby was in distress, and that I needed to have a cesarean. Though I was depressed about having a cesarean, I was so exhausted that I actually felt relieved that the pain would be over.

RICHARD: When the doctor told us Gina needed to have a cesarean, I thought, "Well, that'll be fine. She's been going through labor for 36 hours. A cesarean means they'll stop all that pain. The baby will be out and everything will be fine." I was glad that someone had made a decision that I could understand. I was totally trusting in the operation.

GINA: During my labor I never once screamed out, but when I got into surgery I cried and cried and cried. I felt totally alone and deserted. It felt really good to cry, to release my feelings of helplessness. For a split-second I thought, "I may not come out of this alive."

COMMENTS: *As with many Lamaze mothers, Gina had worked hard to "stay in control" of her labor—not to cry out, not to make noise—to do labor "right." It was not until she was in surgery that she allowed herself to lose control. According to many childbirth techniques, losing control is often looked upon as defeat and failure. However, if Gina had permitted herself to let go of the controls—to shout out, to scream, to cry—to make whatever sounds she needed to make during the labor, perhaps she might have released herself, her labor, and her baby. Her labor might have progressed, and her baby might have been born more easily.*

And contemplating the possibility of our own death is a common experience for everyone being prepped for surgery. For many of us it is the first time we have ever been so close to the possibility of our own death. For some of us it is the first true acknowledgment of our own mortality, the first true test of our spiritual beliefs about life and death.

Though such a questioning experience may be frightening, it may well be one of the most emotionally healthy outcomes of the cesarean experience. If we had lived in other times in other cultures, the possibility of death would be a part of everyday existence. We would have faced the death of loved ones and the possible death of ourselves within the context of life itself. We would have faced the possibility of death in the process of childbirth itself—not simply in surgical birth. Perhaps we might have entered the birth experience having much greater knowledge of the interrelationship of birth and death in the cycle of life—an inner knowledge which might more easily facilitate the letting go necessary both in birth and death.

GINA: I was treated as a piece of meat. They scrubbed down my belly with ice-cold Betadine (an antiseptic), which would be uncomfortable for anyone. But for a woman in labor, it was horrifying.

Then they shaved me. They stretched out my arms and stuck me with needles. While they did this to me they talked as if nothing were happening. Then they covered me with layers and layers of cloth. I felt I was being buried alive. It was one of the worst experiences of my life. Then the anesthesiologist said, "You're sailing," and one . . . two . . . three . . . I was out.

RICHARD: When I first saw the baby, it was in a little cubicle coming out of the operating room. I felt lost. I didn't know if this was my baby, or whose baby it was. Something was happening, but I didn't know what I was supposed to do or feel. I was totally unprepared in every way.

GINA: They woke me in the recovery room with the news that I had a girl. I didn't see my baby until 24 hours later. I held her hand for just a moment, and we were all crying—saying how beautiful she was. But I felt very separate from her—distant, as if I just had a bad dream and there she was. I couldn't really relate that she came from my body.

It wasn't until 36 hours later that I got to hold her. But by that time I was too sore and weak to hold her. She just sort of lay next to me.

RICHARD: It must have been days before I held my baby. I felt so helpless and alienated from the whole process. It was my own fear which had kept me from participating from the beginning.

GINA: I planned to nurse, but they told me I couldn't nurse. So, I thought that if I bottlefed that would get Richard more involved. But my husband hardly ever held or fed her anyway.

The pain after having a cesarean is pretty incredible. I was very depressed. I felt very lonely and empty, without any support. My husband didn't come to visit me in the hospital because it was 60 miles from our home.

After 5 days I wanted to come home. But I kept thinking, "How am I going to take care of this baby when I can't even take care of myself?" During my pregnancy, my mother had told me she would come to help me, but just before I went into labor she told me she would not be able to come. I continued, however, to hope that she would help me anyway. I even believed that when I arrived home from the hospital, that she would be there waiting for me. But she didn't come. It was very disappointing—just bad all around.

I forced myself to become very strong very quickly. I didn't want to have to deal with my scar. I didn't want to look. Although my upper abdomen hurt to gentle touch for two years, at two weeks I was doing sit-ups.

COMMENTS: *We all want our partners and our mothers to love us, care for us, and support us when we are having our babies. When the support and love is not freely given, we may unconsciously go to greater and greater lengths to get that attention. Perhaps Gina's difficult labor and surgical birth were unconscious attempts to get the attention she so desperately needed. Unfortunately, her attempts to get their attention failed. She still did not get what she needed from either her husband or her mother. She even gave up nursing to get her husband's involvement with the baby. She sacrificed her birth experience and her nursing experience.*

Her decision to rely upon her own strengths post partum was probably the first step in attaining her VBAC.

RICHARD: Neither Gina nor I communicated about our feelings during Lia's early life. I'm sure there were enormous amounts of Gina's feelings that I did not understand. I wasn't aware until years later how disappointed she felt about separation, not nursing, and not being able to be conscious during her birth.

I thought, "That's just the way things happen in the hospital." I wasn't able to communicate with her about my feelings because I felt so ambivalent and confused. I was embarrassed because there was a whole well-spring of feelings that I couldn't even identify.

The cesarean was just an extension of where we were at the time. Unfortunately, I didn't learn anything from this experience for quite a while. Eleven years later I learned that we had to take responsibility for our own experiences, including birth experiences. We can't blame anybody else. A cesarean is the result of not being involved or informed, and allowing ourselves to be led by the nose in very important matters. I'm not angry. I'm not disappointed. I consider that the cesarean was the result of our inexperience, our immaturity, our lack of responsibility.

GINA: I was convinced that if I wanted to have another baby that I would have to have another cesarean. I believed there was something wrong with me. I was diagnosed as having CPD, uterine inertia, and fetal distress. I never wanted to have another baby like that again. I would look at pregnant women and feel almost sick to my stomach, thinking, "I never want to be pregnant again." I didn't want to have another baby for years.

COMMENTS: *Sadly, many many women have a cesarean and never have another baby because they never want to have another cesarean. The conflict between wanting another baby and fearing another cesarean may become so deep that they may become pregnant unintentionally, and have unwanted abortions to avoid the fearful experience of another cesarean. Others bury their fears, decide to become pregnant and force themselves to undergo the surgery they feel is necessary for them to become mothers. All women should know that unnecessary cesareans can be avoided, and that even when they are necessary, having had one cesarean does not mean that you must have more cesareans.*

GINA: When Lia was about five years old, I somehow rediscovered myself as a woman. I decided I did want another child, even though having another cesarean was horrifying to me. But Richard didn't want to have another child. He wasn't prepared. He had just changed jobs. He wanted to wait. One year, two years, three years, four years passed. I felt that I probably would never have any more children. I put it off for five years. And it pained me to do that.

When we moved to Arkansas I met a supportive midwife, Francoise, and began to learn from her about natural birth. I asked my husband again, "Could we have a baby?" He was afraid, but I told him I knew

Francoise would help me to have the baby naturally at home. This time he agreed full-heartedly, and from that moment he put all his energies into it.

RICHARD: I originally didn't want to have so much involvement. I was somewhat scared, especially of having a home birth. I was a little bit apprehensive for her health, but I believed in her conviction and knowledge. I was trusting her judgment. Later as I became aware and informed of the natural process of having a child, I realized how easily natural home birth fit into my basic philosophy in the natural order of life.

I felt very strongly that Gina could do it. She is a very strong person. That's one of the reasons I became involved with her. I admire her strength, especially in something that is as natural to her as having children.

COMMENTS: *With this pregnancy, Richard faced his fears early. Even though he felt scared, instead of choosing not to participate, he sought the information he would need to vault the hurdle of his own fears.*

GINA: Marriah was conceived and I must say that at first I was obsessed with, "Will it happen? Will it be OK? Will the baby be OK?"

I went to a doctor for backup, and he told me a horror-story about how my uterus was going to rupture, I would hemorrhage, and the baby would die. Then, I felt, "Am I doing the right thing, am I endangering my life and my baby's life? Maybe I'm asking for too much. Why can't I just be happy with the baby and not have a vaginal birth?"

But Francoise put all those fears to rest. She was always very positive. Finally I did find one doctor locally who said, "Go for it!"

COMMENTS: *With this pregnancy, Gina got the support she needed when her own fears arose. With the support of Francoise, her midwife, Gina was able to overcome her own fears.*

GINA: From the very beginning of my pregnancy, I did a lot of visualizations. I planned how I wanted my labor and birth to be. I dreamt about it. I prayed about it. I was teaching classes with Francoise; I took classes with Francoise. I felt that I did everything I could possibly do to prepare for it. I came to feel after all my preparation, that if it wasn't going to be a successful VBAC, then it was just meant for me to go through another cesarean.

COMMENTS: *Gina took control of that which she could control, and let go of that which she could not control, which is the secret of safe and simple birthing.*

RICHARD: I also took the classes, and I attended and took photographs of a couple of home births.

FRANCOISE: The first home birth that Richard actually saw was my delivery of my third son. Gina was my attendant at that birth, and at the time Gina was five months pregnant.

RICHARD: For me becoming involved and aware was more of a learned experience, where I feel my wife has a more intuitive understanding of labor and birthing. She has learned a lot from her studying, but she seemed to intuitively understand a whole lot more about these matters than I did.

I saw my role as supporting Gina's efforts, recognizing the positive steps she was taking, providing encouragement, and giving her all the support that she needed.

Gina Berquist in labor, with Francoise checking dilation. Support comes from husband, mother, and sister. Note hot compresses on her belly.

Linda Wright Photograph

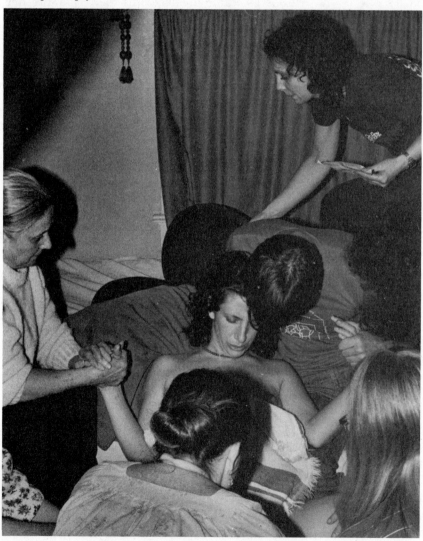

GINA: I got a lot of support from a lot of good people, and I think that's what got me through it. Although I had a hard pregnancy, my husband and my family were all very supportive, and helpful the whole time. Even though my mother was afraid, she did support me. She never questioned or doubted for a moment that I could do it, that we could do it. Francoise and the other midwives supported me thoroughly. I think you need lots and lots of support—people telling you that you can do it, and believing that you can do it. With all their support, I didn't feel so alone—although ultimately I was alone with this decision.

RICHARD: My expectations of the second birth were far different from the first. I knew I was going to be involved. I knew I was going to be taking more responsibility. I was becoming more conscious of the risk. I was becoming more informed.

GINA: I looked forward to my labor. It began one morning with very mild contractions that were about three minutes apart. I went swimming and out to lunch with my mother and sister. I just took a leisure day, thinking that this would be the day that my baby would be born.

RICHARD: Gina's labor started and she was just doing her normal routines. I thought it was wonderful that she was feeling that good about herself. Labor was so mild. I knew it was going to get more intense. I didn't get too involved until it did get intense, and then I was totally absorbed in it.

COMMENTS: *How very different from the first labor! Gina was not desperate to get the baby out. She didn't need to induce labor or rush labor. She was willing to flow with nature's timing, and flow through her day. She integrated labor into her life as an everyday event, and all those around her supported her in doing so.*

GINA: About 5:00 in the evening, my contractions were still mild and three minutes apart. Then my membranes ruptured.

RICHARD: When the waters broke, and appeared to be slightly discolored with meconium, there was some question as to whether or not the baby might be under some stress. The hardest part was making the decision that the baby was really all right, and we shouldn't panic about that.

COMMENTS: *Discolored fluid is not necessarily a sign of distress. It is simply an indicator that the health of the baby should be closely observed. The fetal heart tones (including beat-to-beat variability) should be assessed carefully and consistently in order to determine whether or not the baby is in distress.*

Meanwhile, it is just as important to remain calm. Fear is catching. If those surrounding the mother seem fearful, the seed of fear grows quickly. If the mother becomes fearful, her fear can actually alter the hormones her body secretes (thus stopping the labor), or constrict the blood flow to the baby (thus creating the very problem about which everyone is so worried— fetal distress).

GINA: I started getting into harder labor about 6:00 in the evening, which is exactly what I had hoped for—to go into hard labor in the evening.

Richard was with me the whole time. He was extremely supportive throughout my labor.

RICHARD: I was much more involved in this birth. I had a lot more expectations. I was much more confident. I was a participant. I was excited and enthusiatic about it. I trusted entirely in my wife—in her knowledge and her ability to be in touch with her body. I was in touch with her body, with her spiritual and emotional disposition. I trusted in everything, and it worked out beautifully. I felt like I breathed every breath with my wife.

GINA: At about 8:00 Francoise and my other midwives came to the house. I was about 3 centimeters dilated. My greatest fear had been that I might not dilate, because I had only dilated to 5 centimeters with my first daughter. However, an hour later, I was 7 centimeters dilated, and an hour after that, I was totally dilated.

FRANCOISE: Gina's sister (who had two sections) was her greatest support and it was relieving watching them work through her labor. Gina was a perfect example of aiding herself through visualization and talking to her baby. Phrases like, "I am opening for you, baby . . . come on baby . . . " She was very vocal about her feelings because that was right for her.

COMMENTS: *Gina had all the support she needed, not only from her husband, but from her mother and her sister as well. Instead of feeling that she needed to have a cesarean because her sister had had a cesarean, she had her sister's full and complete support for a natural home VBAC. Instead of needing to beg for her mother's help after the baby would be born, her mother gave her her support and assistance from the beginning of the pregnancy. Instead of feeling hurt that her husband chose not to be involved with the pregnancy, Richard chose to take complete responsibility. Instead of trying to stay in control she gave herself the freedom to be as expressive as she needed to be. She let herself go as she let her baby go.*

GINA: I was standing, kneeling, and squatting throughout my whole labor, which was only about 7-1/2 hours. I didn't want to lie down. I felt that if I squatted in a position that I felt was the most natural position for women to have babies in, that my pelvis would expand to its greatest size, and that my baby would be born.

RICHARD: I physically supported Gina so that she could be vertical and allow gravity to help push the baby through the birth canal. I knew that the reason she had had a cesarean originally was because she was lying down.

FRANCOISE: The supine position for Gina was literally impossible. She had a calcification on her sacrum, which altered the "normal" shape of her pelvis, narrowing its front-to-back diameter. Therefore, considering the position which was forced upon her during her first labor, it is quite possible that her cesarean for CPD (cephalo-pelvic disproportion) was actually necessary.

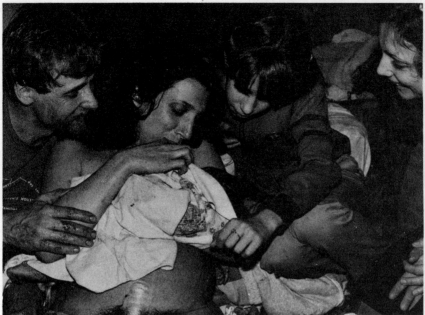

Linda Wright Photograph

The family admire newborn Marriah. Note the cesarean scar.

RICHARD: So we planned that she was going to be vertical, and that gravity would help a whole lot, and it did.

GINA: Although Francoise had told me that in her opinion the calcification combined with the supine position had caused the CPD, it seemed to me that my first baby had been stuck much higher in my pelvis. So I didn't let myself believe that I had a deformity. I just kept believing that I could do it.

FRANCOISE: I was very aware as I did perineal massage, that the descent of the head hesitated a bit as the baby passed over the calcification.

RICHARD: It was very enjoyable helping Gina, touching her, supporting her. We both felt strong together.

GINA: My baby was born at 1:25 am. Marriah was and is incredibly alert and beautiful. She weighed 7 lb. 7 oz., and her head circumference was 13 and 3/4 inches—bigger than my first baby.

FRANCOISE: Marriah's face did appear to have molded around the calcification during the birth process. The right side of her face from her eye down to her chin was slightly compressed. Gina had overcome what had appeared to be a physically impossible situation. She taught me that a woman's belief in herself is more powerful than any physical hindrance. This knowledge has allowed me to help other women have VBACs when it has appeared that the reason for their cesarean may have been physically necessary as well.

RICHARD: The difference was night and day between my first daughter's birth and my second daughter's birth. Everything seemed easier and more enjoyable because we were acting out of much more knowledge.

GINA: My labor, to me, seemed easy. Although contraction to contraction, you know it's hard and something you have to deal with, it seemed so easy to me after having had labor for 36 hours with my first daughter.

RICHARD: Our birth experience reinforces our beliefs and the values about life and the natural order of things—proof that when you get involved and accept more responsibility for your own life, your own health, and your own experience that things can be much better. As we mature, all the significant things get better. It gives us encouragement to continue in those beliefs, as a basis for future decisions about similar things.

This experience added enormously to the richness of our relationship as a family, as a husband and wife. Being involved in the birth of my own child, having participated fully, was in a way a climax to my sex education. Now I can't imagine sex education being complete without at least witnessing the birth experience. It's a wonderful climax, and it's a very healthy experience for the process of family.

Lia was fully involved in the pregnancy, labor and birth. I can't imagine a healthier experience for a girl her age. Witnessing a successful natural birth will reinforce her belief in the natural order. I'm sure it will stay with my first daughter for the rest of her life.

Lia Berquist dresses her newborn sister, Marriah.

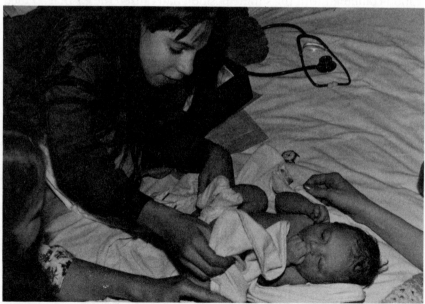

GINA: I felt as if it was an incredibly beautiful dream that turned out to be reality. Everything went exactly as I had planned, and exactly as I had visualized and prayed for. It was perfectly beautiful. I had no depression after this birth. I was in total ecstacy. I smiled for a week after my baby was born.

RICHARD: Seeing the baby when she came out was wonderful! Catching the baby when she came out, touching her, putting her up on Gina's belly, seeing Gina look at her, seeing her healthy, seeing all the people touching with a wonderful sort of communion—was a spiritual and emotional high. I was actually witnessing a miracle, and the miracle extended far beyond just the baby. Marriah's birth was probably the most emotionally fulfilling event of my life.

NANCY (GINA'S SISTER): Every time I recall the experience of my niece being born, the same feeling of excitement, yet calmness, comes back into my being. It's an experience I'll never forget. No words could describe my feelings when that tiny head appeared, and then the body came forth from Gina's body. What a beautiful experience! I do believe sharing this experience with my sister and her family has brought us all a bit closer—to feel the calmness and peaceful teamwork we all shared— no one can remove that from us. The energy is so strong.

The realization of life—how we all have come into this world—how I came into this world. Somehow I never really thought that I was born like that, too! It really is pitiful how ignorant we all are about life.

Post-Script: The Birth of Sierra

GINA: After Marriah was born I thought about having another baby. But I was stalling, I wasn't sure if I was strong enough to raise another child. Richard would jokingly say that when he made his first million we could have another child.

But I became pregnant by surprise in May, 1985. I had mixed emotions about it. I wanted another baby, but because it wasn't a conscious decision I was feeling depressed. Richard was feeling angry, questioning how he could have lost control of his life. A lot of that anger spilled over onto me.

I was nauseous for 3 1/2 months—not feeling well physically. But after the nausea passed, I felt better about the pregnancy. As I felt stronger, Richard became more supportive.

In the back of my mind, I worried about how this labor would go. My main concern was not whether or not this baby would be delivered vaginally, but whether I would be strong enough to care for this baby. I felt more dependent upon Richard than ever before, a feeling which connected Richard and I even more during this pregnancy.

My baby was due February 9, and this time I had planned my birth to be a more intimate experience between Richard and I. I had chosen a midwife, Kate Conway. In addition, the only other people present

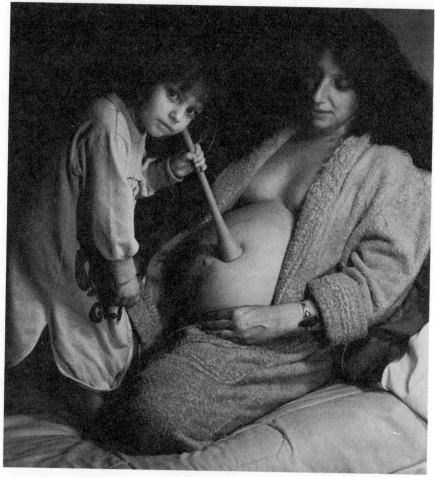

Listening for heart tones with a wooden fetascope

were my friend, Debbi, and my children. I had planned it all out, visualized it, and written it all down. I had planned to spend some of my labor in the bath, alternating with other upright positions.

I went into labor while in the morning of February 20, 1986, with very mild contractions about 5 minutes apart. As the day progressed, there was much commotion in my house, and the contractions stopped. Later in the afternoon as the atmosphere calmed, the contractions returned.

My oldest daughter, Lia, was home from school that day. We spent the day together talking and joking, and planning what was going to happen that evening. Lia and I set up the household for the birth, and then about 4:00 P.M., called Richard to tell him to come home, "This was it!" He arrived about an hour later. At that point my contractions were very close together, getting a little stronger, but not long in duration.

At about 5:00 P.M. I called Debbi to come over. Then at 6:00 P.M. I said, "Maybe we should just call Kate, to have her come to check me." I was just curious about how far dilated I was. When she arrived I was about 5 or 6 centimeters. I was thrilled. Although the contractions had felt mild, I was already well on my way!

I did not want to lay or sit. Richard sat on the bed, and I was kneeling facing him. As I was having a contraction, Richard would lift me up and I would just let everything fall. It seemed to open all my lower vertebrae. This was the intimate experience I had been wanting with Richard. We felt very close.

An hour later Kate checked me and I was 8 centimeters. The baby was definitely coming, and Richard kept saying, "Do you want to get in the bathtub?" Barely able to mutter, I tried to tell him there wasn't time. The contractions were coming very close together and were very intense. Kate said, "Gina, it sounds like you're pushing." And I said, "No, it's not me. I'm not the one who's pushing. It's happening by itself." So Kate said, "Well, let me check you. Maybe it IS time to push." Hearing her words, "You're full dilated!" felt really good. During Marriah's birth I had been trained not to push, but just to blow the baby out. So this time it felt really good to push.

At that point we changed positions. Richard got in front of me so that he could catch the baby. I turned around, and my friend, Debbi, held me up from behind as I let everything drop into a squat. Then I started to push. I was pushing hard. The only thing I had forgotten was the mirror, so that I could watch the birth. But I was pushing with my eyes closed, so I might not have seen anyway.

Gina with her second VBAC baby, Sierra

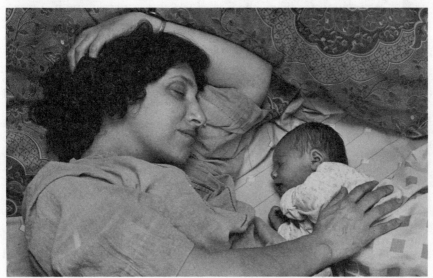

Marriah was already in the room with me. But Lia was in the kitchen preparing the birthday cake. I called to her, "Lia, the baby's coming!" I didn't want her to miss the birth. The head was born. Then I pushed hard twice, but the shoulders needed help. Kate reached in and guided the shoulder out. The rest of the baby slipped out at 7:40 P.M.

I will always remember hearing Marriah shout out, "Now, I'm a big sister!" I wanted to find out who the baby was, Sierra or Jackson. It was Sierra, a girl! Richard knew it was a girl. He makes girls.

Lia called my parents, and they came right over after the birth. Then more friends arrived, and we had a party. We had a birthday cake, and sang happy birthday to the baby.

I took an herbal bath with the baby, which felt great. Throughout the night I had many strong after-contractions, and Richard was there for me the whole night.

I never thought I could feel as wonderful as I had felt with Marriah's birth, but all those same wonderful feelings of joy and satisfaction came back again with Sierra's birth.

15

You Could Have Died

KARYN AIKIN

Karyn had had two previous cesareans. The first was a vertical incision for twins, the first of whom was presenting in a transverse lie. (The baby was lying sideways in the womb and therefore could not be born vaginally). The second cesarean was due to lack of support for a VBAC. The doctor who had initially supported a VBAC changed his mind at the last minute, and told her if she didn't have a cesarean, both she and the baby would die. So prior to labor, Karyn consented to another cesarean, and a low segment transverse cesarean was performed within hours.

With her third pregnancy, Karyn searched once again for a birth attendant. Once again, she heard nothing but horror stories from the doctors. She did find a midwife who was willing to attend her birth. But as a welfare mother, she had very little money, and the state does not pay for the services of lay midwives. So she decided to give birth alone in her hut in Hawaii.

However, her labor was very powerful from the onset. The power of these contractions frightened her, so she called her social worker, and asked her to meet her at the hospital. When she arrived at the hospital, she was fully dilated, and the doctor who had previously told her she would die if she had a vaginal birth, consented to deliver the baby "from below." Karyn was thrilled with her vaginal birth, thrilled that her body could do it, and thrilled with the baby. But she was not at all thrilled with the way that her baby was treated in the hospital— early cutting of the cord, the bathing, the silver nitrate, the vitamin K shot, the separation.

So with her next pregnancy, Karyn wanted to have a home VBAC. Once again she was told that with her history of a two incisions—one vertical and one transverse—she should have another cesarean. Apparently the doctors believed that her history of a previous VBAC was insignificant. However, Karyn's previous successful VBAC was exceedingly significant to herself. Since she had once before endured the "pains of labor" and her body had pushed out her last baby without a problem, Karyn had more faith in herself, in her body, and in God (who was her major support person). Once again Karyn was without a practitioner willing to attend a home VBAC, and once again Karyn planned an unattended home VBAC.

KARYN: I needed supportive input, so I leaned on God. Every time I had a sincerely heartfelt fear of birthing, assurance was there in answer to my prayer.

However, I stopped attending church because people were keeping such close tabs on me, expecting a hospital birth, *of course!* So, I dove into the Bible for home birth support, building up my faith that all would be OK, seeking the kingdom of God, loving God above my own life, and understanding how death lost its sting by Christ's sacrifice for us.

I awoke at 12:15 A.M. with contractions, and prepared the play room for the birth. The baby was born at 3:15 A.M. The placenta came out easily. I got up peacefully and looked in the mirror. Yes, I had torn. So I called the babysitter and went to the hospital for stitches. The doctor massaged my uterus (ooooch) and told me I didn't tear badly, so I wouldn't need a lot of stitches.

I refused to allow the hospital to wash the baby. I weighed him and washed his poopy bottom. I moved slowly and gently, and he didn't cry. The nurse started putting soap on his face. I reminded her that I had said that I wanted to wash him, and whisked her hands off him, as if I were shooing off a fly.

When the doctor realized that he had seen me prenatally, and that I had refused a cesarean, he said, "You could have died!" I said nothing, but I was reminded of how fear of death is used on pregnant women to convince them they need repeat cesareans.

COMMENTS: *When a woman faces the most frightening possibility in birth— death—moving through those feelings with faith (in God, in herself, in nature, in whatever powerful source she holds as her center of life), then she moves into birth with great freedom to allow the natural process to take place. She lets go and her baby is born with ease.*

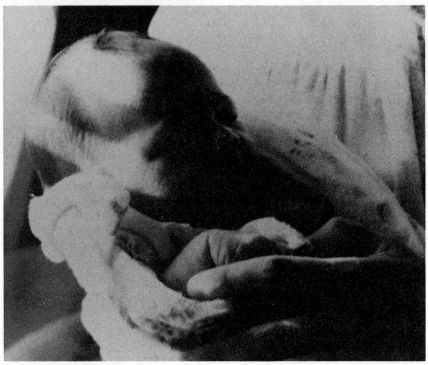

Paul Samuel Aikin (3½ days)

Though giving birth alone is not recommended from the point of view of physical safety for the mother or baby, sometimes a woman is forced to choose between a cesarean and an unattended home VBAC. Given these choices, most women choose a cesarean, as they do not feel confident enough in themselves or in the process to feel safe with an unattended home VBAC. Yes, it is true that Karyn's birth could have been an unattended disaster. And, she could be judged irresponsible. But who is more irresponsible— the mother who decides to birth at home alone because she believes that her body was made by God to give birth naturally, or the practitioner who refuses this woman her God-given right to birth her own baby?

16

From ICU to Empirical Midwifery

APRIL ALTMAN

The Birth of Rivka

APRIL: When I was pregnant with my first baby, at about 24 weeks gestation, the doctor told me that my baby was breech. I said to him that most babies were breech at this time, but he said, "Well, we better do a sonagram and check it out." Then he tried to turn the baby without telling me what he was doing, and it was very painful and unsuccessful.

COMMENTS: *Turning a breech baby requires cooperation on the part of the mother. She needs to feel relaxed. Her uterus must be relaxed to allow the baby space to make the rotation. Practitioners who are highly successful in turning breeches have found certain factors that assist the rotation, and usually have developed a system that permits the version to be both physically safe and psycho-spiritually positive. (See* Breech VBAC Without Pelvimetry *by Leo Sorger, OB/GYN).*

APRIL: Then I asked the doctor about delivering a breech baby vaginally, and he said, "It's very dangerous, and you don't want to hurt the baby." I got a few other opinions from other doctors who concurred with my first doctor.

I let the doctor plan a cesarean for me. It was very frightening, but I did not want to harm my baby. Two weeks before my due date I went into the hospital. I was very scared. But as a neonatal ICU nurse I was trained to follow a doctor's orders. I trusted him.

COMMENTS: *Even though all of us as little girls growing up into women have learned to give our trust to the doctor, nursing training intensifies this belief. Nurses are strictly trained to obey the orders of the doctor. Therefore, perhaps for more than any other sociologic group within our culture, it is most difficult for nurses as mothers to question the authority of a doctor, and place their trust in themselves and in their own intuition.*

APRIL: Once I survived the cesarean, my recovery was fine. But it took me a while to realize how upset I was about my cesarean. At first I was anxious to have another baby. But then later I became so afraid of having another cesarean that I didn't want more children.

COMMENTS: *Whenever we are confronted with trauma, in order to protect our psyches, denial is the first response. April denied her feelings about her cesarean until her psyche was ready to deal with those difficult feelings.*

The Birth of David

APRIL: Finally, I felt that I could somehow handle another cesarean. I was ready, so I got pregnant. I was very excited when the doctor said I could try to have a vaginal delivery. As the pregnancy progressed he said that everything was great—the baby's head was down.

Then about two weeks before my due date, the doctor said, "I didn't want to tell you this ahead of time and get you nervous, but after the baby is born, I am going to do a uterine exploration. It is very painful and I will have to knock you out." I envisioned that I was going to be on a respirator—really knocked out.

COMMENTS: *Since April is a nurse she understood all the potential risks of anesthesia. In her experience as a neonatal nurse, she daily witnesses babies struggling between life and death on respirators. Imagining herself in this state of powerlessness was intensely frightening. Perhaps we should all be more concerned with the risks of general anesthesia related to routine uterine exploration following a VBAC.*

According to guidelines for VBAC set forth by the American College of Obstetricians and Gynecologists (ACOG), immediately following a VBAC the doctor should explore the woman's uterus to determine whether or not the scar is still intact. Uterine exploration is normally indicated only if unexplained or uncontrollable bleeding occurs. Why should the guidelines for VBAC be different? Even if, in rare occurrences, a separation of the scar tissue (not a rupture) were discovered, what course of action would follow? Usually, the risk of major surgery to repair this benign separation (technically, a dehiscence) is greater than the risk of allowing it to remain untreated.

APRIL: The night after I saw the doctor I sat crying and crying, "I can't have this baby. It is going to be too much and I can't do it."

My due date came and went, and the doctor said, "The baby is getting too big and it's getting too late." He wanted to operate. He told me that I had to have the baby by Monday otherwise it was section time. He was going to Hawaii, and no other doctor would want to take me on now as his backup. I had to have this baby before he left.

That day I went jogging, and I took a little bit of castor oil, which started some contractions.

COMMENTS: *Taking only a small amount of castor oil rarely induces active labor. A castor oil induction usually involves at least 2 full ounces of castor oil, and as much as 6 ounces are often necessary.*

APRIL: The labor was not very strong, but I was terribly frightened. I kept thinking about the uterine exploration. When we finally called the doctor I felt like I was in transition. I was shakey and nauseous. The doctor said, "Go to the hospital." I was examined and told, "Oh, you are in labor. You are two centimeters."

Then the contractions stopped. Totally stopped. The nurses told me that I had to stay in the hospital, to keep me monitored. I asked if they could let me up because the labor had stopped, and they said no. I said that I had to go to the bathroom. They said, "Use the bed pan." Then the nurse came up to me and said, "Did you get your pill yet?"

I said, "For what?"

And she said, "For your gas."

I said, "I don't have any gas."

She said, "You will after your C-section."

I said, "I am not having a C-section."   She said "Yes, you are."

Craig and my doctor had to fight with the nurses and the head of the unit to get permission for me to leave the hospital. I had a cesarean scheduled for Thursday and this was Monday. Finally they let me go.

I took a little more castor oil the next day and I had a few contractions, but nothing big. I slept through the whole night, and then the next afternoon (Wednesday) I had to go to the hospital to be admitted. It was awful.

That night as I lay in the hospital bed (without any induction) my labor began. I had back labor, and was rubbing my own back because I did not want the nurses to know I was in labor. I was very sad.

The next morning I had my epidural (regional anesthesia) and cesarean, and I was still alive. Afterwards, the doctor told me that the baby was too big and that it would never have fit. The baby weighed 9 lbs. 4 oz. I was so mad at the doctor. I said to Craig, "The baby wasn't too big. It would have fit. He just didn't give me a chance." Craig said that we did everything we could, but I felt disappointed.

The Birth of Johanna

APRIL: When I became pregnant again, I was so excited. I was determined to have a VBAC. I immediately ran to the same doctor, and he told me, "If you want a VBAC you have to listen to me, because I am in charge."

I was very disappointed. I cancelled my next appointment. I had to look for somebody else. My doctor was a very good surgeon. But I knew that I didn't want more surgery.

Then I went to the VBAC workshop with Lynn, and that is when I decided that home birth was what I wanted. I really wanted a VBAC and from the workshop I realized that I needed to stop trusting doctors so blindly, and learn to trust my body. I did a lot of reading, and it seemed that the greatest cause of uterine rupture was misuse of pitocin. The doctors were causing the very thing they feared the most—uterine ruptures! I decided that I didn't really have to have that fear.

I knew that home birth sounded good to me, but I had to convince Craig. I knew that if he did not feel good, then I would not feel good. The first thing he said was, "Can the midwife come to the hospital?" He liked the idea of having the security of the hospital. I said, "No, you either have it at home with the midwife or in the hospital with the doctor."

He was still very nervous about it until we took Lynn's VBAC classes. At first we did not think that we needed them, because we had done a lot of reading. But it was through the classes that we realized how strong our bodies are and how much fear we have to release. As we took the classes, Craig became so convinced about VBAC that he would say, "Have your home birth, no sweat."

There was only one person I worked with at the hospital that I could share my home birth plans with. I had to keep my home birth plans a secret from everyone else. I told them that since I couldn't have a VBAC at the hospital where I worked because I wouldn't get the support I needed, I had found a good doctor, and was planning a hospital birth at a different hospital. They were very excited that I was going to a nice hospital, and told me I should be OK, as long as I was in the hospital.

The nurses and doctors at the hospital wouldn't have understood my home birth plans. They would have thought that I was very crazy. To them having a home birth would be putting myself and the baby at risk.

Even though I worked with sick babies, I still believed that I would have a normal healthy baby. I was well nourished and healthy, and I was convinced I would not have a premie. The ICU was my work, and I left my work there. I was able to separate myself from what I did for work.

During my first pregnancy there seemed to be more of an attachment between my work and my personal life. Even though I would *say* I wasn't worried about the health of my baby, I think on a subconscious level I was really quite worried. I remember a nightmare during my first pregnancy in which my baby was very abnormal, very sickly. I was at the doctors, and I was trying to take care of my baby. It was very frightening.

This time it was different because I felt very good about myself. I felt my body was strong. I was planning on a normal healthy newborn.

COMMENTS: *April's change in attitude toward the authority of the doctor, the authority of the hospital, and the probability of an abnormality permitted her to plan a home birth. I was afraid, however, that after such stringent training, somewhere deep inside of April there might be a fear of having her baby at home. I had known other women who had felt in conflict about their choice of birthplace. They had planned home births but developed complications that "forced" them to have hospital births. I consistently reminded April throughout the pregnancy that if at any time she felt she wanted to have her baby in the hospital, I would support that decision in any way I could. I wanted her to know that she always had the option of choosing to have a hospital birth, and didn't need to develop complications in order to justify a hospital birth.*

APRIL: Everything was going well. The baby's head was down. At the next prenatal visit, Lynn, my midwife, told me the baby was breech. I immediatly started sweating. I went home and cried. I told Craig, "I can handle a VBAC, but I cannot handle a breech." Then he told me that I could deliver a breech baby, that it wasn't that hard. I said, "That's because I am doing the work and you are not." I was really frightened.

At the home visit my baby was still breech, and Lynn asked me what I had decided to do if the baby remained a breech. She asked me to think about why my baby might be breech, and to do the breech turning exercises.

COMMENTS: *Whenever a woman has a breech baby we can approach this situation with two different attitudes. We can believe that the breech is a signal that something is wrong that needs to be righted, or that everything is fine and just the way the baby needs it to be.*

I usually try to present both points of view. I ask her what in her life feels upside down, and also ask her to spend some time with her baby finding out what it is that her baby needs from her. Why is it that her baby needs to feel so close to her heart? Why is it that this baby might want to be born sitting down, or with his feet on the ground? I find that trying to force the baby to turn around is not usually as effective as helping the woman to direct her energy toward an inwardly safe resolution. Often, once the woman feels safe the baby settles into a safe position—whether that position be vertex or breech.

APRIL: A few days later Rivka, my oldest child, said to me, "Why can't you have the baby in the hospital like you did with me?" I think she was feeling that her birth was wrong, that she had done something wrong. At first I wanted her to feel all right about herself and her birth, so I told her that the cesarean wasn't so bad. But then I realized it was bad, and I didn't want her to grow up thinking that she should have her babies by cesarean. But I wanted her to know that the birth wasn't her fault.

I said to her, "The cesarean was very upsetting. But the doctor didn't know that it was OK to deliver you vaginally. Both the doctor and I thought that this was the best thing at the time for you because we didn't know any better." I let her know that I was very happy when she was born, that I could hold her and love her, but it wasn't the way I wanted the birth. Afterwards she seemed to feel better.

COMMENTS: *Clearing the guilt and pain from the cesarean with Rivka was a very important step in making a vaginal home birth with this next baby possible. Sometimes out of loyalty to our cesarean-born children, we may subconsciously choose to re-enact our cesareans. Similar circumstances appear seemingly miraculously, and unless we consciously choose to heal those cesarean guilt feelings toward our children, we may find ourselves heading down the road to another cesarean. April's honesty and clarity with her daughter, Rivka, not only made it possible for Rivka to feel better, but made it possible for April to move into this next birth having cleared the psychic birth trauma between Rivka and herself.*

APRIL: On February 19 at one of our prenatals, Lynn guided me through a visualization in which she said, "How does the baby feel?" I said that the baby felt comfortable. It sounds silly, but that was the biggest turning point of the pregnancy. Suddenly, I knew that if the baby was born breech, I would be able to do it, and the baby would be all right. It was OK to be breech. I was hoping it would be head down because it would be easier, but I wasn't frightened the way I had been the first time. I stopped working, and was spending time alone with the baby.

Lynn and I talked about where I would want to have the baby if the baby were to remain breech. The backup doctor (who didn't know he was a backup for home birth) told me that I could very easily deliver a 9-1/2 lb. baby. My other doctor had led me to believe that I didn't have a large pelvis, that I could only push out little babies. So I felt more confident about having enough room to deliver a breech baby. If the baby remained a breech, I was planning to stay home and see how things went. I didn't feel that I had to go to the hospital for a breech delivery. However, if I needed to go to the hospital, even if the baby were a breech, the doctor would not be doing an immediate cesarean. He said that if the baby was still breech when I went into labor, he would turn it. He said you should never plan a breech cesarean. So he was different than the other doctor, and I felt I could trust him.

I went home from my visit with Lynn feeling so good I was singing in the car. I felt very secure about this delivery. Either the baby would come out breech or it would turn before labor.

COMMENTS: *April's realization of her safety and trust in both of her practitioners in regards to breech presentation allowed her to feel intellectually safe in having a breech. However, her connection to her baby, her intuition, which came forth so beautifully during the visualization allowed her heart to feel safe. Although information is helpful in intellectual decision making, the safety of birth comes from the heart.*

APRIL: My sister-in-law, Barbara, had wanted to have a home birth. But the midwife she chose could not deliver the baby at her house because she lived too far away from the backup doctor. So Craig and I offered our bedroom for the birth. When I got home from my prenatal with Lynn, Barbara was in labor at my house. It looked as though she was going to have the baby any minute. The contractions weren't that close together, but they looked very intense. She was moaning with each contraction while her husband and support group massaged her.

Barbara was in our bedroom all day. I told her to get up and run around the block, to drink something. But she could hardly walk at all. She would walk from my bedroom to the bathroom and back to the bedroom, which is not very far. And that was the extent of her walking. I felt so strongly that she needed to get out and walk. I wish that her midwife had told her to walk, but she didn't.

This went on all day and all night, and after all that time she was only four centimeters. In the morning they transported her to the hospital because she was so dehydrated. From what I had learned from my reading and from my VBAC classes, I just felt that the whole thing had been mismanaged.

I wasn't going to let that happen to me. Craig was going to make me drink, put a tube down me to force fluids if I wouldn't drink. He was going to make me walk, whether I wanted to walk or not. We agreed that it definitely had to be done.

After Barbara was at the hospital for a while, they wanted my brother to sign papers for a cesarean, and he refused. Then they called up Barbara's mother to get her to get my brother to sign the papers and she said no. So, Barbara's mother came to the hospital and massaged Barbara, and upon the advice of my Lynn's apprentice did a "Logan Basic Contact." Within one half hour Barbara dilated from four centimeters to eight centimeters.

COMMENTS: *A "Logan Basic Contact" is a chiropractic technique that manually releases the ligaments and muscles of the pelvic floor.*

APRIL: So the doctor said, "What ever you are doing, keep doing it, because it's working." Then they gave Barbara pitocin, which made her go crazy, and she started asking for a cesarean. Finally they turned the pit down to a slower drip, and she gave birth.

My brother was so glad that he thanked the doctor for not doing a cesarean. Then the doctor said to my brother, "You do not know what damage you have caused your child. He is not in college yet, so don't thank me." Both my brother and sister-in-law were in a state of shock, "We damaged our child?" They were really upset that the doctor would talk to them like that. There was no medical evidence that the baby had been damaged in any way, and the baby has been fine and has developed normally in every way. But the doctor threw guilt on them because they did not follow his rules.

Shortly after Barbara's birth my baby turned around. I had still felt that it was OK to have it be a breech. But the baby was ready to turn.
— Near my due date, the doctor seemed to be getting a little nervous. He said, "I don't want another big baby. You have a tendency to have big babies."

I said, "You told me on examination that I could easily get out a 9 or 10 pound baby!"

He said, "I did?"

I thought, "Oh, no, this doctor's trying to scare me, too now."

He said, "Well, I just don't want a big baby. It's just more problems. So, on your next visit, I'll see if I can stimulate labor." So I promptly cancelled my next visit.

I found out that he was planning to strip my membranes. So the next time I went to see him, I kept all my clothes on. The nurse said "Take your clothes off since he's going to do an exam."

And I said, "I'll talk to him first."

When he walked in the room he said, "I guess you don't want an internal."

I said, "I'll only let you do an internal if you promise not to strip my membranes."

He said, "I feel it's important to do that because it's getting late."

I said, "I don't feel that it's important because what if you stimulated labor and my body wasn't ready? After 24 hours you're going to section me. I don't want that."

He said, "It usually doesn't throw you into labor."

I said, "It could."

So, he said, "All right, I won't do it. I don't agree with you, but I will let it go. But I want you to have a non-stress test next week."

Then we, Craig and I, sat in the doctor's office and discussed our birth plan with him. He read it and he said, "Well, I have to use a fetal monitor. I don't need to see you til you're five centimeters, but you really can't walk around with a fetal monitor. And I have to do a uterine exploration . . ."

So I said, "What would you do if you found that I had a "window"?"

He said, "Nothing."

So I said, "Why are you doing an exploration?"

He said, "I just have to do it."

I didn't accomplish much because he said he still had to do all the things I didn't want. But I was happy that at least he knew my requests. I decided that if I needed to have a hospital birth, I would refuse to sign for the uterine exploration.

With this pregnancy I knew a lot more, so I was more able to stand for myself. I was able to know what I really wanted, and I felt good about it, so I wasn't afraid.

COMMENTS: *Refusing to allow the doctor to strip her membranes was a powerful act of change on April's part. During her previous pregnancies whenever the doctor had said something that frightened her, April had succumbed to the power of the medical authority. Through visualization we healed April's feelings by changing her responses to the doctor's demands during her first two pregnancies. Through role playing we prepared her for her confrontation with the doctor over the issue of stripping of the membranes. These exercises empowered her to stand for what she needed and to take the responsibility for her birth. Although planning a home birth was a step along the path of change, confrontation of the authority figures was April's final step in freeing herself to give birth trusting her own instincts and intuition.*

APRIL: I went into labor April 2. It began with three very good contractions. They were strong, and I said, "If this is beginning labor, I'm in big trouble, cause this is very uncomfortable." I had an appointment with Lynn that day. She did an internal, but the contractions had stopped, and there was no cervical change.

I was cleaning the house for Passover, but by 5:30 P.M., I couldn't do any more. Craig came home and I was lying on the couch. The kids were running around, the house was a wreck, there was no supper . . . and I said, "I think I'm going to have a baby." He said, "You always think you're having a baby."

So we put the kids to bed at about 8:30. Lying down with Rivka the contractions became more uncomfortable. But I didn't want to get too excited because I was afraid they would stop.

About midnight I took a relaxing hot bath. Then I realized that it must be labor.

COMMENTS: *Baths are a good tool for relaxation. Often if a woman is unsure as to whether she is experiencing true labor or just prelabor contractions, taking a bath can be a designating tool. If it is not labor, the contractions usually will disappear in the bath. If it is labor, the contractions do not go away. They may feel more comfortable, as a result of relaxation, but become more consistent. The contractions may even intensify—come faster and stronger while in the tub. This may be especially true if the woman has been holding up the labor from tension or fear.*

APRIL: Then I started throwing up. So I said, "Oh, I'm in early labor, and I'm nervous."

COMMENTS: *Vomiting in late labor is a physiologic response and is sometimes even beneficial because it often appears to help to complete the dilatation. However, usually vomiting in early labor is not as much a physiologic response as it is a psychologic response of fear and/or tension.*

APRIL: Around 1:00 A.M., we called Lynn, and she told me to try to rest.

COMMENTS: *Since April had told me that with her last labor she had had what seemed to be strong transitionlike contractions but had only dilated to two centimeters, I felt that the best advice I could give her was to attempt to assure her that she could rest and relax through the labor, that she could really do the labor herself. I felt that if I stayed away for a while, that she would find the coping mechanism that was right for her.*

APRIL: I was trying to rest, but I just couldn't. I was still throwing up, with the dry heaves. So I said, "Something must be bothering me. I'm still in early labor, and it's getting intense." So I was sitting up with pillows all around me, trying to sleep, and throwing up. Craig brought me drinks, and I told him to sleep because it was going to be a long night.

Craig was sleeping on the couch and I was sitting downstairs. The kids were sleeping. During contractions I was trying to relax, trying to let it be like a wave, letting it come and go. I didn't feel that I was doing a very good job because I was still having dry heaves. I got up a few times and took baths, and went to the bathroom. Then in the morning I took another bath, but I couldn't relax as well as I had before. By this time it was about 7:00 in the morning. David, my two year old came in and said, "Are you puking?" And I said, "Yes, I'm going to have the baby." And he said, "Were you drinking Juicy-Juice?" (Juicy-Juice used to make David vomit.) So he didn't seem bothered that I was just laying in the tub with my head hanging over the side.

Then about 15 minutes later my daughter woke up and came in. I said, "We're going to have the baby today, I think." She didn't really say anything, she just looked very frightened.

COMMENTS: *I was called again at about 8:00, and was told that the contractions were definitely getting stronger. I said that I would be leaving shortly. I sent my apprentice on ahead of me.*

APRIL: Then Craig called my sister, Dale, who arrived around 8:15. I took another shower. Soon after, I yelled, "I have to poop" I sat down on the toilet and felt this pressure, this scraping feeling. I jumped off the toilet.

Dale grabbed my head, and said, "Breathe with me." Then she timed contractions, which were about 1 minute apart.

There was no midwife there yet, and Dale wasn't going to let me push. She kept breathing with me. And I thought, "If I'm only 2 centimeters, I want to go to the hospital, get knocked out, and have a cesarean. This is too much."

Before I gave birth I could never understand why people would want a woman coach, but after this I understood. Craig was doing everything he could. But he couldn't know what I was going through. Somehow I had envisioned that he would rub my back and feel the contractions with me. But it wasn't like that. I think he was frightened for me, nervous seeing me so weak and overwhelmed with the contractions. It was a lot for him to deal with the kids and take care of me,too. I'm very glad my sister was there with me.

Lynn's apprentice came at about 9:30, examined me, and said, "You're 10 centimeters." And I felt like yelling, "Of course I'm 10 centimeters!" But instead I said, "Are you sure?"

So then they just propped me up, squatting with one leg over my husband, and one leg over my sister, and I started pushing.

COMMENTS: *When I arrived the baby's head was visible, and it was quite clear why April had been experiencing intense contractions so "early" in labor. April had an intense labor because she had a fast labor. Yet, even more amazing than the relative speed of this labor as compared with her other labor, was April's ability to cope with her labor almost completely unassisted. Her belief that this was still early labor and that she just had to find a better way to relax was to her great advantage. For once a woman begins to tune into herself in labor, finding the coping mechanisms that work best for her, she moves more freely into the labor, allowing it to take over, allowing herself to let go into the experience. Thus, with letting go comes efficient powerful fast labor.*

My apprentice was already doing perineal massage (deep massage of the tissue and muscles between the vagina and the rectum, done to prevent tearing). I set up the instruments quickly, while trying to keep the atmosphere calm and quiet.

APRIL: The perineal massage hurt, felt uncomfortable, but it seemed like it was the right thing to do. I felt like I naturally knew the right way to push. I always thought that when I was pushing I would be afraid that my uterus would rupture. But that was the farthest thing from my mind. I didn't even consider that I had ever had a cesarean. It just seemed very natural. My body was doing what it was supposed to be doing. In a few more pushes the baby's head was out, and then she was born. She looked very pale to me. They put her on my lap and I was so exhausted, I just wanted to look at her.

COMMENTS: *The awe the mother experiences after giving birth often requires a moment of hesitation, a blank timeless space during which she settles into the reality that she has a baby in her arms. Often I find that encouraging the mother to massage her baby not only encourages the baby to breathe but helps the mother to cross the bridge between the relatively passive role of pregnant mother to the quite active role of mother of a newborn.*

APRIL: We just rubbed her and she pinked up. Everybody was happy. I got into bed and nursed my new baby.

COMMENTS: *Then I noticed that small gush of blood that signals the separation of the placenta.*

APRIL: Lynn said, "You have to push out one more thing. It's an easy push." And I said, "No. No more pushing." And she said, "Oh, this is an easy one. This doesn't hurt."

COMMENTS: *I have noticed that sometimes a woman may have a "retained" placenta because once she is holding her baby in her arms, she doesn't want to have to do anything more. She doesn't want to feel the sensation of pushing again, the sensation of contractions again. I have found that depressurizing and at the same time supporting the woman to birth her placenta is often a significant factor in the completion of the third stage. Letting her know that letting out the placenta is the easy part allows her to feel relaxed and yet powerful. This is precisely the combination of feelings that are often needed for the hormones to properly release the placenta and yet contract the uterus to prevent further bleeding.*

APRIL: So I agreed to try to push out my placenta, as long as it was an easy one. And it did just push out very easily.

COMMENTS: *After the placenta was born, all the children climbed in bed with April and their new baby, and we took family pictures.*

APRIL: I felt totally exhausted. I had envisioned these home births where everyone jumped into bed, looked great and felt great. But I just wanted to nurse the baby and then go to sleep.

COMMENTS: *Nature usually knows best about the energy that is needed between a mother and her baby. Most women feel "high" for a short time after the birth, while the baby is wide awake and ready to bond. But just as the baby's natural quiet-alert period ends (two hours after the birth), usually the mother, too, wants to lie down, cuddle with her baby, and get some much-deserved sleep.*

APRIL: After the birth one of the nurses I worked with called me. She was excited that I had had the VBAC, and said to me, "People say you planned this at home. But I know that you are more responsible, and you wouldn't take risks like that." I just laughed because I could never let them know that, yes, this was planned. They could never understand. When I go back to work it's going to feel very different. I no longer feel that all we do in the ICU is always so necessary. My thinking now is so different from the way I was trained. I'm into nonintervention, and where I work it's constant intervention .

I was thinking of changing my specialty in nursing—going into labor and delivery. But at the hospital where I work it would just be doing

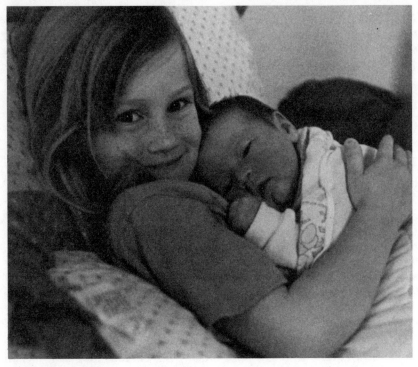

Rivka (5½) and Johanna (hours) Altman

cesareans or helping mothers deliver flat on their back, with IVs, monitors, and episiotomies—all the things that I don't think are necessary or even good for you. So I'm kind of stuck unless I go to work for Dr. Odent or become an empirical midwife. Giving birth was the most intense thing I ever did. I can do anything now.

COMMENTS: *April is now taking my midwifery skills course. Perhaps she will one day be part of a growing number of midwives who have come to this profession as VBAC mothers.*

APRIL: When I first began to consider VBAC, I never would have wanted an empirical midwife to attend my birth. Now, I wouldn't have anyone except an empirical midwife attend my birth.

17

Twice a Cesarean: The Birth of Onna Chunaha

ALICE JORDAN

ALICE: Onna Chunaha was born in the fall of 1980. The meaning of his name is "Morning Circle." The inspiration behind naming him came from his peaceful arrival into this world one crisp early morning, where he was welcomed by a small but special circle of friends.

How different was this birth by candlelight, to that of my first-born, six years ago in an Australian metropolitan maternity hospital. There I had arrived, in strong labor, nervous to be sure, but with a course of Lamaze instructions fresh in my mind and my mate beside me. I believed I was prepared to give birth naturally, with a minimum of fuss. I was greeted at the hospital entrance by two brisk and efficient nurses, separated from my husband and forced into a wheelchair. Then, dressed in a hospital gown that revealed all, I was expected to juggle bureaucratic red tape, while endeavoring to concentrate on my 1-minute-apart contractions. I then had to cope with an enema; I was shaved of my beautiful pubic hair, and hitched up to a bleeping machine that spewed out reams of computerized data. At one point I had nine men in my room, none of whom were my husband. I was knocked out 4 hours later for an "emergency" cesarean section, allowed to see my new son 18 hours after that, and to hold and nurse a further six hours later. After nine days I left the hospital with a sleepy infant, who, after the drugs wore off, sprang to life with such severe colic I didn't know what had hit me. The emotional scars from Mahaya's birth, and the resulting forced separation, are indelible.

Newly arrived in the United States and 4 months pregnant with our second child, we found a "liberal" doctor who was said to give women the type of birth they chose. I presented him with an optimum birth letter, to which he agreed with everything listed, including allowing me to try for a vaginal delivery.

Around noon on the day I began labor, we set off for the hospital, again my contractions were strong and fast. The atmosphere in this smaller hospital was quiet and peaceful, but as soon as I was hooked up to the fetal monitor, my contractions slowed down, and 4 hours later had practically come to a standstill. It was as if the electronic power interfered with my own energy. Its mere presence with its relentless bleeping was disconcerting to say the least, and this coupled with the frustration of being restricted to my bed resulted in the diagnosis, "failure to progress."

Our daughter was born late that night by cesarean section. The lights in the operating theatre were dimmed, the room pleasantly warm. As soon as her apgar score was taken, she went with her father for skin-to-skin bonding until she fell asleep in his arms two hours later. Two days after her birth we were home tucked up in bed together.

My VBAC

Our third child was born at home, and a strong motivating factor for this choice was the experience of two unwanted, and probably unnecessary C-sections. But the most more important motivation was my belief that the birth of a child is an event commanding deep reverence. I had, through my previous birthing experiences, developed an intense dislike and mistrust of hospitals and the medical profession. I felt strongly against the attempts by the average obstetricians to overpower women during the birthing process. I personally refused to be manhandled by doctors I'd never see again, once I had delivered.

In the process of taking charge of my own birthing experience, I began to rely on myself and my intuition. I began to walk in my own light.

The spiritual power of a pregnant woman is recognised in many cultures. The native people of this land are not alone in their unwillingness to allow pregnant or menstruating women to participate in ceremonies and rituals, for fear that the female power will usurp the power available to the men. In modern obstetrics our own great white doctors paternally patronize us in the behest that "doctor knows best." The most devastating image we have of a woman completely out of control is that of the mother sheeted, supine, drugged, and strapped down at the very moment she is bringing life into the world. A cesarean section is the obstetrician's last opportunity to play God.

With my medical history of two classical cesareans, it would have been extremely difficult to find a doctor in the conservative climate of central Oklahoma who would be confident and unbiased enough to respect my judgment and personal views on the birthing process.

Another important reason for my decision to have a home VBAC was a personal one. For some years now, I have been endeavoring to be a strong, self-reliant person, who accepts responsibility for my own actions. I thought that this was my opportunity to strengthen my will and, at the same time, to prove that freedom and determination do concur.

In a political realm, I felt that I would be providing information to my sisters-at-large. For the benefit of other women it would be worth pioneering a vastly neglected area to dispel the myth of "twice a cesarean, always a cesarean." A study done at the University of Malta indicates that women with a past history of two C-sections should be allowed a vaginal delivery, since good results are demonstrable hysterographically (by taking a "picture" of the uterus) in 72% of the women studied. The article points out that this margin of safety may be increased appreciably if both sections were carried out after the onset of labor, and if the interval between the two sections exceeded two years. There was no mention as to which incision was more favorable—transverse, or classical. In my case, my incision was apparently classical, but upon careful study of my medical records, I noted the *uterine* incision was transverse.

Both the above points applied to my circumstances, and I was also encouraged when I remembered having been told by the obstetrician who had performed my first cesarean, that he could see no reason as to why I would need subsquent C-sections. The statistics for his hospital (Mercy Maternity, Melbourne, Australia) for repeat cesareans was, in 1975, 12%. Australia, like Europe, holds repeat cesareans as the exception, not the rule.

COMMENTS: *In this country the overall repeat cesarean section rate is 99%.*

ALICE: Through further research I learned that cesarean section was apparently performed in the days of Hippocrates, but in the old sagas, and through the poets, the fact has been expressed that in the olden times extraordinary deeds were expected of a person who had been "cut out" of his mother's body. Shakespeare undoubtedly thought it was quite a special destiny to be born by a cesarean. He made this motive decisively important in his great tragedy, MacBeth. When MacBeth, having all the dark forces on his side boasts before his duel with MacDuff: "Let fall thy blade on vulnerable crests, I bear a charmed life, which must not yield/To one of woman born." MacDuff, with strength and purity of character answers: "Despair thy charm;/And let the angel whom thou still hast serv'd/Tell thee, MacDuff was from his mother's womb/Untimely ripp'd."

Today there is nothing mystical or even slightly special about being born by cesarean. Indeed, judging by the range of unhappy and negative feelings expressed by "sectioned" women, one needs no poets' license to substitute "ripped out" with "ripped off!" The very word "sectioned" leaves one feeling more like a grapefruit than a human being.

In the case of a subsequent C-section, one must keep in mind the words of prominent obstetrician Barry Schiffin: "If a repeat section is chosen over a vaginal delivery, the woman should be informed for medical and legal reasons that she has chosen the more dangerous of the two alternatives."

Unfortunately, such open-mindedness is rare among obstetricians, so, very often it is up to us, the dissatisfied sectioned women to dispel this myth of "twice a cesarean." In our pioneering efforts we turn to those who can and will support us, and in many cases, the support comes from midwives.

I set my goal from the first week of pregnancy and my task was not to falter. It was not always easy, as the oppositions were many. Each day I aligned myself with my own soul, and with the great Mother. I am fully satisfied that there is a great cosmic female deity. I definitely linked with Her energy, and towards the time of birth, so did my husband.

The power of the Goddess and her presence is always near, more consciously so during the time of pregnancy and childbirth. There were times when discouragement would seep through me. It was always such a comfort to give myself over to a higher being each night, and to imagine Her soft blue shimmering cloak enveloping me gently and lovingly. Each morning I would awake refreshed, with renewed conviction that the goal our family had set could be fulfilled. I found that the blessings are there for the asking, and I encourage all women to use their spiritual alignments to their advantage.

The negativity I encountered when going against mainstream obstetrical practice was staggering. I found that the fewer people who knew of my decision, the less time and energy I spent defending my beliefs and convictions. Everyone thinks you're crazy, or downright stupid, not to mention dangerous. I told only those who cared deeply for me, and who shared my convictions. Actually, as time went on and I became more sure of myself, my positive attitude quite often influenced those who had been rather ambivalent, if not negative.

There were three midwives in Fayetteville, Arkansas. Two worked together, and one worked independently. I approached the team about assisting us with our delivery, but as I did not plan to deliver in that town, they graciously excused themselves. The other midwife, being more alternative in lifestyle as well as in her practice of midwifery, said she didn't consider me high risk.

FRANCOISE (MIDWIFE): Alice had a lot of confidence in herself as a woman. She felt she had been belittled twice, and was not going to let that happen again.

ALICE: Francoise suggested teas to drink, such as raspberry leaf, comfrey leaf, and alfalfa, and told me to read Sheila Kitzinger's, *The Experience of Childbirth*. My husband James practiced quite a few of Sheila's relaxation exercises, along with a perineal massage, and we felt they were helpful. I especially appreciated the nonverbal relaxation exercises. Relaxation is definitely the keyword during labor.

When we moved to Oklahoma, I contacted one of the two midwives here in Stillwater, who upon hearing my story and request for assistance was aghast and said that she couldn't even "condone" such a decision!

"Well, looks like James and I will just have to do it ourselves," I said to myself. (In all seriousness, had I decided to do it with just the help of James, he would have! He never doubted my capabilities.)

Later the local midwife phoned back, and said that she and her partner would like to meet me. So they came over and before long they seemed convinced that I was doing the right thing, although their eyebrows went up and down a bit when they heard that I'd had two "classic" sections. They volunteered to do my prenatal care, but were hesitant to attend the birth. They felt that it had taken them so long to establish their reputation as responsible midwives in this very conservative town. They thought it might jeopardize the work they'd done, if they took on a "high-risk" woman. They were direct and honest with me, and I with them, and it wasn't long before a friendship developed between us. Eventually, one of them, Lynn, said she would like to come to my birth, but she didn't want to be "first in command," as she didn't feel she had the experience to handle my kind of complications (should they arise).

In the meantime, the midwife from Fayetteville wrote to say that she felt perhaps I wasn't getting the support I needed in Stillwater. She asked if I would like her to come over for the birth. So eventually it was decided, that it would be Francoise from Fayetteville; my close family friends from Arkansas, Marsha, Berri, and Gene; Lynn from Stillwater, and of course our family.

My pregnancy was fairly uneventful. I walked 2 miles most days for the first 6 1/2 months, then the heatwave forced me onto the couch, gasping in front of the electric fan until late September. My diet is always centered around whole grains and vegetables, I just stepped up the protein somewhat. I gained 20 pounds and had no excess weight after the baby was born. I don't smoke anything, and I drank no alcohol or coffee during pregnancies. I took a calcium supplement, plus iron and folic acid and the aforementioned teas. In the last three weeks I included a Dr. Christopher herbal (capsule) combination. I was quite regular with daily kegels (exercises designed to focus upon and strengthen the pelvic floor). I do feel that if I was to take responsibility for my body and birth that I must do it on every level. I placed emphasis on good nutrition, and exercise.

COMMENTS: *Taking responsibility is* not easy. *Taking responsibility means doing your own research, making your own decisions, and doing everything in your power to tilt the scales of outcome in your favor. This means doing everything you can do for yourself and your baby on a physical level (nutrition and exercise), on an emotional level (getting in touch with your feelings and seeking out resolution and acceptance), and on a spiritual level (finding spiritual connections that bring you grounding and peace). Taking responsibility also means that if the outcome is less than you had hoped for, you are willing to realize what part you play—not to lay all the blame on the doctor or the midwife, or your mother, or your partner. Taking responsibility is the most difficult task we are given in life. Why should it be easy in birth?*

ALICE: About 10 days before the birth, the fetus swung into a transverse position, and the midwives thought I should perhaps prepare myself mentally for the possibility of a C-section. I said, "Sure," but I thought, "NO" and refused to entertain the idea. What a cruel cosmic joke that would be!

Still, it was something unexpected that I hadn't reckoned on, and I had to work hard at keeping my vision clear and unfaltering. The midwives suggested an exercise used for turning breech babies: I would lie on my back, head down, buttocks up at a 45 degree angle, twice a day, for 15 minutes. Quite uncomfortable as it threw the fetus against my diaphragm which caused a shortness of breath. However, I wasn't in a position to trust luck so I persevered.

Not too much happened for a few days and the anxiety of outside influences began to creep in. I am a firm believer in the efficacy of the Bach Flower Remedies and as I have the set, I put together a couple I knew would be strengthening.

COMMENTS: *The Bach Flower Remedies are based upon the connection of the emotional state of a person and their physical health. The specific remedies are chosen according to a person's emotional and spiritual needs, and are taken by droplets into the mouth. In addition to taking each of the remedies, particular affirmations may be said to enhance the physical and psycho-spiritual connection. I have found them to be quite effective, especially if the primary "cause" of a physical symptom is psycho-spiritual in nature.*

ALICE: James and I decided to try a "laying" of hands. I never asked James about the energies he contacted but he did comment that he experienced an alignment with the Mother energy.

Three days before I went into labor, the fetus swung down and right past the birth canal, lodging in the opposite transverse position. The midwives wondered if the reason for the head not engaging could have been because of placenta previa. They urged me to see a doctor for an ultrasound to determine the position of the placenta. I phoned their backup doctor, who did not seem to me to be the most progressive of thinkers. My appointment was for Monday, October 13 ("Labor Day" and James' birthday).

I spent those last few days before the birth in deep prayer and meditation. Indeed, I just handed it over to those working for me in the spiritual realms!

My waters broke an hour and a half before my doctor's appointment, which brought about a quick decision not to keep the appointment. Inwardly I knew all along it would be disastrous for me to attend a doctor, although I'm not suggesting that all women should take the path I chose.

Labor was mild. It began around 9:30 on the 13th. I was able to straighten the house and cook the evening meal in advance, so I'd be relieved of any (self-inflicted!) obligation to play hostess. I prepared the bedroom for the birth.

Everyone arrived from Arkansas by suppertime. Gene and my neighbor pooled childcare over the next 15 or so hours. Stillwater midwife, Lynn, came by around 8:00 P.M., with her youngest daughter. She suggested I take a brisk walk to get things started. I walked for a couple of miles while the others put the children to bed.

Contractions were good and strong later that night and I was about 5 centimeters dilated. Around 1 or 2:00 A.M., James said he thought we would have a dawn birth. I thought, "Hmm, not if I can help it," but it was to be. My support was terrific. Loving, sleepy women padded in and out of the bedroom with warm oil and backrubs. James felt like a part of me. I seemed to flow into transition.

FRANCOISE: Alice's labor and delivery were very peaceful and very natural.

ALICE: Suddenly we discovered that the head was presenting. There was a shift of gears as we all prepared to "push on." Actually, that excluded me. Francoise was adamant that I allow the baby to do the pushing.

FRANCOISE: Having no experience with a woman who had two previous c-sections, my feeling at the time was just to let the uterus do it's own work without the woman forcing the birth.

COMMENTS: *Some midwives feel that not allowing pushing is advantageous to easing the birth process and the stretching of the soft tissue. Others believe the body generally indicates what it needs to do, and if pushing is what the body is asking to do, then the woman needs to follow her own body.*

However, there will always be times when the midwife needs to tell the woman not to push when she wants desperately to push, or on the other hand tells them they have to push when their body didn't seem to be wanting to push at all. Some women never want to push. Others seem to want to push prematurely. Pushing is like riding a bicycle built for two—for two because the woman and the baby must push together. Once you feel its balance, you never have to think about what to do to make it happen. Every person feels pushing a little differently, describes it a little differently. Pushing is a very delicate balance with which each woman, her baby, and her attendant(s) must work as a team.

FRANCOISE: I remember putting my hand on Alice's scar as the baby was descending into her birth canal, as a subconscious security that her uterus wouldn't rupture. But I felt very calm, and sure that the birth would happen well.

ALICE: Berri and Lynn concentrated on massaging me with warm oil as Lynn stretched my perineum (the tissue and muscle between the vagina and the rectum). I was concentrating on not pushing. Francoise began blowing along with me, to keep the rhythm. All of a sudden her face was transformed with a wonderful light. Her whole countenance was just radiant. I couldn't stop looking at her. I kept thinking, "My God, Francoise, you look so beautiful!" My gaze was fixed upon her until the birth. This was a tremendous help to me. Just breathing rhythmically along with another person greatly facilitated my concentration.

FRANCOISE: As we were breathing together, I recall that one of Alice's support people asked me if she wanted her glasses to be able to see the birth of the baby. Alice responded, "I can SEE!" She could see more than we could see. We were talking to her on the physical plane but she was seeing way beyond us.

ALICE: My birth experience confirmed something I'd read before I had children, that the World Mother is present at each and every birth. Until that moment I'd believed that to be so, but now I realized it. Some days later, Lynn, the other midwife remarked that she endeavored to be a "vessel" for that spiritual energy. What wonderfully high work you midwives have chosen.

COMMENTS: *Though we may not all call the spirit by the same name, almost everyone who has ever attended a truly womanchild centered birth (at home or in the hospital) becomes touched by the presence of the spirit of God, of birth—*

of a power far beyond those present in the room together. This spiritual power, of course, can be ignored. Unfortunately, most practitioners have never been taught to acknowledge its presence. Yet, if we all could find that place within our hearts and souls where we realized that the power of birth is not simply in our own hands, then the tremendous egopower struggles that can ensue over the decisions at a birth could be let go. Doctors and midwives could step off their pedestals, and parents could gently assist them in doing so. We could all come to birth equal, open, trusting in one another and in the power of that great spirit, ready to learn and to grow.

ALICE: Mahaya and Imantia, our two children, slept in our bedroom peacefully through the night, and woke just as the head was crowning.

I think my immediate reaction at the moment of birth was, "Well, I certainly won't do that again in a hurry!" But then, that sweet moment of triumph, "We pulled it off!"

FRANCOISE: Alice's ecstatic pleasure that she had done it was shared, and I don't believe I could explain it. It was a very memorable experience. Alice, I truly love the woman that you are.

ALICE: The word Onna is Choctaw for dawn. (My husband is Choctaw, hence the reason for the choice of our childrens names). We named this special little boy Onna Chunaha—Morning Circle as he was born into a very special circle of friends.

No doubt everyone will think you are crazy for attempting a VBAC. It is still viewed as "the impossible." Shortly after the birth of Onna I began corresponding with a woman, Judy Twist, from North Dakota, who was expecting her third child. According to the eight doctors with whom she had consulted, she should have been expecting her third cesarean. Instead, she chose the alternative of a home birth, and of course was considered "crazy." With good health, the right support and information, and sheer determination, yet another "crazy" woman managed to have the birth of her choice. She delivered a healthy son at Christmas-time in the privacy and serenity of her family bedroom. We are almost a movement!

18

The Movement Continues

JUDY AND ALLEN TWIST

JUDY: My story begins almost six years ago when I was pregnant with my first child. I, like most American women, thought that my doctor would take good care of me, so I did everything he told me. My pregnancy had its ups and downs, mostly downs. I had nausea—he prescribed anti-acid pills. I had edema along with probable "risk" of toxemia—he prescribed a diuretic, told me to leave salt alone, and to limit my weight gain.

COMMENTS: *Judy was the victim of medical misinformation. Clearly, her doctor realized that excessive vomiting was not healthy for a pregnant woman. He also correctly associated excessive weight gain and edema with toxemia. However, he did not realize that vomiting could be most easily controlled by positive nutritional changes. He also failed to recognize that the excessive weight gain and edema were only symptoms, not causes of toxemia. Dr. Tom Brewer, OB/GYN has spent many years studying the causes and cures of toxemia. His research has shown that malnutrition is the primary cause of toxemia—that most pregnant women need 80-100 grams of protein a day, 2500 calories a day, salt to taste, and drink to thirst. Unfortunately, since most medical doctors have little to no information about nutrition, many of them have not yet acknowledged the value of Tom Brewer's work. Many still dangerously advise pregnant women to watch their weight, cut out salt, take diuretics, and sometimes even advise amphetamines to control weight gain. Practitioners who have become more aware of the value of good nutrition usually can help pregnant women avoid serious complications of pregnancy, such as toxemia. Had Judy been given positive nutritional counseling, her "risk" of toxemia and her "need for a cesarean" would most likely have disappeared.*

JUDY: In order to avoid the "risk of toxemia," my doctor said he would induce labor if I did not go into labor naturally in two weeks. Two weeks before my due date he took x-rays of my unborn child and told me that I would need an immediate cesarean because of "risk" of cephalo-pelvic disproportion.

My husband and I were shocked, disappointed, and kept asking, "Why?" But the only answer we got was that I or my baby would die if I didn't have a cesarean. The doctor also told me I would never ever be able to have even a three-pound baby vaginally.

COMMENTS: *It is difficult to assess just why the doctor might conclude that the size of Judy's pelvis would be so inordinately small. Perhaps the x-ray was distorted, and the diameters could not be correctly measured.*

HARLAN (CHIROPRACTOR): An x-ray film is produced by directing radiation at a person. The person's bone and/or soft tissue structures will be highlighted on film because these structures are absorbing the radiation, producing a "blank" or "white" area on the film, which is placed behind the area to be x-rayed. The greater the distance between the structure and the film, the more distortion is evidenced.

In addition to the distortion of x-rays, it is important to note that the body is a dynamic structure. When an x-ray is taken, it represents a moment (and a distorted one, at that) of time in the dynamic situation of birth. Because there are many ligaments that have been hormonally prepared throughout late pregnancy for birth, this static x-ray cannot possibly account for the body's ability to stretch the pelvis in order to accommodate the passage of the baby.

It is understandable for a physician to conclude that a woman with a marginal pelvis would not be able to deliver a large baby if she were hormonally and physiologically unprepared. However, neither an x-ray nor a clinical exam could possibly determine how much accommodation the soft tissue (ligaments and muscles) can permit.

COMMENTS: *However, it is also possible that the doctor was using the cephalopelvic disproportion as an "excuse" for doing the cesarean in order to avoid frightening Judy with his fears of toxemia and its worst outcome—the possible onset of convulsions and death of mother and baby. Most medical training implies that proper management of a potentially dangerous situation would be to get the patient to do what is medically necessary without disclosing your real fears. Proper management is "protecting the patient," "keeping the patient calm."*

If such "management" were the real motive in telling Judy she had such a disproportionate pelvic diameter, it is sad, indeed, that Judy had not been given the true diagnosis. Telling a woman that her pelvis is so deformed, so inadequate, has deeply psychologically destructive implications. A woman not only carries this feeling of inadequacy with her into her next birth, she carries it with her into her feelings about herself as a mother, as a woman, for the rest of her life. Practitioners must realize that though the truth may be frightening or painful, the truth is far better told than a conjured up diagnosis which carries such personal confusion and heavy psychological weight. We must be extremely careful about the "psychological seeds" we plant as practitioners, as mothers, as partners, or as friends.

JUDY: So, of course with those dire warnings, we consented that I would have a cesarean. I did not go into labor, and I was put into the hospital the night before surgery. My sister had two cesareans and I had also had other surgeries, so I knew how terrible I would feel after surgery. I absolutely DID NOT want a cesarean. My first thought was, "If only I could get out of the hospital and go home . . ."

I had an absolutely terrible night. The next morning at 9:02 I had a cesarean under general anesthesia, and did not know until that afternoon that the doctor had delivered a healthy, beautiful 9 lb. 12-1/2 oz. baby boy. His head, chest, and abdomen were all 14 inches, and he was 23 and a half inches in length.

The nurses and my husband were trying to wake me up for a long time, but all I wanted to do was sleep. At about 3:00 P.M. they brought the baby (Justin) to me. My husband held him while the nurse was getting him all "hooked up" to nurse because I was still too groggy. Believe me, I came around fast when it felt like they had brought in a vacuum cleaner instead of a baby. I begged them to take him away because I hurt so much. (Months afterwards I was glad he had such a strong sucking reflex because I wouldn't have had the strength to keep a sleepy baby interested in nursing).

That night three nurses came to my room and wanted me to walk a little bit. Now, it takes a few minutes after abdominal surgery to stand up straight from a laying down position. But the nurses were in a big hurry and I was on a fast walk, being told to stand-up straight and quit acting like a baby. I really felt like the nursing staff was not supportive of cesarean mothers.

Whenever I thought about birth, it seemed dangerous and terrible. I felt I had been cheated, that deep inside there had to be a better way to give birth.

When I was pregnant with my second child two years later I asked three doctors if I could have a vaginal birth. I was told it was too "risky" and it was crazy to even think of it. I received all of the horror stories, and was told how we modern women "just aren't strong enough to birth our babies." I was very angry because of the implication by doctors and lay people alike that some women are just *weak*. I'm a very healthy, active person. I was a cheerleader for 4 years, played basketball, and ran track. After I married I stacked hay bales, and fed cows by lifting 50 lb. bags of feed over the fence. I drove steel posts into the ground for fencing. I helped build our log home. I had a huge garden. I also exercised and ate good food. People said I was *weak*??!

In our church of forty people, nine are young women. Five of us had cesareans and four had vaginal deliveries. Did God really goof us up?? I asked our pastor and other women, but no one gave me a definite answer. I really felt God gave us breasts to use for our babies food and comfort. Didn't He also make us to birth our babies naturally, without all this danger everyone talked about?

We were always told in our prenatal classes that the doctor was always right. We were not to ever listen to anyone else (like friends, mother, sister, or aunts) about our health or the health of our child. So I figured that I had asked too many questions already.

COMMENTS: *"Ask your doctor" is the phrase most often used to connote absolutism in health care. Such beliefs which became prominent in the forties when our mothers were having children, were the seeds of distrust from generation to generation that discouraged breastfeeding and natural childbirth. For generations prior to this scientific era, mothers learned the skills of labor, birth, and mothering from their own mothers, aunts, sisters, and grandmothers.*

Many childbirth educators who are either hired by the doctors or the hospitals are bound by fear of losing their jobs to teach that the doctor is always right and that hospital policy is "for your own good." These classes do women a tremendous disservice. They remove the power of giving birth from the women themselves; they remove the power of the woman's intuitive and instinctual knowledge; they remove the power of the extended family in assisting the woman to make the transition into motherhood—and give all this power to the doctor and the hospital! No wonder so many women have cesareans! It is imperative to interview and search not only for a good practitioner, but also for a good educator—an educator who will empower you, not the doctor!

JUDY: I was told there was a new machine in the hospital, called ultrasound that could determine the due date of the baby within 7 days. Three months after I had ultrasound, I needed to have amniocentesis, because the doctor couldn't tell when I was due. (Great new ultrasound!) The doctor needed to know so he could do another cesarean two weeks before I went into labor, as that is the standard practice at our hospital.

I went into labor 3 weeks before my due date. My doctor almost had a fit! He told the nurses to have me "prepped" and into the operating room in 20 minutes. The doctors proceeded to do the operation, discussing golf, their dinner the night before, and other assorted topics. I wondered why my husband couldn't be there, since birth is one of the most important events in a woman's life. I needed to share it with my husband, the man I loved, instead of a room full of masked strangers who didn't care and just needed to get the job done.

The doctor pulled the baby out and told me I had a baby girl. But there was no crying and I panicked. I kept asking if she was breathing. They finally told me they were resuscitating her. It seemed like an eternity before I heard the beautiful cry.

COMMENTS: *Judy's baby would have been more likely to breathe spontaneously and less likely to need the resuscitation had she been "allowed" to give birth vaginally. Birth through the vagina prepares the baby's upper respiratory system for breathing by clearing the mucous from the airways, and by the surge of catecholamines (stress hormones) which prepare the infant to survive outside the womb.*

JUDY: The nurse laid her on my face for a few seconds before they took her away. I could not touch her with my hands because my hands were tied down.

When my legs "unfroze" from the spinal, I vowed I would never go through that again. Many of the mothers in the hospital and some of my friends were envious of the cesarean birth, and told me so. Their idea was that you didn't have to go through any pain to get the baby into the world. I invited them to witness the period after birth when the mother was coming out of the anesthesia and to follow her home for recovery. Strange, I did not have any takers!

COMMENTS: *As Barbara Brown-Hill, experienced VBAC educator and birth assistant writes:*

> *Childbirth is PAIN! It can be the healthy normal pain of labor and birth. Or it can be medically "painless birth" through anesthesia and/or cesarean with subsequent weeks to months of painful recovery while struggling to care for our newborn babies.*
>
> *There is no escaping the pain. The choice we have is to work with the pain and experience the satisfaction of birthing our babies, or to fight the pain.*
>
> *It's unfortunate that in our society we have come to view childbirth in only one of two ways: "painless childbirth," or "horrendously painful childbirth." We don't have a word to express the healthy pain of labor.*
>
> *The healthy pain of labor is natural, and a realization of our own personal power as women and mothers. It should be viewed as a milestone to be embraced, a rite of womanhood. The pain of major abdominal surgery is unnatural pain (a signal from our body that something is seriously wrong), and usurps our own power as women and mothers. It should be viewed as something to be avoided.*
>
> *Anesthesia introduces a substance into our body that can alter the course of our labor, and harm the health of our babies as well as ourselves.*

It might allow us to temporarily escape the pain. But anesthesia can cause
temporary or permanent harm. Thus the price of escape may be paid by our
bodies or our babies.

Anesthesia causes many women to feel that they have lost something.
They may seek to recapture the experience of what transpired while they
were numb—the physical and emotional sensations which represent the
connection between the pregnancy and motherhood. Many women spend
the rest of their lives looking for the experience they have lost.

We have choices about pain, but we cannot escape it. We can pay now,
or we can pay later. . . .

JUDY: I was able to have my baby (Elissa) with me sooner than I had
had Justin after my cesarean with him. The hospital finally had rooming-
in, so Elissa and I just snuggled in bed day and night.

After my second child I did not want to ever get pregnant again.
But . . . I did, and I was scared. I really did want another baby, but I
didn't want to have a cesarean, no matter what! I started reading about
vaginal birth after cesarean (VBAC). I was really amazed that in other
countries in the world the doctors let and want their women to go into
labor. Even if they know that the birth will be another cesarean, it is
better for the baby and for the mother.

So I began to interview the doctors. Three of them were in my
hometown. Some were 150 miles away. I talked on the telephone to one
that was 500 miles away. I went armed with many articles, all written
by doctors. I had articles on VBAC after two cesareans, articles from
the National Institute of Health on guidelines telling doctors that vaginal
birth for women who had previous cesarean was as safe or safer than
another cesarean. Other articles pertained to the risks of cesareans for
mothers and babies. I had spent hundreds of hours of research on the
subject of birth and cesareans. I asked the doctors if they would please
read the articles (many of them underlined in red, so that it would not
take too much of their time), but *not one of them would read the articles.*
They told me I would die, and that I was crazy. One walked out of the
room and would not come back.

ALLEN (Judy's husband): When presented with facts from the National
Institute of Health revealing a higher risk and death rate for mother
and babies for repeat C-section than for VBAC, they would say, "That
doesn't pertain to your case."

JUDY: I asked them who it did pertain to, and they ignored the question.
While I was having my internal examinations I asked if they thought I
was ample to have my baby vaginally, and what position the baby was
in. They told me I would not need to know the answers to the questions
I had asked because I would have another cesarean.

One doctor bragged about how he had helped change many of the
attitudes of doctors toward birth, and how he had helped get rooming-
in, fathers in the OR, and breastfeeding on demand in his hospital. I
asked him if he would change the attitudes on cesareans by letting me
have a vaginal delivery. He told me he would help me only if I had

another cesarean. He said the hospital policy would not allow what I wanted. I asked him who made the policy, and he told me the people of the community did. I said I would like a change since I was one of the people of the community He then told me the doctors have to vote on it, and it wouldn't change. It sounded to me like "passing the buck"!

COMMENTS: *Hospital policy is the law of hospital heaven. No one ever seems to know just where it comes from or how to change it. Everyone (including the nurses and doctors) is intimidated by it. And no one ever seems to feel they have the power to change it.*

Unfortunately, as long as we all continue to maintain this belief system, our beliefs will be manifested. The hospital policy will not change as long as we continue to believe that no one has the power to change it! However, if we as consumers, nurses, and doctors decided to empower ourselves with the decision to do what we need to do to make the changes, the changes can and will be made. With knowledge and determination comes the power to make the changes we believe are necessary for the good of ourselves and our families.

JUDY: Whenever I asked the doctors questions about risks, they seemed to feel I had to listen to them, but they didn't have to listen to me. Yet we were still supposed to be a health care team! They all wanted to take my baby 2 weeks early, and there were 5 opinions on my due date within a range of 6 weeks. I asked them if they could assure me of my due date. I asked about the consequences of taking the baby too early—the risks of hyaline membrane disease (respiratory distress caused by lack of surfactant in the lungs, also known as respiratory distress syndrome) and other problems of induced prematurity. I was told I would have an ultrasound to determine the due date. But what are the long term effects of ultrasound on babies?

COMMENTS: *Ultrasound has not been sufficiently studied to determine its long-term effects. There is some evidence that the high-frequency sound waves of ultrasound might effect cellular changes or cellular replication in the long term. Since cellular change is a pre-cancerous state, ultrasound might be a carcinogen. Changes in cellular replication might affect the testes or ovaries of our unborn babies, thereby affecting generations to come. Ultrasound has not been studied long enough to answer these long term questions. Our babies, and our babies' babies are the "test groups" for long term study. We can only choose to be part of the "sample" (those who are exposed to sonagraphy), or part of the "control" (those who are not exposed).*

Though the medical profession generally insists that ultrasound is safe (and they obviously must believe it because they order at least one if not four or five ultrasounds per pregnancy), we must remember that the medical profession also insisted that x-ray was safe. It was considered so safe in the fifties that x-ray machines were used in the shoestores to check the fitting of children's shoes. Can we trust so blithely the routine indiscriminate use of ultrasound in pregnancy with our unborn babies, on the basis of such claims of (unstudied and inconclusive) "safety" by the medical profession?

In Judy's case, the question of safety was enough to push her into an entirely different set of choices for her birth.

JUDY: In addition to the ultrasound, I would have to have amniocentesis, and x-rays. That is when I walked out of their offices, saying, "NO, thank you," and knowing I would never come back.

ALLEN: After confronting several doctors and gettng no satisfaction, Judy began to diligently and prayerfully look for an alternative that would give both of us a little more peace of mind about our child's upcoming birth.

JUDY: I finally found a midwife.

GARNET JONES (MIDWIFE): It was early in October that Judy Twist called me and asked if she and her husband could come over to have a pelvic exam. She wanted to know if her pelvis was large enough to give birth vaginally. Her former doctor had given her a cesarean because he said her pelvis was too small. And now, no other doctor she contacted within 150 miles would even measure her pelvis. So, Judy, her husband Allen, and her sister Kay all came to my house for a visit.

JUDY: Garnet had me get my medical records.

ALLEN: We found the doctor contradicting himself on reasons why Judy's first cesarean was necessary. And the reason for the second cesarean was simply because she had had the first. The more we learned, the less it seemed necessary for Judy to have another cesarean.

JUDY: Throughout my records it was written that I had a "risk" of toxemia and a "risk" of cephalo-pelvic disproportion. We all have a "risk" of a car accident when we drive on the roads. We have a "risk" of our house burning down sometimes when we are gone from home and cannot call the fire department. But should we stay at home forever afraid to do anything?

Why was I not allowed to go into labor the first time to see if I really did have cephalo-pelvic disproportion? Why was I not allowed to continue my natural labor with my second child to see if I could have had a natural delivery? I was not told of the "risks" of a cesarean. I was not told of the "risks" of not having a nutritious diet. I was not told the "risks" of the medication I was supposed to take. Why?

GARNET: I explained what measuring the pelvis entailed, using books and diagrams. Then I measured her pelvis.

JUDY: My midwife examined me and found that I was adequate to have a vaginal delivery. I was very glad, but cautious because my family thought I was crazy.

KAY TWIST (Judy's sister): In spite of our six and a half year age difference, Judy and I have always been close. We agree on many subjects, but when Judy told me she wanted to try to have a vaginal birth after her two cesareans, I told her she was crazy. I wondered if she had *really* listened when I told her about my first baby's "birth". It took months to recover from my long labor and cesarean, and I couldn't imagine why Judy *wouldn't* learn from my experience. Fortunately, Judy didn't give up!

ALLEN: My first thought of a home birth was that it was far too dangerous in our particular situation. I must admit I was very skeptical, but we had been praying and looking for an alternative, and this was another possibility.

GARNET: When I measured Judy's quite ample pelvis, I instructed Allen about how he could measure her also. He also felt how roomy it was, and perhaps this helped him to be more supportive of Judy's wishes to attempt a home birth.

ALLEN: We told the midwife of our confrontations with the doctors, and their refusal to consider a VBAC. She admitted having never been involved in a VBAC before, but was willing to read any available information, and to contact other midwives about it.

GARNET: Being an empirical midwife, I was a little apprehensive that Judy and Allen were not able to enlist the help of any doctor who would listen to their concerns and allow a trial of labor. But that worry was overshadowed by the positive aspects of working with this couple. After reviewing Judy's previous hospital birth records and seeing the dimensions from her pelvic x-ray, I was reassured that she was capable of giving birth vaginally. The couple were intelligent, had a very strong desire to have a vaginal home birth, had done lots of research, and were concerned about maintaining a relaxed atmosphere with safety from drugs and surgical procedures. Their concern was for the baby's and mother's health and happiness, but they were determined to try a VBAC no matter what the outcome and were willing to assume full responsibility.

COMMENTS: *Taking responsibility is perhaps the most difficult aspect of birthing. Though it is easy to talk about, it is not always easy to do. The responsibility of the parents is often the deciding factor for a midwife as to whether or not to take on particular clients. Taking co-responsibility—parents and practitioners together—needs to become the focus of both legal and philosophical changes in the practice of obstetrics if that practice is to benefit all involved.*

ALLEN: The midwife's greatest concern seemed to be the possibility of uterine rupture. When she read Judy's medical records, she found that the doctor had commented on the apparent strength of the uterus, and also that a horizontal cut had been made in the uterus which greatly reduced the possibility of a rupture. Seeing the midwife's caution turn into confidence and enthusiasm was a great encouragement, and gave me a peace of mind I needed.

COMMENTS: *A truly supportive professional, such as Garnet, is of the utmost importance for the comfort and relaxation of all involved. Especially once seeds of doubt have been planted by other less supportive professioinals, it is imperative that VBAC parents find a professional who will not only* allow *a VBAC, but who will* support *a VBAC! We often look to the professional as the guide for our feelings. If professionals approach your VBAC with positive support, they set the tone of the pregnancy, labor, and birth. The feelings are contagious. Just as an unsupportive professional can plant the seeds of doubt and failure a supportive professional plants the seeds of confidence and empowerment.*

ALLEN: Our confidence in the midwife and in Judy's ability to give birth naturally was boosted by the midwife's dietary advice and exercise suggestions.

COMMENTS: *Unlike the focus of obstetricians (complications and disease), the focus of midwives is on health care within a natural process. Therefore, it is not at all surprising that most midwives have educated themselves quite highly about nutrition and exercise. Most have done much reading on the subject, taken workshops, and even developed their own systems of nutritional analysis, supplementation, and exercise plans for pregnancy and labor preparation. Most midwives ascribe to the theory that many many complications can be prevented through good nutrition and exercise. Such an emphasis is a primary difference in the quality of prenatal care given by midwives as opposed to the care given routinely by obstetricians. Often when parents first experience the prenatal care of a midwife, they are surprised by the possibly extensive nutritional changes they are asked to make. But usually any doubts they may have had about the advice of the midwife are dispelled by the marked positive changes in their own health and the health of their babies and children.*

GARNET: Judy and Allen talked over their wishes with me in detail. We planned who should be present, what their jobs would be, and we discussed an emergency backup plan just in case she would need to be transported to the hospital 25 miles away. The only others to know their plans were her sister and mother and my husband.

KAY: As Judy gathered information, she shared it with me, and it wasn't long before I saw that I had been the one who was crazy. Judy was the only sane one around! When Judy and Allen decided on a home birth, I asked if I could be there, and they so generously said they wanted me there.

JUDY: The midwife taught us about the birth process, which also encouraged Allen. He started reading many of the articles that I had read, and that really helped him to decide.

GARNET: Judy and Allen met regularly with me to discuss normal birth and home birth, problems that could arise and what we would do. Exercises to prepare for birth, relaxation practice, the stages of labor, and coaching were all discussed and practiced in these prenatal visits.

ALLEN: By the time the day of birth came, I was confident that all would go well.

GARNET: I prepared mentally for giving Judy a lot of emotional support and encouragement. I was not fearful of a bad outcome, for I *had much confidence in Judy and her ability to give birth normally.* Her diet had improved considerably since her first pregnancy, and she was preparing herself positively with reading and exercises. I thought that this birth should be handled like any other first birth, except that I would be more watchful for uterine rupture signs, checking the abdomen for tenderness.

Because of uncertainty about conception and a slight spotting-type period, and conception while breastfeeding, the due date was uncertain. I visited Judy and Allen at their home on December 15th, and it appeared to me that she was almost ready to give birth, and I wondered if she would go until January 23rd, which had been set as her due date, based on her last (slight) menstrual period. So I was not surprised when, on December 23, Judy and Allen called and said she was in labor.

JUDY: On December 22nd I went into labor, and on the morning of the 23rd, Allen called the midwife, my sister, and my mother.

GARNET: It was a blizzardy day with lots of ground drifting and very cold, so my husband drove with me the fifty miles to their home. I was glad not to be out on the road alone.

JUDY: It was so nice to be with my children and family in familiar surroundings. I had emotional and physical support throughout my entire labor. My husband never left my side.

GARNET: Judy handled labor well. I knew that she was an excitable, expressive person, full of life and love. I expected her to be somewhat vocal during birth, and I thought she might need to express negative feelings about her previous birth experiences.

During first stage, Judy relaxed beautifully. Her mother and sister were around, in and out throughout the day, caring for the children, and preparing meals. Late in the afternoon, things began progressing, and Judy settled into strong active labor. She was quite expressive during transition and second stage. She expressed doubts, fears, negative feelings, mixed with worries and positive statements, too. She needed frequent reassurance that all was progressing normally.

Judy's sister, Kay, rubbed her feet and was very encouraging with great anticipation. Her husband Allen was loving, attentive and encouraging. Her own mother prayed, offered love, comfort and support by her presence and assisted with the children and household duties. I had spoken with her mother earlier and told her she was welcome in the room at all times as long as she did not say anything negative. She was wonderful!

JUDY: My mother had said that she would never be able to see a birth, much less her own daughter's, but she did beautifully, and was excited about it! She had been with both my sister and me after our cesareans (5 cesareans, in total), and she said we looked like "death warmed over." She hurt for us just as much as we hurt. She was always with us rubbing our feet or cooling our brow after our cesareans. So I knew she would be with me during my VBAC, because she did believe the natural way would be better. Just as the rest of my family needed nine months to get used to the idea of a home VBAC and needed to read important information, she did also.

COMMENTS: *Grandmothers at births are a wonderful support, if, as Garnet clearly realized, they convey positive energy. Garnet was wise, indeed, in setting the stage for positive support for Judy from her mother. The recognition of the need for a supportive attitude thereby actually created a more positive experience not only for Judy, but for Judy's mother as well.*

KAY: During Judy's labor I relived my labor with my first baby. At times I could hardly keep the tears back for the sympathy I felt.

GARNET: I listened for the baby's heart rate periodically, encouraged Judy to urinate, and timed contractions as usual. Labor progressed rather slowly, so vaginal exams were kept to the minimum so as not to be discouraging or to interfere with relaxation. Our focus was comfort, relaxation, and encouragement.

I observed closely to be sure that everything remained normal. All decisions were made by Judy and Allen as they found what was comfortable for themselves.

ALLEN: Even in the final stages of labor, when the contractions came hard and fast, I felt quite confident.

GARNET: It was quite intense during birth, with Judy making strong effort, and Allen wanting to help.

Judy's mother was peeking in at the door, afraid to say the wrong thing. Then she came over to see the baby's hair as the head was crowning. Kay was excited to tears, so glad the birth was actually happening and going so well.

JUDY: At 10:02 P.M. *I delivered* a beautiful 7lbs. 3 oz. baby boy. His head measured 13-1/2 inches and his chest was 13 inches. There was no tearing.

GARNET: The baby had quite a lot of vernix (white creamy covering on the baby's skin), but his ear formation and general development appeared to be that of a full-term baby, not a 4-week premature baby.

ALLEN: When our son came into the world and took his first breath, our joy and excitement was indescribable. It was great to witness this wonderful miracle of birth, and I will never forget it.

KAY: When Kirk was born, my mother and I realized that Judy and her baby were both fine. We hugged and danced in a circle, and cried tears of joy and relief. We had just witnessed a miracle!

JUDY: My mother-in-law and father-in-law brought our other children over to our house immediately after Kirk was born. The children and grandparents were able to hold and love the baby right away, which makes such close bonding. Justin (4-1/2 years old) hurried into our room, and sat down beside us. Kirk was still attached to me, and everything was *wet!* Justin rubbed Kirk's back and head, and said to him, "Hi I'm your brother, Justin. How are you?" Kirk looked at Justin, and Justin was so excited, he kept saying, "The baby looked at me!"

After a while, Allen clamped and cut the cord.

KAY: Less than an hour after Kirk was born, Judy had a nice warm bath. She walked better than she would have three days after a cesarean.

JUDY: While I was in the bath Kay was holding Kirk. Justin said, "I *still* didn't get to hold my brother." Kay sat Justin in a little rocking chair, and put Kirk on his lap. They were both so content to sit and rock, as Justin quietly talked to Kirk. That was so precious to me.

After my bath I walked back into the bedroom and delivered the placenta. Allen made me the very best meal—a peanut butter sandwich—and we had a party!

Allen and I just lay on the bed and admired each other and our new baby, Kirk. Our daughter Elissa was two years old and she was so glad to have her mommy with her all of the time. She just snuggled down with us, and patted her brother's hand. Elissa keeps asking if she was born at home like Kirk was. And when I say, "No," she always wants to know, "Why not?" Elissa and Justin ask if we could please have another baby at home. Our children are still very bonded to each other.

COMMENTS: *Bonding is an elusive butterfly. Though many studies have tried to analyze it, because it is a spiritual and emotional phenomenon, no study can describe it. Unfortunately, most cesarean families have been deprived of this experience. And though it is certainly still possible to love our children, even though deprived of "bonding", it is a priceless indescribable experience that lasts a lifetime.*

The spiritual energy and openness of bonding is not restricted to the bond between the mother and the baby. All those present at a birth who are open to these energies can experience this lifetime bonding. Children who are bonded to one another may still argue, fight, and feel jealous of one another from time to time. But the bonding is the glue that holds them to one another. Judy's children may be too young to understand what bonding is, but they have experienced it, and they liked it so much they want to keep experiencing it. Their spirits and hearts will know what to seek when their own children are being born—a bonding birth.

JUDY: I believe the bonding is so close between Kirk and me because I delivered him—not the doctor—and I was able to see and nurse him right away. He and I were always home!

There are days I want to cry for my first two children because of the beauty of birth I missed with them. I have always loved all my children deeply, but the home birth of Kirk helped me to regain the bonding I had lost with my other children.

COMMENTS: *Though it may be difficult to understand how the birth of a baby can heal the pain from the losses we have endured with our other children, the answer is quite simple. Birth is a healing. We can heal ourselves, our relationships with our partners, our children, our sisters, and even our mothers. It is a timeless moment that is indelibly imprinted upon us. If we are open to its healing, miracles can occur.*

Birth is a new beginning. We can choose to use the birthing energy, its bonding spirit, to let go of the anger of the past, forgive the pain, and move on from a center of love and life. We can use this miracle as a tool to further enhance the love and life of the family.

JUDY: In retrospect, I have learned many things from my cesareans and home VBAC. I think we should ask many questions of our doctors when they tell us we need a cesarean. We ought to be informed enough about cesarean so that we know we ABSOLUTELY NEED ONE before we consent.

GARNET: We, as women, need to gather our strength from our own intuitive wisdom, research facts to back up our instincts, and emit confidence in our womanhood. Through this process we will strengthen other women, our children, our husbands, and extended families, as well as ourselves. I feel that my role as a midwife and childbirth educator includes helping others to trust their bodies, go with their instincts or intuitions, and develop confidence in themselves and their families. Throwing off the shackles of ignorance and intimidation, and believing in the innate goodness of our bodies and selves, can help us to reach our greatest potential.

KAY: Judy succeeded in having a natural home birth after two cesareans. No medication, no cuts! Between us, Judy and I have had 6 babies—5 cesareans and 1 VBAC. Because I supported her and because I was there, I also share her victory. There was healing for me in her birth. I've wondered why women all the way back to Eve have been able to give birth and why I was so inadequate. Judy accomplished the "impossible."

JUDY: A good birth experience can have a great effect on a woman's life. I am more content with motherhood now. I am also a more patient mother. I have three wonderful children and a very supportive husband. I don't feel like I have to prove myself to the world and compete with the men.

A birth can bring tears of sorrow or tears of joy. We can ask any grandmother about her birth experience and she can remember in detail things that happened fifty or more years ago. I am so happy my Creator made me the way I am and that I was able to fulfill the Master plan.

ALLEN: As I'm writing this I can look out of the window and see the red glow of the sunrise in the eastern sky above the North Dakota prairie. I'm comparing in my mind the similarity between the sunrise and a birth. Both are a beginning, both are beautiful, and both have been designed by God to happen naturally.

19

How I Became a Feminist

KAREN DIESSEL

KAREN: During my first pregnancy I had prepared in the usual Lamaze fashion. We were taught to rely on our doctor's judgment. By staying *in control*, we could *help* our doctors *take care* of us, and *coached* by our husbands, we could be *part of the team*. If we were particularly *nice* and did not antagonize the doctor by being too demanding, he might *let* us do some of the things we wanted. A *well-trained* Lamaze *patient* got to *watch the doctor deliver* the baby in the mirror. It was emphasized to us what a privilege it was to have this opportunity, and not to abuse it by being *uncooperative* with hospital personnel.

When I got to the hospital in labor I was having a lot of what was never spoken of in my Lamaze class—*pain!* I decided I must be doing something wrong and worried how I was going to get through the rest of the labor.

A nurse repeatedly asked if I wanted medication, finally saying, "It would be a pity to lose control just because you were too stubborn to take medication." That remark, carefully aimed, penetrated my consciousness like a knife.

"Am I losing control? She thinks I'm losing control. I must be losing control," I concluded nervously. I was being uncooperative—misbehaving. The nurse won.

I was medicated for the remainder of my labor. Eventually, I was invited to try a few pushes. Half sliding, half being pushed, I was transferred to the delivery table and my legs laced in the "leg rests." I pushed a few times while the doctor and my husband scrubbed and gowned. I found myself involuntarily raising my legs up out of the stirrups and sort of waving them in the air like a turtle on its back.

The nurse asked if I wanted to watch the birth in the mirror. "Yes," I exclaimed emphatically, hoping to get a little closer to this intimate event that suddenly seemed so remote. The mirror was wheeled into place, and the nurse pointed out the baby's head, now visible in the birth canal. I felt as if I were watching TV, somewhere at the foot of my bed, miles away. This didn't seem to be happening to me. The bottom half of my body was covered with sterile drapes that we had been scrupulously taught not to contaminate by touching. The area where all the action was taking place was off limits to me, and now belonged to these strangers bustling around me. The business of the birth was now in their hands, their job, their chance to "show their stuff," and take the bows.

Finally, after a large episiotomy, I looked in the mirror just in time to see the baby explode from my body like a cannonball. It was 11:15.

After 16 hours of hard labor, I had nearly missed the birth in the few seconds I inadvertently closed my eyes to push.

It was over. The contractions mercifully ceased, but there were no raptured thrills. I lay there like a wounded animal, too exhausted to move. Considerable embroidery of my derriere awaited me. The baby was wrapped in a receiving blanket and shown to me briefly before being whisked away.

The next day, I began to brood over the events of the birth. I was embarrassed that I had not "performed" very well during labor and felt somewhat substandard because I could not have my baby without being cut. Something seemed to be missing, but I didn't know what. After all, I had had natural childbirth. Why did I feel like I missed the birth?

The Birth of Caroline

When I became pregnant with our second child two years later, I investigated the possibility of having a home birth. But I could not find any doctors or midwives in the area willing to attend one. I briefly considered having the baby at home, unattended. When I tried to visualize the birth, however, I couldn't get the baby past the perineum (tissue and muscles between the vagina and rectum). I could not give birth. Therefore, I quickly discarded the idea of an unattended home birth and reluctantly decided to go to the hospital.

On leap year day, I awoke to mild contractions, that seemed to fade when I was not up and moving. I assumed that this was not real labor. Later, my husband and I took a walk. The contractions increased in strength, and were 5 minutes apart. When I arrived at the hospital I was 6 centimeters. While the doctor was still in the room, I had a really heavy contraction that left me nauseous and wondering if I was going to be able to give birth.

I took a deep breath and greeted the next contraction with my usual breathing routine. Midway through, however, I heard my breathing interrupted by the deep gutteral sounds I recognized as second stage. The doctor and nurses heard it too, and they all came flying back into my room.

I was on my way to the delivery room. My elation soon turned to disappointment as the delivery was almost an exact replica of my first birth. I watched, straining to drink in every detail, while the baby took her first breaths in the doctor's arms. Finally, an hour later I was given my newborn. I felt her wriggling warmth beneath the receiving blanket and wondered what her naked little body would have felt like next to mine.

My Miscarriages

A little more than 2 years later we conceived again. We were excited and hoped to experience a truly natural childbirth. A few days before leaving to visit relatives in Germany, I noticed that my early pregnancy feelings had pretty much faded. I couldn't quite rid myself of a nagging fear that something was wrong.

The day after I arrived in Germany I started spotting, so my sister-in-law took me to her gynecologist, who told me that the baby had died. This was sad news, but it confirmed what I had suspected all along. I had felt my body had been returned to me. That familiar pull was gone.

I telephoned my husband back in New York. It was hard giving him the news long distance. I so wanted to be in his arms and cry my heart out, but instead, I had to maintain control. It was difficult swallowing all those tears, so I wrote to a friend:

> *The worst is not having the luxury of my own home to stomp around and scream in. Instead, I have to walk around with dead tissue inside me and pretend to enjoy the vacation. It really doesn't help very much either to be reminded that I already have two healthy children and of all the work a third would entail, and that I am luckier than most. All of this may be true, but before I can get to that point, I need to feel miserable for a while.*
>
> *My anxieties right now center on my future childbearing potential. Is this just a one-time accident of nature, or the beginning of a pattern? Am I simply getting too old to turn out viable eggs, or is there a monster lurking in my womb, waiting to snatch up potential offspring?*
>
> *If I were ten years younger, maybe I could take it more in stride, but at my age, I really don't have time to waste on such nonsense. Also, I have such long infertile periods while nursing, who knows how long it will take to re-establish my menstrual cycle if it ever does re-establish? And if I have a D & C, who knows what havoc curettage will wreck on my uterus—will the fools miss with the knife and remove my liver?*

I decided to tell my oldest daughter, who was then 5, and had been very much looking forward to the baby. She burst into tears and wailed, "I knew it was something bad, but I never thought it would be *this* bad. No baby? What will I do with all the little clothes I've been collecting for the baby, and all the things I planned to make? This is terrible." We cried in each other's arms.

Over the next couple of days, the bleeding became heavier, and I began to have some light cramping. One evening I went to the bathroom and felt something slither out onto the sanitary pad I was wearing. When I investigated, sure enough, there was a medium-sized clot and something transparent shimmering through. As I retrieved it, I saw what I already suspected—the embryo still enclosed, intact in the amniotic sac. It was about the size of my thumbnail. I cast a half-reluctant glance, fearing to perceive some horrible, deformed creature. To my astonishment, however, I recognized first the curvature of the spine, and beheld to my wonder, not the random growth of cells as I had dreaded, but the human form, in miniature.

With trembling hands, I brought it closer to the light and gazed with a mixture of cold, scientific interest and utter humility. What I saw was, as far as I could tell, a perfectly developed embryo, about 4–6 weeks into life. The arms were there and fingers were forming on the hands. It still had a fishy looking tail when viewed from the side, but when viewed from the back, it remarkably resembled a baby, curled up. The most impressive feature to me was the perfectly formed, tiny fontanelles, visible on the top of the head.

For a moment, I got a start when it seemed to move inside the amniotic sac, then I realized that the tiny body was only floating in the fluid.

I couldn't stop looking at it. I was so awed by its perfection and beauty. My initial reaction was, "It's an embryo," and then, "It's human. It's my own flesh and blood, potentially one of my children."

Suddenly, I felt very protective. I knew I couldn't flush it down the toilet. I thought for a few seconds about burying it under a tree, but how could I explain that urge to my relatives? Could I smuggle it outside in the moonlight? What would passersby think of a crazy woman in her nightshirt poking away at the earth at 2:00 A.M.? Finally, I decided to place it in a bottle of water and take it to the lab for examination the next day.

For a while after the embryo had been passed, the bleeding slowed down, and I thought it was over. The following day, however, I began having a lot of cramping and started passing massive blood clots. After a couple of episodes, I became so weak that my sister-in-law had me transported to the hospital.

At 9:00 A.M., the next morning, two wooden-faced doctors appeared at my bedside and briskly took a medical history. I was told I would have to have an emergency D & C. I was dumped off like unwanted cargo into the operating room. I shook uncontrollably with cold and dread. I was obliged to place my legs high up into the stirrups and my legs and arms were strapped down with thick leather straps. I felt like I was about to be executed. As the doctor prepared to lace the syringe in my vein containing the substance that would render me unconscious, I panicked.

"No, no, I can't do it. I won't do it," I repeated over and over again. The doctor asked me why I was afraid, but I couldn't tell him. I understood and spoke German, but I desperately wanted my own language. It felt like I was on a different planet. I mourned for my two little children, asleep in their beds, whom I did not want to leave motherless. I never felt so powerless. But I knew I was trapped.

The next thing I was aware of was the anesthesiologist standing over me and saying, "Open your eyes, Frau Diessel, open your eyes. It's over."

I was still alive! I couldn't believe it. The recuperation was slow. I waited anxiously for the results from the laboratory to which I had sent the embryo. I wanted to know everything possible about the baby. I now realize that this was not merely a morbid preoccupation, but an effort to give the baby some identity so that I would have something tangible to grieve for. But there was not much the laboratory could tell us, and so the baby's identity remained a secret.

After this experience it took a long time to shake the feeling that I was not dead. My belly felt violated and I was very anxious about my ability to bear future children. I kept looking for reasons as to why this had happened, but nobody could tell me anything, not even my doctor.

This miscarriage was not to be my only one. A few months later another soul came into my life momentarily, and left quickly. I came to peace with this experience as I walked with my husband through the beautiful spring blossoms—that it was to be a part of the natural process.

The Cesarean Birth of Benjamin

Our third child, Benjamin, was conceived immediately following my second miscarriage.

In about the sixth pregnancy week, we went on vacation. My parents lent us their camper, and we camped along the shore of Lake Huron. Having already experienced two successive miscarriages, I was very anxious about the pregnancy. However, as the weeks progressed, the familiar sensations of pregnancy increased and were reassuring to me. While camping one day, I became so nauseous that I had to lie down. I remember complaining happily to my husband about being sick in my stomach. Then, the very next morning, I woke up in a panic. I had lost the feeling of pregnancy. My body felt strangely quiet, as if something had "unplugged."

"It's gone!" I wailed to my husband.

My husband and I had been looking forward to a rare opportunity to spend some private time with each other. Now, I couldn't even enjoy it. All I could do was sit on the shore and cry into the waters of Lake Huron. I felt so childless. Something inside me had died and my two daughters were away with their grandparents. I missed them terribly, and felt a desperate need to hold them in my arms. We cut our camping trip short, picked up the girls, and headed home. As we arrived at home, I noticed the sensation of pregnancy returning somewhat.

"Strange," I thought to myself. "Could I have had twins and one died and the other is growing?" I speculated, trying to make some sense out of the conflicting messages my body was sending.

A few days after we were back, I went to see my doctor, who brushed aside my anxieties, telling me that everything checked out all right. One week later, with no warning whatsoever, I suddenly started bleeding bright red blood clots. I was sure I was miscarrying, but we had to wait until I could be scheduled for a sonagram the next day. If fetal death were confirmed, then I was to have a D & C. The next day, in the ultrasound room, I was upset but resigned to the idea of miscarriage.

"Well, it doesn't look all that bad," one of technicians said as they viewed the ultrasound.

Then suddenly, there was a flurry of activity in the ultrasound room as more technicians and the heads of the department were called in. They disappeared to "confer," reappeared, pointed at the screen, asked each other, "Do you concur?" and buzzed around in a huddle. Finally, after considerable excitement, they approached me with their findings. "We have found evidence of two amniotic sacs," they informed me. "One contains a viable fetus with a very strong heartbeat. The other is empty. We feel that your bleeding is due to your body's efforts to eliminate the nonviable twin. It is very unusual to make this discovery as early as the 8th week."

I was stunned. This unexpected happy news overwhelmed me and I started to shake and cry.

"Then *feed* me," I demanded, wiping away my tears.

The uncertainty dragged out over the next five weeks with episodes of heavy bleeding. I elected to maintain strict bed rest the whole time in a desperate effort to preserve what was inside me. I felt as if two forces were at work in my body; one trying to hold on, and the other letting go. I agonized over which one would win out.

Finally, one night I started passing large blood clots. We inspected each one carefully for evidence of fetal tissue, but there was none. My husband carried me down the steps to the car, and I rode into the hospital with my feet up on the dashboard, determined to keep the baby from "falling out." At the hospital, I was obliged to go through the routine admission procedures and to supply them with information that I was told they would need for the death certificate. It sounded so final, but I accepted the idea with grim resignation. However, the bleeding tapered off during the night, and the next day, a sonagram revealed a lively fetus of 11 weeks gestation.

"If I can just make it through the first trimester," I thought hopefully. In the sixteenth week, the doctor picked up fetal heart tones. From that point on, the pregnancy normalized beautifully, though I always had an uneasy feeling.

I began counting the days until "viability." Finally, by the 34th week, I thought we were home free. We bought a few baby clothes and some baby toys and I called a meeting of my birthing team. Since everything seemed fine, we decided to go ahead with plans for a very much dreamed of home birth that would include the older children and some dear friends.

The day after the meeting of our birthing team, I felt a sudden gush of water. My membranes had ruptured. My heart sank. Fearful of what might happen in the hospital, I called my midwife to ask about the criteria for a cesarean section with a premature baby. I assumed I was going into labor. She reassured me that as long as the fetal heart tones were good, there was no need for a section.

When I got to the hospital, nobody knew what to do with me. When my doctor appeared, I was not in labor, although my membranes had quite obviously ruptured totally. Since ultra-sound was busy, the doctor ordered x-rays to determine the presentation of the baby. I was both surprised and alarmed that the doctor proposed to x-ray the whole baby. When I expressed my misgivings, however, the doctor pooh-poohed my concern. I felt like I was being trivial, so I gave my (uninformed) consent.

(I have since learned that children exposed to x-rays in utero run a 50% greater chance of developing leukemia.)

The baby was found to be vertex, after all, but I was still not in labor by the end of the first day. The doctor said that about 90% of all women go into labor spontaneously when the membranes ruptured, but he seemed to think the extra time in utero would be good for the baby since I was only 34 weeks pregnant.

But the next day he began to express concern about infection and called around to some colleagues for opinions on how to handle the situation. He presented those to us. (Meanwhile, I did some calling around myself, but could find no one who had much information about premature rupture of membranes.)

Most doctors felt I should be sectioned at once. The more conservative suggestion was to perform an L/S ratio to determine the maturity of the baby's lungs, and if positive, try to induce labor.

COMMENTS: *The L/S ratio is a test of fetal lung maturity, done through amniocentesis. When the ratio of lecithin (L) to sphingomyelin (S) is greater than 2:1, then the fetal lung surfactant is said to be present, and therefore the fetus would be viable outside of the womb. In making the decision as to whether or not to perform such a test, the risks of amniocentesis must be balanced against the risks of proceeding without the knowledge of the test results.*

KAREN: When I suggested the possibility of monitoring my temperature, we were told that the baby could get sick and die before the mother ever registered an elevation of temperature.

COMMENTS: *The medical protocol for preterm premature rupture of membranes without labor is unclear, which is why there had been such indecision regarding Karen's case. At term, the protocol is usually induction and/or cesarean, if labor does not occur spontaneously after 24 hours following rupture of membranes (R.O.M.). However, traditionally, preterm women were told to stay in bed, eat, drink, take precautions to aviod infections (such as no intercourse, and no baths, and no vaginal exams by anyone) and hope that labor did not occur spontaneously until term. Doctors tried to keep the baby in as long as possible, not get it out as fast as possible. Karen's doctor was obviously initially following the traditional protocols.*

However, in recent years with the development of the L/S ratio and the increased success rate with preterm infants in the intensive care nurseries, medical management of preterm premature rupture has become more aggressive. Fear of infection has received greater and greater attention. Infection, especially in the hospital setting, is a growing problem. Many bacteria that were once controllable with antibiotics are now developing resistant strains. Fear of infection now overrides fear of prematurity, and therefore, induction and/or cesarean has become commonplace even with preterm pregnancies.

Basically, three choices were available to the medical personnel and to Karen:

1. She could go home and take precautions to avoid infection. Home is the place of choice in this instance because her body is used to the bacteria of her home, and has most likely built a resistance to them. She would take the traditional precautions of routine bed rest, no baths, no internal exams, and no intercourse. In addition, she could take high doses of vitamin C (to prevent infection) and/or other herbal remedies that stimulate the lymphatic system (such as echinacea). Some practitioners would recommend prophylactic antibiotics as well. She could take increased doses of vitamin A, because vitamin A strengthens the mucous membranes, and the amniotic sac is most certainly a mucous membrane. She could be monitored for possible infection by taking her temperature every 4 hours and by taking a white blood cell count every day. Her baby's heartrate, too, would be an excellent indicator of infection. If any of these monitoring methods showed an elevation, then the baby would need to be born immediately.

2. She could have the L/S ratio done and have the labor induced, if the test showed that the baby's lungs were mature enough to be born; or

3. She could have the L/S ratio done, and choose an elective cesarean.

Karen had heard of the less interventive method (the wait and see method) of "managing" her situation. However, unfortunately, she did not have enough information to feel confident when her doctors tried to undermine the theory. She was faced with a very difficult choice, indeed.

KAREN: We had the L/S test. Finally, about 60 hours after the rupture of membranes, I was informed that the test was positive, my baby's lungs were mature, and the doctors would soon start the induction. I thought sympathetically of the innocent baby in my womb, unsuspecting of the shock that lay before it. The baby was still high in the uterus, and I knew it was not ready to be born. I also knew my body was not ready to give birth. There was nothing auspicious about this day. It was a day like any other day in pregnancy, and yet this was the day my baby was supposed to be born.

For the first time in three days of strict bed rest and a conscious effort to "keep" the baby inside me, I stood up, and tried to "will" the baby to come out. Mindful of the rigors of labor, I walked to the bathroom, splashed cold water on my face and arms, did some neck and shoulder exercises, and tried to refresh my body as best I could. My heart pounded with a mixture of dread and hope as I waited for them to wheel in the IV with the "pit." I knew that the artificial contractions produced by the pitocin could be excruciatingly painful and I was afraid. I was also afraid that no contractions would be produced, and of course I was afraid for the baby.

The nurse and doctor appeared with the pitocin and I gave my (uninformed) consent for the induction. (I have since learned that when the baby's head is not engaged, use of pitocin is contraindicated for labor induction.)

COMMENTS: *Pitocin induction is contraindicated when the head is floating (not in the pelvis) because the risk of fetal distress is greatly increased. If the head is not "engaged," there is no indication that the proportion of the fetal head and the mother's pelvis is adequate. The pitocin contractions may thereby force the fetal head into the bony pelvis. Though it is unlikely that Karen's baby's head circumference would be too large to pass through her bony pelvis (especially in light of the fact that she had previously delivered two term infants vaginally), the premature baby's head is much softer and less tolerant of head compression than is the head of a term infant.*

Not only is the head of the preterm infant softer and more sensitive to pressure, the preterm cervix is not nearly as soft as a term cervix. It is firm and rigid, and unlikely to dilate, even in the presence of pitocin.

In addition, if the head is not "engaged" the force of the pitocin contractions could cause an even more dangerous situation to develop—cord prolapse. Cord prolapse means that the baby's umbilical cord is being pinched between the mother's bony pelvis and the baby's presenting part. When cord prolapse occurs, the baby is deprived of life-sustaining oxygen through his cord, and if the situation is not remedied quickly (usually by emergency cesarean), the baby will die. Thus a pitocin induction when the head is still floating is clearly medically contraindicated.

Therefore, in analyzing the risks and benefits of the traditional management of preterm premature rupture of membranes (the wait and see approach), versus the current management (induction in the face of a nonripe cervix with a floating presentation), it would appear that the risks of the induction far outweigh the benefits that could be gained from such an attempt.

KAREN: The pitocin drip was started, but I felt nothing. The dosage was increased while I waited hopefully. Still nothing. Again, the dosage was increased and I experienced light, fleeting contractions. I clung to them expectantly, joyfully, savoring the sensation of labor, only to have them fade away. As the pitocin was increased to its final dosage, the doctor looked on skeptically. Two hours had elapsed.

"I'm not impressed," he stated flatly.

I started to cry as the doctor explained that now since we had intervened, we were committed to getting the baby born soon and therefore, he would have to do a cesarean section.

COMMENTS: *Approaching the situation more intuitively, and a bit less medically, it is easy to see that Karen's intuition about her baby's need to stay inside her had been absolutely accurate. The baby was not yet ready to be born. Had the baby been ready, he would have naturally dropped into position with the gush of the waters rupturing. Had he been ready, Karen would have had contractions without the aide of pitocin. Had he been ready, the pitocin would have been much more effective in stimulating contractions.*

Had the medical personnel been trained to value their own and the mother's intuition (in addition to the use of medical technology), they might have been more willing to follow the signs of nature. Actually, her doctor's initial response to her ruptured membranes—his own intuition to let well-enough alone, and hope that the baby would not be born for some time—would have probably been as medically safe a course of action as the course he was advised to follow by the experts. But the more interventive approach was legally much safer for him. With the rate of malpractice suits rising each year, more and more doctors are following the legally safe course of action, even if the medical outcome using an alternative less interventive approach would be as medically safe or even safer than the legally safe approach.

Practitioners and consumers must seek another solution for getting optimum health care, besides malpractice suits and the practice of legally protective medicine. We must seek a different system, legally and medically, that redefines the responsibility of the practitioner and the consumer, that supports the use of intuition (as well as science) in decision making, and that allows for the natural processes of both birth and death.

KAREN: Conflicting emotions whirled through my head. "I'll get even. I'll reject the baby," I resolved angrily. Then I melted. "Well, I guess I love my baby enough to give up everything I wanted, even the birth itself," I relented. "OK, let's get it over with," I said resignedly as I gave my (uninformed) consent to the cesarean section. (No one explained the risk of C-section to me).

Then the doctor pleaded with me to be "reasonable" and have my tubes tied at the same time he did the cesarean, as throughout my pregnancy he had been outraged that I would be pregnant at such an age—39. My husband refused, as he knew my desire to have more children.

I was prepped in the usual manner, and the rest of the surgery proceeded normally. When the baby was born, my first awareness of him was his cry. How small and out-of-place it sounded in that highly technical world. The room was very still, as the pediatrician examined the baby.

"He's fine," he confirmed.

The baby weighed in at a bouncing 6 pounds, an impressive weight for a baby 6 weeks early. The doctors marveled at his good appearance.

I kept straining my neck for a look at the baby. Finally, he was wrapped in a blanket and given to my husband to hold. I tried to make some contact with the baby, but it was very awkward. His eyes were glued shut, but his mouth was open. I instinctually wanted to nurse him. However, I was told I couldn't because the anesthetic would go through to the baby. (Later I found out this was nonsense.) It took a long time for me to be sewn up, but the baby remained with us and accompanied us to the recovery area.

COMMENTS: *Nursing on the operating table, having the baby with you throughout repair of the incision, and throughout recovery are requests that are often made by cesarean mothers. Unfortunately, very few mothers succeed in getting their requests fulfilled, unless they make these arrangements in writing in advance. I would advise everyone to plan for the possibility of cesarean for each and every birth—and in so doing make your requests known to all the medical personnel who might be involved if your birth were to occur via cesarean.*

KAREN: When I was taken to my room, the baby went to the nursery for observation. As I was in a great deal of pain, I lost interest in the baby. By the time I felt well enough to nurse, the baby had become dehydrated and too weak to nurse. By the second or third day, it was obvious the baby was becoming jaundiced and was losing weight. Fortunately, I had recuperated sufficiently from the surgery to make more of an effort to get him to nurse. But he would just take a couple of weak sucks and then fall asleep. It was very frustrating.

As his weight continued to drop, and my breasts became engorged, I realized I was going to have to resort to more aggressive measures. With the aid of an electric breast pump, I pumped enough milk for one or two feedings from a bottle with a premie nipple—just enough to keep up his strength while I continued my efforts to get him to nurse from the breast. He was so unlike my other full-term babies. For even though he weighed a robust six pounds, he seemed very unripe, very detached. Eventually, my efforts to get him to nurse paid off, and he began to regain his weight. But he had to be coaxed and feedings required much patience for the next several weeks.

COMMENTS: *Premature babies are oten quite jaundiced, as their livers are even more immature than the livers of term babies. Jaundice can make even a term baby become lethargic. But premature babies can little afford the weight loss and subsequent dehydration that often accompanies the jaundice. Karen's commitment to nursing her baby assisted him to move through this difficulty to regain his vitality and health.*

KAREN: My days in the hospital were filled with many emotions. I felt as though someone just handed me the baby from out of nowhere. The feelings of dissociation were incredible. Every time I held the baby, I kept looking at him and asking him incredulously, "Where did you come from?" Something seemed to be missing.

For a long time after my cesarean, I grieved. I grieved because even though I had three beautiful children, I had never experienced birth, and probably never would experience it due to my age and cesarean scar. Each year as the anniversary of the "day he came into the world" arrived, I had a hard time calling it a "BIRTH day", and my celebration was wistful and ambivalent.

COMMENTS: *"Birth days" are often difficult for cesarean mothers. Each birthday is a reminder not only of the joy of our child's life coming into our lives, but also of the pain, frustration, sadness, failure, the loss of the birth of which we had dreamed, and the loss of our self-esteem as women and mothers. The birthday is an anniversary not only of a birth, but of a death, as well—the birth of our child, but the death of our dream birth, and the death of our sense of ourselves.*

KAREN: I questioned the necessity of the cesarean. It was bad enough if fate had dealt us a bitter blow, but the thought of having had an *unnecessary* cesarean was outrageous, unbearable. For a long time I preferred to think of my cesarean as necessary. When I began to entertain the idea that maybe my cesarean was not necessary after all—and perhaps neither were my two episiotomies, nor lying down on the delivery table, nor the ridiculous stirrups, nor being coached on how to give birth—I *became angry!*

Finally, I realized what had been missing from *all* my births—it was my dignity, my sense of autonomy and control over my own body and pride in my own performance. I became a feminist in the deepest sense of the word. I grew up.

The Birth of Katharina: Home VBAC

Shortly before Benjamin turned 3, while living in Germany, I conceived again. We were ecstatic, but cautious in our optimism. No doctor ever failed to remind me that I was 42 years old, and of course I was advised to have an amniocentesis. But we had decided against it because of the risks and because we did not feel we could accept an abortion.

COMMENTS: *The risks of amniocentesis include placental separation, injury to the fetus, premature labor. It is also important to remember that an amniocentesis cannot be performed until the second trimester of pregnancy. Therefore, if the results of the test show that a fetus has genetic anomalies, medically a saline abortion is the only possible abortion. When a woman has a saline abortion she experiences labor and delivery of a dead fetus. Not every saline abortion is successful. Some babies are delivered viable, and must legally be transferred to the ICU and placed upon life-sustaining apparatus. Other attempted saline abortions may not result in actual delivery, and a cesarean (called a hysterotomy) must be performed. And perhaps most traumatic, due to the error rate of the test, a few saline abortions performed on the basis of amniocentesis result in the stillbirth of a genetically perfect baby.*

Though amniocentesis is often done routinely for pregnant women over 35 years of age, it is of the utmost importance for parents to carefully consider all the physical and emotional risk factors of the test, balancing them against the risks of delivering and caring for a defective child.

KAREN: Early in pregnancy, I sought prenatal care from a doctor on the staff of a nearby hospital. I would have preferred care by a midwife, but I wanted to have some medical contact in case I had a miscarriage and required a D & C.

Doctors in private practice in Germany do not attend the births of their patients. Births are handled by doctors on the hospital staff. Thus, a woman does not meet the doctor who will "deliver" her baby until she arrives in labor at the hospital. This was a scene I hoped to avoid.

I had been planning this birth in my mind for a long time. Ever since my cesarean I was preoccupied with the idea of THE NEXT BIRTH. From the first time I shuffled to the bathroom clutching my wounded belly, my thoughts centered on what tidbits I had read about vaginal birth after cesarean and how I could get more information.

Vaginal birth after cesarean is routine in German hospitals, but so are a lot of modern technical interventions. We contacted a German midwife whom we had heard was doing home births in the area. Independently practicing midwives are practically extinct in Germany now as nearly all births take place in hospitals. Although she never really felt comfortable with the idea of a home VBAC, after much persuasion she did agree to attend me at home. And, although I never really felt comfortable with her philosophy of birth and feared a power-struggle with her, I compromised some of my most deeply-felt beliefs because the American midwives whom we had hoped to import for the birth already had previous commitments to other birthing women.

The midwife suggested that we switch to a doctor in private practice who could come for suturing, if necessary. When the obstetrician examined me, he felt the baby was rather small compared to the amount of amniotic fluid and concluded that I had polyhydramnios (too much amniotic fluid). He suggested a sonagram. Although we had refused the usual routine sonagrams, we agreed to this one because we were left to speculate about the grave implications for the baby (twinning, diabetes, or spinal anomalies). We decided, under the circumstances, to have the sonagram done so we would know what to expect and how to prepare for the birth.

Two days later, we were back in the doctor's office for a sonagram. We watched anxiously while our baby manifested part by part on the screen. First came the heart and head—thank God it was all intact. The size of the head was measured and the scanner insisted it was 35 weeks, although I was in the 39th week of pregnancy. As the doctor checked the bladder and kidneys, they were found to be abnormally enlarged. Then the back was located and the doctor proceeded down the spine. I saw a cloud pass over his face and I glanced at the screen. He pointed out an obvious hole at the base of the spine with the characteristic sac above it. Spina bifida (a developmentally defective closure of the encasement of the spinal cord, through which the cord and meninges may or may not protrude). I had seen it a hundred times in pictures, but never expected to confront it so intimately.

I hardly focused on the rest of the exam. The doctor showed us fingers, toes, and what seemed to be a penis. It all seemed so irrelevant. The doctor suggested we go to the university clinic in Bonn the next day where they have more sophisticated equipment in order to confirm the diagnosis and assess the extent of the problem. This would also provide information as to whether the baby should be born by cesarean section! We were stunned.

We drove home in relative silence. Our baby had spina bifida, kidney problems, was retarded and Lord knows what else. So this is how it was to have a handicapped baby. Somehow I felt a sad but calm acceptance of the situation. Other parents had faced this, too. I recalled the touching birth stories I had read in which they shared ther pain and drew strength from them. I did not feel alone.

When we tried to explain about the baby to the children, the two older ones, aged 10 and 7, became hysterical. Our 3 year old was bewildered. My husband broke into sobs. Seeing the children so heartbroken was the most difficult part for me. Somehow we got them calmed down enough to sleep.

My husband also fell asleep but I spent most of the night making myself cups of chamomile tea and struggling with my emotions. My husband kept repeating, "Poor baby," but I kept thinking, "Poor me." I dreaded the next days. I wanted to get it all over with, wanted the baby outside my body (a reflection of my desire to escape the problem, no doubt), wanted to run, but the baby was always with me. It seemed so futile, sustaining this being that was possibly near death anyway.

Should I have had an amniocentesis, an abortion? How would I get through the birth, possibly another cesarean? How would the baby be? Would it live? What kind of life would it have? What kind of life would we have trying to care for it? I hoped the baby would die.

On the drive to Bonn the next morning, my husband and I discussed the baby's funeral. I wanted the baby baptized. Neither of us is officially connected with a church, but I felt baptism would entitle the baby to a proper funeral and be a comfort to the rest of the family. We also discussed how to nurse and care for the baby should it live.

As we entered the clinic, the emotional numbness that gripped me was melted suddenly at the sight of pictures of smiling babies in the otherwise drab waiting room. I fought back the tears as we waited silently for our turn. After what seemed an eternity, we were called.

My husband handed the referral papers to a sober, young technician and the scanning process began all over again. This time I looked away while the long arm of the machine rolled this way, that way, over my bulging abdomen. My husband and I clutched each other's hands while the technician continued to stare at the screen, without expression, without comment. I assumed he was taking various pictures of the defective spine. Finally, my husband broke the silence with the remark that there had been a suspicion of spina bifida. Suddenly, the technician acknowledged us for the first time and asked, seemingly surprised, "Really? Where?"

In my wildest fantasy, I never dreamed of the possibility of an error.

Hardly daring to hope, we poured out the episode of the previous day in the doctor's office. What had we seen so clearly on the screen? "Artifacts, subcutaneous fat, perhaps," we were told. The head of the department was called in. He could find no evidence of any abnormalities whatsoever. No spina bifida, no enlarged kidneys, no excessive fluid, and no growth retardation. As a matter of fact, the baby already had a lot of fatty padding, chubby cheeks, probably weighed 9 pounds and incidently, was a girl, not a boy.

How could the obstetrician have been so wrong? Our joy was indescribable. It was like coming back from the grave, and yet I couldn't quite rid myself of the nagging fear. Frankly, I think this experience will always be with me. In a way, I still feel as though I had had this baby, almost to the extent of grieving for it as if it had died. Perhaps I had already started to love this little boy with the hole in his back.

At our follow-up appointment with the doctor, he shared our relief, but doubted the baby would be as big as estimated. He also voiced some concern (which he shared with the midwife) that due to the large amount of amniotic fluid and the vast number of children I had borne (3), my uterus was overstretched and would not contract effectively for the birth. Something always seemed to be wrong.

Nevertheless, we stayed in touch with our midwife and went ahead with plans for a home birth. We had been through so much during this pregnancy. It would have been helpful for us to have some reassurance and support from her, but in order to get her assistance, it was necessary for us to camouflage our own anxieties and reassure HER.

COMMENTS: *Unfortunately, when we are talking our practitioners into attending our VBAC, we cannot share our deepest concerns with them because they might back out if they hear that we have fears.*

KAREN: My due date approached and passed. All my accumulated anxieties began eating at me. Maybe I never would go into labor. Maybe the doctor was right. Maybe my uterus was old and overstretched. The possibilities for something to go wrong seemed infinite. I had lost some mucous and was leaking fluid. I was afraid it was amniotic fluid and that I would be faced with another PROM (premature rupture of the membranes) situation. But the midwife thought it was only runny mucous.

COMMENTS: *Many women experience the fears that had haunted them from the previous pregnancies as they move into their VBAC labors. Confronting these fears often seems to be a necessary step in giving birth.*

KAREN: During the latter part of the pregnancy I often experienced sharp, shooting pains just over the pubic bone that seemed to be aggravated by gas. I had never experienced them with my other pregnancies and, of course, wondered about its possible connection with my uterine scar. I was never fully able to shake the paranoia of the possibility of uterine rupture.

COMMENTS: *Many women who have had a previous cesarean experience these sharp shooting pains during their next pregnancy. Most of them feel as Karen did—frightened that their incision might be rupturing. And unfortunately, very few of them summon the courage to ask anyone about the pains. They live with the fear locked inside of them. Of all the women I have worked with who have experienced these pains, myself included, none have had ruptured scars. In exploring these pains further, it would seem possible and even probable (though not documented) that these pains are due to the breaking of surgical adhesions when the uterus stretches in subsequent pregnancies. This theory is further supported by the fact that women who had felt these pains with their first VBAC pregnancy, seem to experience significantly less pain with each subsequent VBAC pregnancy.*

KAREN: The night after my last doctor's appointment, I was lying on our bed when suddenly my membranes ruptured, sending gushes of water everywhere. It was 8:30 P.M. We called the midwife to give her the good news and said we would call back when labor was well established. About an hour later, the contractions came on—very strong and concentrated uncomfortably on one spot in the lower abdomen. We called my two sisters-in-law who were coming to help out with the kids and lend a little festivity to the event. I really missed my close friends from America, and wished they could have been with us at this time.

Meanwhile, I got under the shower and sprayed warm water over my abdomen which was the only thing that seemed to help me relax and stay on top of things. These were much different contractions than I had experienced with my other births. From the beginning, they came on every 2 minutes, and though somewhat short, were very intense.

There was no gradual buildup of the contractions or the labor. It was just upon me. I could not do the slow, relaxed breathing that had helped me in previous labors, and was only comfortable standing and walking.

We called the midwife to let her know the contractions were two minutes apart. My two sisters-in-law arrived at 11:00, the midwife arrived about 12:30. After examining me, the midwife announced in a rather peeved tone that I was only 2 centimeters dilated, that I (my cervix) was rather tense, and if this continued we might as well drive directly to the hospital. My heart sank. I felt humiliated, abandoned in my hour of need.

I found the contractions to be unusually painful and difficult to work with. They were so close together and so intense. There was no time to enjoy the labor. What was most overwhelming was not the actual pain, but the dilemma of being caught between two forces simultaneously— the intense labor and a rejecting midwife.

The midwife thought I was not relaxing properly and should lie down and concentrate more on slow, deep breathing. She said the pain in my lower abdomen was due to the cesarean scar, and not unusual in her experience. She recommended a homeopathic remedy—caulophyllum and gelsemium—to help relax the cervix.

COMMENTS: *Caulophyllum is a homeopathic dilution of blue cohosh, an herb that stimulates contractions, and furthers the progress of labor. Gelsemium is used when the os of the cervix feels rigid.*

KAREN: After receiving the injection, I tried to relax lying down. This did not work for me and slowed down the contractions, so I climbed back into the shower and stayed there until the contractions became so overwhelming I could not keep my weight on my feet. Then I walked up and down the hall supported by my husband and leaning against him during contractions. As the force of the contractions increased, I began taking more and more of my weight off my feet, until eventually, he was holding me completely. He would say, "Let go," and I would let go not only of my body weight, but would just surrender to the whole process.

After about an hour and a half (around 2:00 A.M.), I began to feel some pressure in the lower back, and was beginning to make some low, grunting noises at the end of the contractions. The midwife was afraid I would cause my cervix to swell by pushing too soon. She had me lie down and try to breathe through a couple of contractions. By the next contraction or so, I was allowed to push.

The midwife put on her apron, and rolled up her sleeves. I was still on my back. This position was apparently comfortable for the midwife, but made me feel helpless and submissive. However, I was so overwhelmed by the force of the birth process, I could not take the initiative to move myself. My husband made an attempt to suggest a different position, but was brushed aside by the midwife. She asked my sister-in-law to get a flat pan to place under my hips so she could maneuver the shoulders when they came out.

So there I was, on top of my frying pan, with one foot pressing against the midwife's hip, trying to push my baby into the world. I feel I would have pushed much more effectively and joyfully had I been in an upright position. I need to have my head above my shoulders to feel in control.

During my pregnancy, I had discussed nonhectic second stages with my midwife. But now she commanded me sternly to push, push, push, harder, harder, harder, and then scolded me because I was not doing it right. Her disapproving comments made me feel I was hopelessly incompetent and that she had to do it for me. She told me that I was pushing ineffectively, that it was all going into my head, and that I was damaging my baby. I think if the midwife had had enough faith in the natural process to back off a bit and give me some space to integrate my sensations, I instinctively would have found the best way to birth the baby, and would have felt it to be more my own achievement.

COMMENTS: *Birth in the "stranded beetle position"—recumbent and passive— was the birth that Karen was trying to overcome. Yet it was also most likely the only birth position with which the midwife felt safe and assured of her skills. Changing anything in life is difficult. Changing a practitioner's sense of safety with birth is a most difficult process.*

In order for Karen to have an upright birth, she would have needed to "stand firm" in her commitment, challenging the midwife's authority at that very moment. However, along with her challenge, she would have needed to accept the possibility that instead of her midwife complying with Karen's wishes, the midwife might have left. Karen would have had to confront the possibility of completing the birth without the assistance of a professional practitioner. She would have had to take the full and complete responsibility of the outcome of the birth herself. Karen made the decision that was right for her at the time, even though she did compromise some of what she had hoped for in the birth process.

KAREN: Slowly, the baby slipped down the birth canal and the head became increasingly visible. I had planned to reach out and touch the baby's head, but somehow, I didn't.

In the small mirror my husband held for me, I watched the head with its long, wet, dark hair begin to push through my vagina. I watched the midwife's hands, busy working on my perineum.

As the baby was crowning, my husband and I spontaneously kissed excitedly, with a force that seemed to be evoked by the force of the birth itself. Everyone made appreciative comments about the baby's long hair. Finally, after about 6 pushes, out came the head. The midwife used the DeLee catheter (a long tube which goes down the throat of the baby in order to remove mucous) to suction the baby. Then came the shoulders, and whoosh, there she was. A perfect baby girl. What a relief! It was 2:17 A.M.

The baby needed some more suctioning and a bit of stimulation so the midwife placed her directly on the bed and used the electric suctioning device and massaged and blew on her to get her going. I reached out and held her hand.

COMMENTS: *Judging from the condition of the baby at birth, it is possible that the midwife became commanding about pushing hard and fast because she felt the progress of second stage needed to be accelerated to assure the baby's health and safety. Breathing your baby out in a quiet peaceful atmosphere is without a doubt an ideal birth. However, progress sometimes may not be made without assertive pushing, especially when the woman is in a supine position.*

KAREN: There was a small gush of blood, followed by the placenta. The midwife was afraid of a big bleed due to the baby's size, so she gave me an injection of Methergine and Syntocinon (pitocin).

After a couple of minutes, the baby perked up and the midwife told me I could hold her. I had always dreamed of a sensitive, spiritual welcoming for the baby, but now, to my surprise I declined, and asked my husband to take her. I continued to hold her hand while the children were called in to admire their new sister. She was beautiful, and already so round and fat.

After a few minutes, I took her into my arms. She opened her eyes for the first time and we exchanged gazes. I prepared to offer her the breast, but before I could position the nipple, she reached out quickly with her mouth and latched on tightly. We all laughed admiringly at what an eager and skillful nurser she was.

The midwife sighed with relief and declared emphatically that never again would she do a home VBAC. It had been too hard on her nerves.

COMMENTS: *Home VBACs can be tension producing for midwives. The legal situation for home birth midwives in most states in this country, and in most industrialized countries in the world is less than optimum generally. But even where home birth and midwifery are legally acceptable, home VBAC is not. If at a home VBAC the health of the mother and the baby do not necessitate a hospital transport, the legal position of the home VBAC midwife is not compromised. However, if further medical assistance were needed, "the authorities" would certainly take legal action against the midwife (even if the complications had nothing to do with the previous cesarean scar).*

If Karen's midwife needed to resuscitate the baby, she must have been feeling some tension about the legal ramifications if this baby were to need hospitalization. She was surely sticking her neck out to give Karen her desired home VBAC. I'm sure she was quite relieved to see the baby nursing so eagerly.

KAREN: Eventually, the baby was weighed (4100 grams—9lb. 5oz.), cord attended to, and dressed. Then we broke out the champagne, sang "Happy Birthday" to the baby. At 6:00 A.M. my husband and I finally snuggled into bed with our new daughter. We were exhausted but happy.

I wish I could say that my last birth, my home birth with a midwife, was the birth in which all my issues were resolved. But having a home birth does not guarantee total satisfaction, or your money back. What most of us are seeking, I believe, is as much a style of birth as a location. Though I came very close, in the last moments of the birth, the midwife in her panic resorted to power tactics, and I in my desperation, succumbed. Both uf us reverted to the old role models, creatures of habit

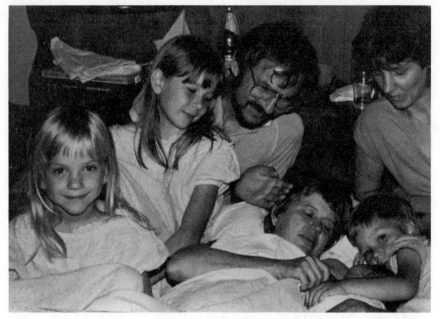

Karen and Hans Diessel, with Caroline (7), Jennifer (10), Benjamin (3), and Katie (1 hr.)

that we are. The system had followed me into my bedroom. Old ways die hard.

Through every action we as women take to reclaim birth for ourselves, we are giving birth to ourselves as capable, complete persons.

My two Lamaze hospital births had left me feeling confused and unsatisfied, but it took the intensity of a cesarean section to open my eyes completely to the oppressive nature of the prevailing system of childbirth in this country. As I struggled to come to terms with the cesarean experience, I gradually came to see that women's natural power in birth had been usurped by a male-dominated medical establishment. Those who were in control of birth had no first-hand experience with birth, and no belief in women's innate ability to give birth naturally. Instead, they sought to rescue women from the experience of birth by active management and a myriad of interventions. Some of these interventions, like shaving and enemas were degrading; others, such as anesthesia and labor induction were downright dangerous; while still others, like routine episiotomy, bordered on sadism. Most were unnecessary, merely allowing the doctor a greater role at the birth while the woman's role was diminished. The woman's presence was rendered incidental, even troublesome. At best, she was converted into a passive observer, her participation welcomed to the extent she could "help" the doctor.

This insight left me feeling cheated and angry—angry at the system that perpetuated such injustice, and angry with myself for going along with it. Then I suddenly recognized that the oppression that existed in the childbirth arena was really a microcosm of the oppression of women in a much wider context. I saw my own passivity in childbirth as an end product of generations of conditioning to passivity and dependency common to all women. How particularly ironic and cruel that women, long denied participation in so many other areas of society considered the domain of men, should also become outsiders at such an undeniably feminine process as birth! I finally realized that the powerlessness of women at birth is simply a reflection of the powerlessness of women in society in general. In order to feel whole, women must be able to function freely as competent human beings at their births, and in all areas of their lives.

COMMENTS: *When we as women take back our power to birth and to live as whole human beings, then we have* become *VBACs*—very beautiful and courageous women!

20

My Brother—I Felt Like I Had Known Him All My Life: A Child's Perspective

THE TAYLOR FAMILY

The Birth of Paul

COMMENTS: *Having prepared in the usual Lamaze fashion, Joanne and Marc entered the hospital in early labor awaiting the birth of their first baby. Exhausted by a 3-day labor, by the time she was fully dilated and ordered to push, her contractions had disappeared. Her attempts to push without contractions failed, and Paul was born by cesarean for failure to progress, posterior presentation, and cephalo-pelvic disproportion (CPD).*

JOANNE: The emergence of Paul into our life was like finding a rose on a pile of dung. The beauty of his existence, the spirit he has, the blessings we experience having him with us, cannot be diminished; but it has been difficult to extract that beauty from the time of his joining us, from all the crap that surrounded it.

MARC: We had some very difficult times surrounding the birth of our son Paul. But I think that our relationship was strengthened overall because we had to work so hard together to avoid the same mistakes in our second birth. Through this experience I learned that ignorance is not bliss.

The Birth of Ryan

COMMENTS: *After much searching and soul-searching, Joanne and Marc finally found Dr. Sorger, the only doctor within three hours of them who would attend her classical-scar VBAC. The following is the story of the birth of their VBAC baby, as told by their first child Paul.*

PAUL: One night we had some visitors over. After they left my mother started having contractions and my father told me Mom was going to have a baby. We went out to the car, and I was real tired, so I went to sleep real fast. When we stopped at the hospital I woke up. My mother and my father and me went to a certain room. But I had to stay out in the hall.

COMMENTS: *Although Joanne had made arrangements with the hospital that Paul could be present for the birth, the nurse on duty when they arrived would not permit him into the labor room. She told him he had to stay out in the hall.*

Joanne Taylor, immediately after the birth of Ryan, with Paul and a nurse looking on

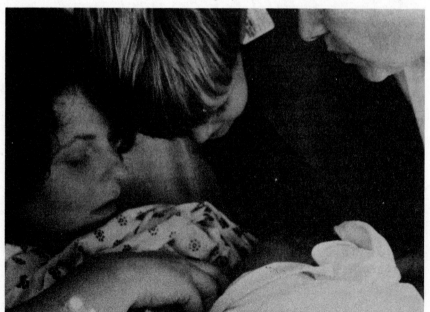

PAUL: But when our doctor, Mr. Sorger, came in he said, "What are you doing out here, honey? Follow me." And I went in and watched everything. After six hours (of pushing) my mother got pushed into a bed with wheels, and we watched her push out Ryan. I felt like I had known him all my life.

The doctor put him in a little bed in a glass cage with a hot light shining on him to keep him warm. We took a rest, then. After a while we went home and called to tell our friends.

JOANNE: After Ryan was born Marc was able to hold him for a long time while I was cleaned up. Paul stood by his side touching Ryan, looking at him and kissing him. They were holding him when Ryan first opened his eyes. There was a very strong bonding between Ryan and Marc and Paul. I feel that we were blessed to be able to have had such a birth and to have known, by contrast, that it was so special.

The Birth of Jeremy

COMMENTS: *With the next birth, Joanne planned a homebirth attended by a midwife, and hoped for a faster second stage. The following is the story of Jeremy's birth as told by Paul.*

Joanne Taylor with Ryan, just after the birth of Jeremy

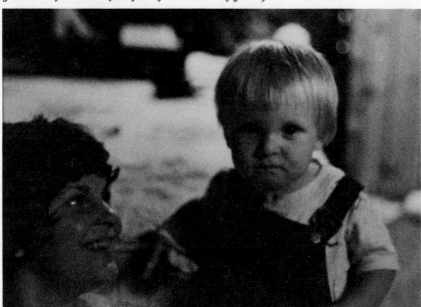

PAUL: One night I had some friends over and we watched a movie. One of my friends said that a lady was here, and I thought she was our midwife. So I asked my father if Mom was in labor. He said she was, so I went upstairs. But Mom said to go downstairs. And then my father yelled, "Get Ryan up here right now!" I was so excited I almost knocked him down. When I got upstairs his (the baby's) head was out, and then he came out. And Linda came over and got us dinner.

JOANNE: For me, this was the way to have a baby. It was *so* right, that there was nothing spectacular. The baby was born, we held him, nursed him, loved him and life went on. There were no discontinuities, no contraptions, no routines, no distractions . . . just the birth of our baby. A miracle, and yet nothing out of the ordinary.

I also realize that this birth experience happened as it did because of things learned through and as a result of my previous experiences. I could not extract this experience from the others. Without them, it would not have happened this way, this time. Without the other experiences this experience would have been perceived differently. I am grateful for each birth, just as I am grateful for each child.

21

Sexual Abuse and Letting Go

BARBARA

BARBARA: I was sexually abused as a child from about the age of 2 until 12, by my biological father. It was not rape. I was not forced into anything. I was seduced.

My father is a great talker and communicator, with a tremendous imagination. He played great games with us. He was like a kid, and it was great being with an adult who understood what it was like to be a kid. My brother was born when I was two years old, and I turned to my father for love and attention. He took advantage of the situation. To fulfill his own needs he used his imagination negatively to devise attractive scenarios for seduction for me and my sister. He set the scene with mood lighting—really went all the way. I guess he had to be more and more creative because I was being more and more resistant. Although he never made me touch him, he suggested it when I was about 10, or so.

My father had a very poor relationship with my mother. She is a very cold person, and rarely let him touch her or be warm with her. The first few years of their marriage, there was almost no sex whatsoever.

She never *enjoyed* him loving her—she only barely permitted it. He should probably have left her. But his own mother always told him that men were all alike. "Don't be like your father—playing around all the time," she repeated to him. He would not be like his father. So he wouldn't leave my mother, and he wouldn't have affairs outside the marriage.

My mother knew about my father molesting me. When I was about 4 years old, I thought it was wrong to keep secrets from my mother. So I told her about what my father was doing. She tried to do something about it. She went to a minister who basically told her that men could do anything they wanted. She really had no place to go. If she had had strong supportive parents, she could have gone with them. But her parents would not have been able to face anything so ugly. They would have rejected her. So, she really couldn't leave.

However, although my mother could not leave, she could have chosen to protect my sister and me. Logically, if you know your husband is molesting your children, if you can't leave, and you do feel that the man does have some redeeming qualities, you make sure he is *never ever alone with your children.* But my mother would go to her board meetings, and she would leave us alone. She would go to church, and she would leave us alone. Whenever she would leave us alone with him, that's when everything happened. She could have taken us to church and bedded us down there. It wouldn't have been a problem. She could have told everyone else that he was working late. She didn't have to tell anyone else why she had brought us along. But she didn't bring us with her. She left us there alone with him. She knew what was going to happen, and I feel that unconsciously she wanted it to happen. She used us to give my father what she couldn't give him, and she allowed us to be in that situation because it was much easier for her. If my father was getting what he wanted from my sister and me, then he wouldn't bother my mother. It was just too painful for her to have to deal with her own sexuality or his sexuality.

In order for me to keep my sanity while I was being abused as a kid, I learned to isolate and control my feelings. I couldn't let go of control, because if I did, I would go crazy. So, though my father could touch me and do anything he wanted physically, he couldn't get into me emotionally at all. I know he wanted me to let go of the emotional controls because he would ask me to say that I loved him while he was doing this to me. But I wouldn't. He wanted me in every way, not just physically. He wanted to have a warm relationship with someone and he was not getting it from my mother.

I married someone who I knew would never do anything like that to my kids, and someone with whom I felt very secure myself. I also married someone who has an infertility problem. The only way I could conceive was by artificial insemination—a procedure that abused me mentally and emotionally. Although it did not actually abuse me physically, it did hurt physically. However, maybe if I weren't so hurt inside psychologically, it wouldn't have hurt so much physically.

We had to go through all the tests related to infertility until the doctor could diagnose the problem. The testing is an invasion of your privacy, and is emotionally and sometimes even physically painful and difficult. Depending upon the conclusions of the tests, sometimes the only way you can get pregnant is through other invasive techniques that are difficult to handle emotionally, as well. In our case, it was my husband's low sperm count and slow motility that was preventing conception.

Therefore, in order to conceive, I had to be inseminated with his sperm through a tube that was passed through my cervix directly into my uterus. That was painful and difficult primarily because I didn't want somebody else (the doctor) "down there" making me pregnant. He was doing something to me sexually that just didn't feel right to me. Conceiving that way is not the loving, tender closeness by which most people conceive a child. The conception hurt me, but I turned off all my feelings and just did whatever I had to do because I knew it was the only way I was going to get pregnant. I handled the emotional abuse that surrounded the conception in the same way I had handled it with my father. I just wouldn't let myself feel emotionally.

I feel my need to stay in control during these early sexual experiences and through the difficulties of conception affected my ability to give birth because even though I wanted to let go of the controls in labor, I couldn't. Deep down, I don't think that there was anything that could have been said or done to make me lose control. I don't know if I'll ever be able to do it right. It's something I don't seem to be able to touch with my mind and make myself change. It's so gut. It's just there.

My labor and birth with my first son, David, began before my body was ready. My cervix was thick—not at all effaced. I was late, and I was feeling scared. My doctor was talking about the possibility that my placenta would stop functioning. He wanted to do a stress test. I became so upset that I told the baby that it was time to come out—*now!*

The labor started and stopped that night, and started again the next day. At midnight I went in to the hospital. I was 5 centimeters dilated. By 3:00 A.M. I was 8 centimeters. Things were going well. Then the contractions stopped. The doctor tried using some pitocin. I was getting a few contractions, so he tried having me push. However, my cervix became swollen. I wasn't making much progress. At 8:00 A.M. I had a cesarean. The baby weighed 8 lbs.

I did not have a hard time with my section. It wasn't hard for me to recover. I learned from an early age to compensate for whatever problems confront me. It's part of my strength—I recover well. I felt sad that I had to have a cesarean, but I was tired of sitting there like a jerk not having any labor.

I would probably feel the need to perform for anybody, but in the hospital for me it is worse. Because I am a nurse I felt I had to have a baby "the way you are supposed to have a baby." When the contractions stopped I felt so frustrated. There was nothing I could do to make it happen. I was frustrated with the nurses and doctors, too, because they didn't know what to do either.

Because I am a nurse, I know what "they" are thinking, even when they aren't saying it. I can just look in their eyes and know what they are thinking, because I know what the procedures are. I knew from the way the nurses and doctors were acting, that they were thinking "section." But I *couldn't* make the labor start again.

The people in hospitals don't know anything about "natural" techniques. They didn't need to do a section "to save the baby." There was no problem with the baby. Maybe if they had let me go home, I might have had him right away . . . maybe just falling asleep would have been enough . . . My body was feeling no pain, and maybe with a few hours of sleep, I would have just let go . . . Who knows? But once you get to 8 centimeters, they aren't going to let you go home for anything, because they are afraid that if anything happens to the baby, it's a law suit for them.

With my second pregnancy, I knew if I planned a hospital birth that I would have another cesarean. It wasn't that I had had such a horrible experience with my section. It was that I had to prove to myself as a woman that I work, my body works, that I could have the baby the "right" way. I wanted to prove to myself that I was "OK." So I planned to have a home birth. The more flack that I got from people, the more intent I was that I was going to have a home birth.

I was going for prenatal care with a midwife (Lynn) instead of a doctor. Her approach was much more psychological. During the pregnancy, we worked on many issues surrounding my own sexuality. I have come to realize that I have a big problem loving men and feeling that there is trust there. However, I also had a need, because my mother had abandoned me to my father, to give and receive love from women.

COMMENTS: *When Barbara first approached me regarding a home VBAC, she told me that she planned to have her baby ALONE, without her husband and perhaps even without a midwife. Barbara was beginning to uncover some of the factors in her previous cesarean. She wasn't sure if she could trust anyone besides herself when she was feeling as vulnerable as she knew she would be in labor. After intensive work on her feelings from her childhood sexual experiences Barbara seemed to be moving toward trust (of her own ability to give birth, of us as midwives, and of her husband as a labor support person). It appeared that as she approached the final weeks of her pregnancy, that Barbara would have a positive home birth experience.*

In addition to working on emotional issues and physical assessment during regular prenatal care, I always require that a backup plan be established. Even though early in the pregnancy I recommended that Barbara use my "friendly obstetrician" as her backup, she preferred to maintain the relationship with her doctor (her infertility specialist).

BARBARA: Of course, due to my infertility situation, my doctor wasn't just someone I had seen once a year for pap smears. I had been seeing him every month for years, calling him once or twice between visits to report my temperature and other vital information. My relationship with him was quite intense. I felt a sense of loyalty to him. I loved him because he had helped me to have my children. He was like a second father. I loved him and felt loyal to him, even though I was in a situation of abuse.

I wanted him as a backup. He agreed and wrote in the chart that I would labor at home until I was about 8 centimeters. In this state you can't really tell certain people that you're planning to have your VBAC baby at home because of the legal risks for yourself and your attendants. So I didn't really tell him the whole truth. I said I was going to labor at home, but I didn't say I was going to deliver at home.

The day after my due date, he asked me if I planned on delivering at home. I said, "Well, I'm ready to deliver at home if we have to. Anyone who is planning to labor at home until 8 centimeters needs to be ready to have the baby at home." During the previous week he had had a run-in with the assistant to the midwife I was using. When he realized she was planning to assist at my birth, he wanted me to sign a statement releasing him from any responsibility for this birth. He called his nurse in to witness and cosign the note. He said, "If you have that woman there you are guaranteeing yourself either a dead mother or a dead baby!" I felt shocked and hurt to the core. I was extremely angry, so I refused to cry in front of him. But I was really ready to cry. I cried all the way home.

I was rejected. My father never really rejected me. I had to reject him. However, this rejection by my "second father" brought up feelings about what I had had to do to end the abuse from my father. I had to bring it up in front of both my parents, and watch their reaction between the two of them. I was 12 years old at the time, and I was afraid that my whole world was going to crumble. When I lost the doctor's support, I had the same feeling that everything (my entire backup system) was crumbling. I'm sure it would have hurt a little anyway, even if he had only been a regular gynecologist to me because I have a thing about authority and I like to be good. However, since I had had such a close relationship with him, his rejection hurt more. That emotional pain carried through to the labor.

COMMENTS: *Barbara called me when she returned home from her prenatal with the doctor. Her voice was tight and she was clearly in much pain as she relayed the story of her doctor's accusations and rejection of her. However, she did not cry. She held her feelings in, as she asked for the name and phone number of my "friendly obstetrician." She made an appointment to see her immediately, so that she would not be without backup for her now post-dated birth. She examined her and agreed to backup her birth, even though she had had a previous cesarean. I felt her decision to support Barbara was clear evidence of her understanding of the needs of pregnant women, of her trust of me as a midwife, and of her commitment to safe and healthy birth.*

Getting the backup Barbara needed was important to her, but she continued to carry feelings about her own doctor. She was intensely quiet and distant. Once again she had trusted and loved a man, like a father, and once again her trust had been shattered. No amount of counsel seemed adequate to lift this weight from her. This rejection was poorly timed for Barbara. She did not have time to identify, process, and resolve her feelings before labor.

Labor began slowly with light, intermittent contractions, that stopped after a few hours and started again the next night. The second morning she came to the office to be examined to assess progress. At that time she was 50% effaced, 4 centimeters dilated and the baby was at about -1 station. She had a light bloody show (small amount of staining). Although her contractions were still mild, she was experiencing intense low back pressure. Harlan, her chiropractor, found that her low back was subluxated (not in proper alignment thus producing pressure on the nerves), and gave her an adjustment. Instead of the usual talkative exuberance most women experience with early labor, Barbara said very little and appeared to be depressed. She expressed only that she needed to be alone with Ron, her husband. I felt Barbara's desire to be with Ron was hopeful. Apparently, even though she had experienced such deep rejection from such an important father-image, she was still willing to give her trust to another man—her husband.

BARBARA: I have a big problem trusting men. Even with Ron it is a constant battle. I really only trust him well when I am in an extreme situation. With this labor I did trust him completely, because I was in an extreme situation. But I don't know if I should have.

COMMENTS: *The labor picked up that afternoon. At 8 p.m. Barbara returned to my office again. She was 6 cms. She returned home again, to be alone with Ron.*
At 11:00 P.M. Ron called. The contractions were coming closer and stronger, and he wanted us to come to help.

BARBARA: Ron was upset. To him, it was time—time for someone to get there. He could see that I wasn't able to talk. I wasn't able to listen to heart tones—I had to trust him. That's when you have to let go and trust. I was letting go of my control, and he couldn't cope with me losing control. I'm the kind of person who normally never loses control. I'm afraid that if I get out of control that I'll overwhelm everybody. I'm a big strong person. I don't know how I'll act if I'm "out of control", and it scares me. So I never let myself lose control. This was the first time that Ron had ever seen me begin to lose control. It scared him, so he called the midwives.

COMMENTS: *Throughout the pregnancy Barbara had been considering the possibility of delivering her baby unattended. However, Ron had not been planning on being the only attendant at the birth. He was not prepared to take on the complete technical as well as support responsibility in the birth of his baby. Therefore, although Barbara may have felt that she still needed more time alone without us (the midwives), from the point of view of the midwife, Ron called us just when he should have.*
Aside from keeping in close touch with a laboring woman, we ask that we definitely be called when a woman can no longer talk or walk through a contraction. Most midwives like to arrive at a birth somewhere between 6 and 8 centimeters dilatation, so that they can ease themselves into the mother's space as unobtrusively as possible, set up their instruments for the birth, and actively monitor the most intense part of labor. I knew that since Barbara had been 6 centimeters at 8 P.M. with mild contractions, that with intense contractions her labor could potentially progress quite quickly. It appeared to us that we needed to be there with Barbara.

BARBARA: I was 8 centimeters when the midwives arrived at 11 P.M.

COMMENTS: *When we arrived at Barbara's home, she was on her hands and knees, clearly in transition. She labored well—changing positions, walking, voiding, sounding, visualizing, drinking and taking honey supplements happily and willingly. She was supported and massaged by her husband and friends. However, by 5:00 A.M. Barbara was still 8 centimeters; by 9:00 A.M. she was almost 9 centimeters.*

We decided that perhaps she needed time alone with just one of us. We dimmed the lights, and everyone else moved to another part of the house.

BARBARA: Nothing really was moving. I didn't know what to do, and I knew the midwives didn't know what to do either when they started asking me, "What's holding you back?"

I could not seem to let go of the control completely and fully. I could not find that "something" that kept me in control—to make it go away. It is almost as if I would have rather died than given up that control. That control is what kept me "together" as a person for all those years as a child with my father. It began at such a young age that I don't know if I could ever find that feeling.

Finally, we went for a walk at the beach.

COMMENTS: *While we were at the beach, I felt very strongly that Barbara's energy was waning. Though I did believe it was possible that she might have eventually delivered her baby at home, it also seemed probable that sometime before the moment of birth either the mother or the baby would lose their energy completely— a situation that might become life-threatening to one or both of them. I was not willing to gamble that a few more hours of labor at home would produce a healthy home birth. The longer I waited to transport, the less energy Barbara would have to continue her labor in the hospital, the greater the probability that she would have another cesarean.*

So, while Barbara continued to walk on the beach, I telephoned the backup physician. Her partner, (whom neither Barbara nor I had ever met) was on-call. I explained that Barbara had been in labor for 24 hours, and her labor had been arrested at 9 centimeters for a few hours due apparently to the head not being well applied to the cervix. I emphasized that although her labor had been arrested for some time, I felt very strongly that she could still deliver vaginally if she were given pitocin and an epidural.

As Barbara finished her walk on the beach, we discussed the transport. We decided to go home and rupture the membranes. I usually do not rupture the membranes unless every other technique to stimulate a labor has failed. Although it sometimes does speed the labor through increasing the application of the presenting part to the cervix, if the labor is not significantly changed by the amniotomy and a slow labor continues, eventually the baby may be compromised because the baby's natural cushion that protects him from the force of the contractions has been removed. However, I knew that if I did not rupture the membranes, they would be ruptured in the hospital without hesitation. If rupturing the membranes would work in this case, we could possibly avoid transport.

BARBARA: The midwives broke the water and there was meconium. It wasn't dark green. It was a brownish color. However, at that point I wanted to go to the hospital.

The backup doctor was a good guy. He listened to Lynn, and followed her advice. My cesarean scar is under the hairline and is very difficult to see. So we didn't bother to mention to him when we went into the hospital that I had had a previous section. He never would have done a trial of pitocin if he had known I had had a section, especially if he had known how long I had been in transition! I was in transition for 16 hours—I guess I can take a lot of pain!

So they gave me pit with the epidural. It was perfect. I got exactly what I needed. The pitocin didn't really seem to change the contractions, but I feel what aided me most in completing the dilatation was the epidural—not feeling the pain. My body didn't have to listen to my brain. Somehow my brain had been telling my body subconsciously not to do it.

I would say that sexual abuse can truly affect a woman in labor — it can make the labor long, and make it difficult to open up. It makes you have a need for control. We have often likened transition in labor to the transition of moving from life to death. The longer you hold onto the controls, the harder it is. When you let go you can "slip away" (into birth, or into death) peacefully. So when it came to that place in transition where I was approaching a death, a different state, I just couldn't do that. I could not let myself approach being "almost dead" with my father. If I had let go I would have lost my mind. I couldn't let go because it was not a situation I could trust. Maybe there isn't a situation that I can trust.

Maybe the epidural made it possible for me to feel dead, to be like dead, and allow whatever happens there to happen. It never really happened in my mind, but at least it happened for my body—my mind no longer had the control to stop my body from reaching that state. The epidural broke the pattern of control. My brain couldn't stop my body from letting go any more.

I was very happy and I'm sure my baby, Jonathan, was happy, too. "Let me out of here, Mom. Come on, How long are you going to keep this up?"

In 2 hours I was fully dilated, and the epidural had worn off. On the way to the delivery room the doctor asked me how long it had taken to push out the last baby. It was then that we had to tell him that I hadn't pushed the last baby out at all— that he had been born by cesarean. The doctor took the news quite well, saying, "Oh, OK. Well, we'll continue with where we're going. Now, I want you to push really hard."

Even though I was fully dilated I didn't feel the urge to push, except during the peak of each contraction. Then I would feel just a little urge to push. Once I would start pushing, I didn't know if the contraction had ended or not. I just kept pushing. It felt good.

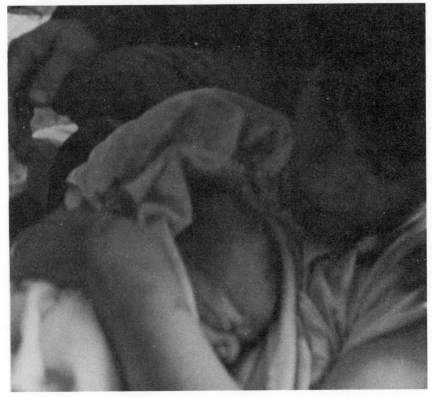

Barbara holding Sara, immediately after birth

When I was pushing, Ron was watching and telling me that I was opening up a little bit. I needed that encouragement. In the end, while I was pushing, the doctor also used the vacuum extractor. However, he let me do most of the work, and just put on the vacuum a little bit to help me out. He didn't leave me feeling that I couldn't trust my body, that my body couldn't push out my own baby without his help. Jonathan weighed 10 lb. 5 oz.— and I only pushed an hour, so I think I could have done it without the vacuum.

But I do wonder, if Ron had just let me go with it, if he hadn't called the midwives, would trusting and letting go have been easier? If it wouldn't have frightened him to see me out of control, could I have let go of the controls myself? Could I have done it without the pitocin, without the epidural, without the vacuum?

COMMENTS: *Although interventions often lead to another cesarean, sometimes those same interventions can actually help to avoid a cesarean. Although interventions often leave women feeling powerless, it is possible for a conscious practitioner to judiciously use interventions while supporting a woman's self-esteem in the birth process. It is not interventions themselves, but rather the abuse of the interventions that we must fear.*

BARBARA: From the psychological work I did during my pregnancy, and have continued to do since then, I have begun to realize the full impact of the abusiveness of the artificial insemination. I have decided not to return to a doctor again in order to conceive. If I am to have another child, the conception will have to occur naturally.

If I get pregnant again, I still want to have a home birth, but I don't know—it may end up being the same way again. I didn't know what to do, and I'm afraid that I'll never know what to do. I don't know who I could trust. If you can't trust your own mother, you can't trust anybody. Maybe I could trust myself, but I don't know if I could let go all the way. It would have to be between God and me.

* * *

Following the birth of Jonathan, Barbara continued intensive self-investigation. She and Ron conceived another child within the next year. This conception occurred naturally out of their own love and affection for one another. Nine months later Barbara let go. They gave birth together in their own home.

22

Having a Vaginal Cesarean

LINDA STELLA ZENTNER

My Own Birth

LINDA: I was born in 1947 by cesarean. I was due in September but I was taken in August. My mother could feel all my little toes through her abdomen. The doctor said her uterine wall was too thin, and I needed to be delivered as soon as possible. My mother told me this damage was all due to an accident she had as a teenager.

Through the years this never made any sense to me because my brother, seven years my senior, was born vaginally at nine months and he weighed over 9 pounds. My mother always told me that I was so frail and white, and I would have been just as nice as Benny if she could have carried me to term.

I've always hated that part of the year that I considered the "downhill" part—from January through summer. I dread summer. In the spring, to this day, I still want to pull down the shades, close doors, and hide until fall comes. When June comes sometimes I feel a real panic, feeling I will be forced to do something soon that I am not ready to do. I always blamed it on the weather. But now I know that part of me feels that I may be born in August instead of September, again. This feeling of not being quite ready is a theme throughout my life. Fortunately, with maturity, I have been able to achieve a greater sense of self-knowl- edge to be able to distinguish between when I am really not qualified for a job (personal or professional) or when it is this other force coming into play.

I have always felt that I was a great overbearing stress on my mother, enough to cause her to reach a breaking point. Yet my brother Benny never seemed to cause my mother this kind of stress. I always felt guilty for making my mother sick and her abdomen look so awful. She had a tremendous vertical scar. And whenever she thought others weren't around, she was always looking in the mirror at her abdomen. She thought it was the ugliest thing in the world.

The Birth of Christopher

LINDA: I found out I was pregnant at 5 months gestation with my first child, Chris. I went to the doctors at about 2 months. But because I was having light periods they discounted the possibility of pregnancy. I was given very potent medications for ulcers and was told to limit my food intake and not be so "nervous." I obeyed.

By February 1970 my fatigue and discomfort became extraordinary and I felt throbbing in my abdomen. I was sure I was deathly ill. I went to an OB/GYN. He didn't tell me what he was looking for but he used some kind of instrument and jabbed it into my abdomen. He told me to get my husband and meet him in his office. I know now that he thought I might be pregnant and the instument was a fetascope. The doctor asked Ron and I if our parents had any grandchildren. He told me to come back in a week. Once I absorbed the shock that I was 5 months pregnant, I knew that the throbbing was my baby's movement!

Come back in one week I did. I was given amphetamines to keep my weight down. In fact the doctor stood up and became quite emphatic about my not gaining weight. I obeyed. I weighed myself every three days to be sure I gained minimally. I took all medications diligently. The doctor praised me for being "so good."

COMMENTS: *Dietary advice such as was given to Linda by her obstetrician is not only torturous to pregnant women (whose bodies are clearly asking for more food), but may actually be life-threatening to both them and their unborn babies.*

Limiting weight gain in pregnancy was thought to be good for the mother. In addition, drugs such as amphetamines and diuretics were given to the mother to help control her appetite and the swelling that often developed from the mal- nutrition. Such dietary restrictions and drug use have since been found to cause toxemia—a dangerous and life-threatening condition of pregnancy. Dr. Tom

Brewer has extensively studied the effects of nutrition in pregnancy, and his wife, Gail, has written several books expounding his nutritional recommendations in pregnancy.

LINDA: My membranes ruptured Thursday morning, June 18. I was so elated that I had to let the doctor know right away. He told me to be at the hospital at noon. I laid flat on my back under the covers at home, passing the 6 hours until noon. I hoped something would happen, but nothing did. I got to the hospital and even then, in all my ignorance, I felt it was kind of stupid to be in the hospital when my labor hadn't even begun.

But, I obeyed all the way. The nurse felt my uterus and said how thin I was and that she expected about a 4-1/2 lb. baby. She told me to lie down on this flat hard "bed" (stretcher). I was so flat my abdomen hurt. She said I could not lie on my side or turn. She gave me what I now know to be a pitocin drip. I was hit with these overwhelming stabbing contractions. It was then, reacting to those first contractions, that I realized that my ankles and my wrists were strapped down. As I look back at these events, I wonder, "Where the hell was I? Where the hell was my brain? Couldn't I have stopped this from happening to me?" After all these years I still wonder how the hell I could have allowed these people do these unspeakable things to me.

I told of the pain I was experiencing. Everyone seemed so big. I thought then that they all seemed so big because I was lying so flat. I know now that I had already been given something for "the pain"— scopalomine. And it was the "scope" that was making everything so out of proportion. Everyone seemed to be deciding what to do with me while I wasn't there.

COMMENTS: *Scopalomine is a drug that was given extensively in the 1950s and 1960s to women in labor. It is an hallucinogenic and amnesiac. Most women to whom it was given have little to no memory of the labor. For others, their memories are nightmares. As with other hallucinogens, such as LSD, some women even have flashbacks—moments when they reexperience the nightmarish trips that were inflicted upon them in labor. Thankfully, most obstetricians no longer use scopalomine. But in some hospitals it is still being used today.*

LINDA: But the torment was only yet to begin. I began to writhe and struggle. I tried to release myself from the binds. I forgot I was human and I forgot I was giving birth. I writhed in this stupor for 6 or 7 hours more.

At one time when I was coming back to consciouness, trying to get my legs free, I heard the doctor say how proud he was of "these girls who kept thin—their labors were so short. Keeping them thin was the trick." Then another stronger dose of the medication put me down again.

I struggled continuously. I had a sense of something extremely powerful overtaking me. But I had no feeling physically, so I just struggled and fought to counterbalance the powerful force. I couldn't achieve consciousness and I didn't know which way to push. I knew someone desperately needed me somewhere. They called my name loudly, and yelled at me for not pushing. But I gave up. I just couldn't get conscious enough to direct any of my efforts.

I was shown a baby 12 hours later. It was in the corner of the room. They told me it was mine. He was dark and olive skinned and big. My baby was supposed to be under 5 pounds. I felt half dead. Where did they get this baby from?

Of course "scope" was not all that went wrong with Chris' birth. The left side of Chris' face was paralyzed from the misapplication of forceps.

COMMENTS: *Whenever a woman was heavily medicated in labor, as Linda had been, the babies were delivered by forceps. Forceps are applied to the presenting part of the baby—hopefully at the edge of the cheekbones to avoiding damaging the baby's brain. However, when forceps are used while the baby is still high in the pelvis, it is quite difficult (if not impossible) to reach the forceps all the way to the cheek bones. When the forceps have been applied wrongly, damaged babies have resulted. Chris was lucky in that his tremendous intelligence does not seem to have been compromised by the forceps with which he was delivered.*

LINDA: I am five feet, six and three-quarters inches and I left the hospital carrying a 7 lb., 7 oz. baby, while I weighed 89 pounds.

COMMENTS: *This is clear evidence of the malnutrition Linda suffered in this pregnancy.*

LINDA: Chris was sullen and depressed for 4 to 5 months. I was in somewhat of a daze for about the same time, if not longer.

COMMENTS: *The effects of drugs in labor are not over after the baby is born. Such depression, lethargy, and disconnection from reality were most likely the long-term unacknowledged effects of the scopalomine.*

LINDA: I was incontinent for almost 2 years. There's so much more that would need pages to describe.

COMMENTS: *Incontinency following a birth is due to bladder damage. This damage may simply be the result of neglecting to empty a full bladder at the time of second stage. Or it may also be the result of the forceps that can damage the pelvic floor.*

The Birth of Andrew

Andrew was born in 1976 when Chris was almost 6. With Andrew I stayed at home in labor for quite a long time. But even though I had changed doctors, my birth experience was once again completely usurped in the hospital. I truly feel more strongly now after all the research I've done that my birth experience was better with Andrew only because I stayed home longer.

After Andy was born my doctor said that my body was just not meant for having babies, that my pelvis was just too small, and he could see why my first birth was so traumatic. He then proceeded to tell me how lucky I was he was there. He seemed to be relieved it was all over.

The Birth of Camille

Twenty-three months later my third child Camille was born. This time I wanted to be really present for the birth. Both my husband and I took Lamaze classes. This time I was given pitocin really late in labor, coupled, once again with a lacing of "scope" in the "pit" drip.

I tried to use breathing for escape, which is the style taught in the coping class instructions. Sometimes we're so stupid that we don't see what's right in front of us. When I look back at Camille's birth, I am aware of how all this "escape" left me not only out of touch and powerless, but once again I lost touch with reality and forgot all purpose of the labor and birth.

The Great Depression

After Camille's birth I felt that all the bad birth experiences I had had were indeed my fault. I fell back into the role of being the frail, white, underdeveloped, not quite finished human being I had been considered as a child. I succumbed to a very serious depression that lasted over two years.

COMMENTS: *Linda had great expectations about the birth of Camille. Because she had taken Lamaze classes, she believed she would be awake and aware at this birth. But, once again, her power had been usurped. Once again the experience she had longed for was lost. But she had no one to talk to who understood what she had lost. She grieved without support, without even understanding that she was grieving, without understanding that at the end of the long dark tunnel of grief, she would find a rainbow. Her fear that if she allowed herself to feel all those feelings that she might never again return to "normal" caused the depression to escalate, allowed the depression to swallow her. Had Linda had even one good friend who understood what she had lost, or simply information that the feelings she was having about her birth experiences were normal, she might have avoided the "great depression."*

The Birth of Shanna

LINDA: Labor with Shanna, my fourth child, began not only in the same way (ruptured membranes) but also at the same time of day, and the same day of the week (Thursday) as my labor with my first baby, Christopher.

COMMENTS: *Linda's labor with Shanna was clearly a working through of all her past labors, but especially her birth with Chris. I was called by Gerri who had been doing labor support for Linda, and wanted to consult with me. Linda's membranes had been ruptured for over 48 hours with no significant labor, and Gerri was becoming concerned. She felt that Linda was perhaps not allowing herself to go into labor because she was afraid of going to the hospital. She asked me to come to Linda's to talk with her, and to ascertain whether or not a homebirth might be feasible.*

But when I arrived, it was clear that we were not going to be doing any talking about this birth. As I approached Linda's window, I heard the familiar sounds of transition.

LINDA: She hesitated to enter the room. But I was longing to see what I would have to deal with now—who would try to steal my baby. I felt vibrations from her even beyond the room. This vibration began to give me peace and power from the beginning. She was the midwife.

The midwife was on the bed next to me. Looking back and remembering her presence then, I described her as "woman of the ages." She examined me once, after asking me if she could do so. She found me to be 8 centimeters dilated.

COMMENTS: *I had been told by Gerri that the doctor had told Linda that she had a small pelvis, so while I checked her dilatation, I did a quick pelvic assessment. Her pelvis was as "big as a barn", and I told her so!*

LINDA: At this point I just didn't want anyone to take me away from my body and I asked not to be examined again. She agreed to my wishes, and told me to do what my body said. Imagine, a professional saying to go with my body—permission to be, to give birth.

My friend, Gerri, did not encourage me to get out of my body and escape. Instead she asked me to get into the contractions, into the opening of my body, and to welcome my sweet baby, for whom I so longed. "Come, baby, come." I came into deeper contact with my body, and she, my friend, became more and more supportive of seeing this in me.

With this child—my fourth—I was entering a world of birthing I had never known before. A world of birthing for which I could not be promised an outcome—for which, in order to be given permission to continue, I didn't have to sign any papers or be a good, quiet complacent patient. (I think it's interesting that good babies are supposed to be the quiet ones.)   Well, do what my body said, I did—four babies worth! All the vocalizing, agonizing, living, giving, pushing, feeling, loving, releasing of 12 years of control.

COMMENTS: *Linda was reliving the scopalomine births. Between contractions she was with us in present time. But during contractions she was somewhere else, physically and verbally fighting off assailants. She released all her pent-up anger and frustration at the demoralization and dehumanization she had received during her past labors.*

When she began to feel the urge to push, she yelled, "I have to push! I have to push!" I responded, "Go ahead, follow your body." But she held her urge to push back, and screamed again, "But I really have to push!" *She was back in the hospital with the scopalomine labors, attempting to obey the authorities and fighting her body's own urges. I drew in very close to her and repeated,* "Go ahead. Follow your own body."

LINDA: With the peace and power that I felt from the midwife, and the support from my friend I became so exquisitely in contact with what was going on within me. I was able to tell when to push very, very delicately and when to push with all my being. I could also tell apart all the subtle variations of feeling in between. And my baby's head crowned.

No!!! This couldn't be! I closed my body up and held Shanna in. I felt that the doctors must have been truthful with me. After all, they said, my body was not made to deliver babies. I had sharp spines, they said, and would surely need a cesarean for this baby to be born. Sure, up until now everything was fine, but there had to be trouble now, or else I had trusted, paid, had faith in, a bunch of liars. So here's where my body had to be built incorrectly. There had to be something—a bone, a tumor, extra tissue, some abnormality, something, that if my baby were to pass through it, it would kill her. I couldn't let her die. I needed to protect her with desperation. I tried to keep her inside me to save her. I had loved her so much for so long, I wasn't ready to lose her.

COMMENTS: *Linda had been standing up pushing, supported by her husband Ronnie and her friend Gerri. The baby had moved smoothly and easily down to her perineum. Then, just before her baby's head was about to be born, suddenly, she pulled her legs together and tightened her entire pelvic floor. I gently stroked her legs, and whispered,* "Open, your legs, Linda. Relax and open your legs." *But she only became more rigid in her stance. A little louder, this time,* "Linda, open your legs." *Still no response. Now, with fear mounting inside me,* "Linda, you must open your legs!"

(This is a time when head compression is very great for the baby, and if the baby is not allowed to be born, the baby could be severely depressed, brain-damaged, or even die.)

LINDA: The energy intensified and filled the room. The midwife demanded my cooperation.

COMMENTS: *Using all their strength, Ronnie and Gerri lifted Linda's knees and her legs were opened.*

LINDA: I needed to push again. This, the most crucial time of this birth, was the hardest push of all, not physically but emotionally. At this moment I had to transfer trust from the doctor to my body. It was also the only push in which I couldn't give my all. I shut my eyes prepared to lose my baby.

Then I felt the sweetness of my baby's body sliding out from within me. I opened my eyes and saw her—my big, beautiful, wide-eyed, alert and vibrant sweet girl. My need for her exploded within me and I asked for her. I held her on my abdomen and named her. How I loved her!

And then the blood of sacrifice and guilt began to flow. I had to sacrifice my life. I'd felt too much love, known more than I should know, lived too much—and now I knew a truth about my body that I had no right to know. *Me—myself—my body—could and did deliver a healthy baby all by myself!* Perhaps I was almost not ready for this truth. This was a blaring truth that I would almost rather die than accept. I had evaded this truth for my whole life. It was a truth that had been passed down to me from my mother, and through the doctors. I had financially and emotionally invested in a lie.

COMMENTS: *Blood was gushing from Linda's uterus, and no amount of uterine stimulation, either naturally or medically, would stop it. I reached inside her vagina, following the cord up to the top of her uterus where her placenta still partially clung to her uterus. I looked at her and said, "You can stop this bleeding anytime you want to." She replied, in amazement, "I can?" "You can. Let go of your pregnancy, let go of your placenta."*

LINDA: At this point the midwife's voice brought me back to contact and responsibility. Her face gave me peace and power once again. I welcomed the peace, and took the responsibility and power. The peace flowed through my entire body and the power hit the top of my uterus. Out came the placenta.

COMMENTS: *And the bleeding stopped.*

LINDA: At last I accepted totally what my midwife and friend had begun to hand over to me at 8 centimeters. The truth of my healthy body and my right to give birth, love with it, and live with it.

My baby, my body, I had it all. And no one wanted to take anything from me. My friend and midwife didn't want anything from me now. They didn't grab my baby and whisk her off. They didn't act like the sights, the sounds, the secretions of birth and love were anything that needed to be whisked away. All of it was for me and Shanna, and Shanna and I loved all of it. We slept all night together, nursing. loving, living.

Shanna and I were both born that night, and our sweet rest together was sublime.

23

Be Thankful for Your Baby, No Matter How She Was Born!

BARBARA CULLIGAN

The Birth of Courtney

BARBARA: On February 9, 1984, I went to my doctor's office for my weekly checkup. I was exactly 40 weeks gestation that day. Dr. Antellan said that she would strip my membranes to help start labor. She would be going away and I was worried that a doctor I did not know would be in the delivery room with me when I delivered my baby. She assured my husband Pat and I that the procedure would be perfectly safe for my baby.

COMMENTS: *Stripping the membranes is a process by which the practitioner sweeps the internal opening of the cervix and part of the lower uterine segment with his/her finger, separating the membranes from the cervix. If done at or near term, this usually weakens the membranes (causing rupture of membranes a few hours later) and/or stimulates production of oxytocin, thus inducing labor. Often stripping the membranes is done routinely during an office exam without knowledge or consent on the part of the woman. The practitioner may simply allude to the intervention, by saying "This exam may help to get your labor going."*

BARBARA: The next day, I lost the mucus plug at about 7:00 P.M. I felt fine—all excited and bubbly. This would be it! I was really looking forward to seeing the little girl I knew I was carrying—who had changed my body and my mind . . . who had made me look at the world with innocent open eyes . . . my own personal miracle.

Since I was told not to eat during labor, dinner on Friday was my last meal. I didn't even drink anything. At about 11:00 P.M. we went to bed. My first pain was at 6:51 A.M. Pains continued throughout the day but they were not gradually increasing as labor pains should. They were close together and very long. Later, I realized they were not labor pains but the severe abdominal cramping associated with staph aureus toxemia (toxic poisoning from a virulent bacterial infection).

We went to the hospital at about 7:00 P.M. They examined me, said I was about 90% effaced, 1 centimeter dilated and sent me home. The nurse said I was in false labor and should not be doing Level 3 Lamaze breathing—I couldn't possibly hurt that much. They said to go home, have an alcoholic drink and something to eat.

161

COMMENTS: *Those who have observed many women in labor have developed a sense of judging where a woman might be in her labor by the way she is responding to her contractions. A woman at one centimeter is usually sociable, excited, and doesn't need to pay much attention to her contractions. While a woman in transition may have difficulty communicating with any words whatsoever, as her contractions overwhelm her. Whenever a woman who is only one centimeter is acting like she is in transition, clearly something is awry.*

Usually what is awry is that the woman is extremely afraid of labor, and is overreacting to the contractions. The solution offered to Barbara by the nurse is a common one to help a woman in early labor relax, get in touch with her body, and find her coping mechanisms. The nurse's response at the time was not unusual. In retrospect, however, if she had investigated the unusual physical pain Barbara was experiencing, the outcome of Barbara's birth might have been drastically changed.

BARBARA: We went home, had a small bite to eat and Pat went to sleep for a while. I dozed intermittently. At 5:00 A.M. I suddenly got the chills, shaking and chattering. Pat got me a blanket and called Antellan. She sounded unconcerned and said maybe we should get dressed and come on in to the hospital.

COMMENTS: *Once again, the chills, shaking, and chattering are all characteristic signs of labor. Though they are most often associated with transition, they can be present when a woman is extremely fearful and overreacting to her early labor. Dr. Antellan was probably unconcerned because she had seen this labor pattern so many times before, without serious consequence.*

However, to avoid making any presumptions, whenever a woman is experiencing symptoms that might also be associated with a fever, the woman's temperature should be taken. This simple procedure will allow the practitioner to know whether to treat such symptoms as "normal labor" or to act quickly with medical intervention to save the life of an unborn baby.

BARBARA: It was pouring rain. I was so cold I couldn't even move and I was throwing up. Pat suggested a warm bath to relax me and take off the chill. We didn't want to go out into the rain while I was still throwing up.

By 6:30 we arrived at the hospital and I was just another complaining woman in labor. They said I had the flu and hooked me up to IV fluids. Before, I had been so adamant that I wouldn't want an IV in labor, but at the time, I was so sick, I didn't care. They also gave me a suppository for the nausea. While I was expelling the suppository, they ran out of paper for the fetal monitor. The nurses at the station weren't even watching it—Pat had to tell them.

COMMENTS: *This situation exemplifies the fallacy of the fetal monitor. Though the monitor may be an accurate (50% of the time) device for assessing the fetal heart throughout labor, there is no value to the monitor whatsoever if a skilled technician is not there to assess the fetal heart pattern. In my experience, the best method of ascertaining the health of the fetus is careful consistent auscultation with a fetascope by a skilled technician.*

BARBARA: By this time they had lost the baby's heartbeat. They broke my membranes and tried to insert an internal monitor. No heartbeat. Another monitor. Still no heartbeat. A third. None.

COMMENTS: *Either Barbara's baby was in very serious trouble, or there was something wrong with the machine. Rather than listening carefully with a fetascope, they wasted valuable time inserting monitor after monitor. Perhaps no one in the hospital was skilled in ascultation with a fetascope (a skill that is quickly being lost because of dependency upon the monitors). Had sufficient attention been paid to the monitor tracings, the stress the baby was experiencing would probably have been detected before the heart tones had disappeared entirely.*

BARBARA: They drew blood and took my temperature. White count of 31,000 (normal is 5,000–9000) and temperature of 102. Antellan arrived and did an emergency C-section under general anesthesia. I awoke and they told me Courtney was a little boy. I thought that was odd since I had always felt that I was giving life to a girl.

I went to recovery. Antellan came in and said I delivered a stillborn girl. I said, "No, you have the wrong baby. They told me mine was a little boy." She said the baby was a girl, and she was not expected to live. I asked if this was the best place for her. She said, "Yes." I asked to see her. She said, "Maybe." I said, "Babies don't die, this isn't the Middle Ages."

COMMENTS: *Having grown up in the age of medical miracles, most Americans have come to believe that having your baby in the hospital with a doctor will* guarantee you a healthy baby! *Unfortunately, there can be no guarantees in birth, no matter where, with whom, or by what means your baby is born.*

In our society where taking control over your life is a primary goal, letting go and accepting death as a possible outcome of birth seems almost impossibly cruel.

BARBARA: Pat came in and I asked him if this was a nightmare—if I really was awake. He held me.

Poor Pat. He was left alone while I was in that room being cut up. Every so often, a nurse would come in and say, "Yes, the baby's out, but we can't tell you how it is or what it is or how Barb's doing." Antellan finally went to see Pat and told him the baby was stillborn and that I was fine. He just sat there for a while. Then he called his mom. When he came back, Antellan was *laughing* with a bunch of nurses.

COMMENTS: *Dr. Antellan's laughter was probably her only coping mechanism. Although doctors and nurses often witness death, they have been trained to remain detached, uninvolved, feelingless. They cannot allow themselves to feel for each and every death. If they allowed themselves to feel, they might not be able to go on practicing medicine. They often have difficulty giving support to grieving parents who have lost their children because they have never allowed themselves to experience grieving over the loss of their patients. They have difficulty understanding the importance of a family's connection to one another, or else they would never separate families, regardless of the circumstances. In fact, if they really understood, they would see to it that* especially when death is a probable outcome, that families would be together.

BARBARA: We later found out that it took them 20 minutes to resuscitate Courtney. She lived almost 6 hours. We saw her once when she was still alive and all hooked up to all these machines. She died when I was holding her. We held her and cried. We looked at her beautiful body— so perfectly formed and so utterly lifeless. She had never cried or moved or nursed or even opened her eyes long enough to see the two people who had created her from the love they shared.

By Tuesday night at 11:00 P.M., the doctors put me on genomicin and cleosin. My white count had risen to 52,000 (over 11,000 is considered higher than normal). Blood and urine cultures revealed staph aureus and Courtney's autopsy revealed that she was grossly infected with it. The doctors kept telling us that my body gave Courtney the disease through the placenta. They were covering Antellan's tail!

COMMENTS: *Though there can be no absolute proof, in all probability the cause of Courtney's systemic staph infection was not transplacental, but through external contamination by the vaginal exam and stripping of membranes at the clinic. Staph is normally present on the skin and mucous membranes of all people, but the growth of the bacteria is usually held in check by the immune system. When there is multiplication of the bacteria, it usually begins as a localized infection on the skin (such as a boil). Unless the host's natural resistance is extremely low, or the organism itself is extremely virulent, staph infections tend to be localized and very slow to progress into a systemic disease.*

If Barbara was a healthy pregnant woman with no history of localized staph infections on the skin (or any other mucous membrane such as the ears, nose, or vagina) then the staph bacteria had to be introduced from an external source. In addition, judging from the rate of the spread of the infection, the bacteria must have been extremely virulent. It is in hospitals and clinics where the most virulent antibody-resistant and antibiotic-resistant strains of staph reside. Therefore, the most likely place for Barbara to have contracted her extremely virulent staph infection (that eventually caused the death of her baby) was from the clinic where the exam and stripping of membranes occurred just prior to her labor.

BARBARA: By this time, my tummy was extremely swollen and the staples holding the wound closed were coming out. Antellan took all my staples out on Wednesday and left the wound open for secondary healing. The following Wednesday, she noticed that the fascia was coming apart so she took me back into surgery and sewed just the fascia (layer of tissue below the skin) back together. She left the skin and fat to heal on its own. It took almost three months before I was completely healed. During that time, I would cleanse the open wound twice a day and repack it with gauze.

COMMENTS: *The length of time involved in healing Barbara's incision is certainly indicative of the virulence of the bacteria involved. However, it does not mean that her scar will not be strong enough to have a VBAC.*

BARBARA: Courtney is buried next to her Grandpa Culligan in Chicago. I hope they're together somewhere now, and that he's holding and rocking her, and singing all those soft sweet lullabies to her—just like I wish I were doing now.

Grief and Healing

COMMENTS: *Barbara first contacted me when she was 7 weeks pregnant with her second baby. Barbara was looking for a way to avoid a recurrent outcome with this new pregnancy.*

Very little time had passed between the death of Courtney and her new pregnancy. She had hoped the new pregnancy would help her to feel better. But she found she felt worse because she was afraid to get close to this baby. She had felt very close to Courtney while she was pregnant with her, so when Courtney died the pain of the loss of their closeness was almost unbearable. Pregnant again, she was trying to protect herself from feeling that pain again (in case this baby died, too) by not allowing herself such closeness. But her attempt at denying her natural spiritual closeness to her unborn baby was excruciating. I made some suggestions to help her resolve her conflicting feelings. Months later she wrote to me:

> *Sparky, our second baby, a boy is due in about 4 weeks. I'm glad we had an ultrasound. It made this baby more real and less like Courtney to see him. It's somehow easier to bond knowing he's in there, and a boy.*
>
> *Now we just have to get through labor and delivery! We're excited, but scared, too. We're going to the nurse-midwives with an obstetrician as back-up in case we can't have a VBAC. The care we are receiving is really good, and it feels good to know that we're not on an obstetrical delivery line. It's very family-oriented. The midwives really care about the women, husbands, and eventually the children they see.*
>
> *I will surely let you know when Sparky makes his grand arrival.*

DONNA MORGAN: (Certified Nurse Midwife [CNM]) We had no reservations about accepting this client. I felt that Barbara and Pat knew what kind of care and birth they wanted.

RUTH NEWCOMB (CNM): They were serious about and dedicated to having a vaginal birth, but not at the cost of safety.

DONNA: They wanted to be sure that we could meet their needs, and they needed to feel that they could trust us. In order to do this we worked on having open communication.

RUTH: Of course, the physical concerns were important, but the emotional concerns were of equal importance. My major concern was for the emotional health of this couple after their devastating previous birth experience.

DONNA: My initial perceptions were that it might be difficult for Barbara and Pat to believe that they had a healthy, living child.

The Birth of Sparky

BARBARA: On Monday, April 8, 1985, at about midnight, after making love, I felt the first pains of labor. They were light, so I tried to sleep for a while. By 6:30 the pains were getting regular, so we decided to go to the hospital. But I didn't even take my suitcase. I was sure they would send me home.

We arrived at the hospital at about 7:30. Donna listened to the baby with a fetascope, and then put on an external monitor to check the contraction patterns. They were regular, so she concluded that I was in labor. I was only 1 centimeter dilated, but she thought I should be admitted. I lived very far away (45 minutes), and this was a VBAC. But the most important factor was that we had lost Courtney. I really didn't mind being admitted. In a way, I felt safer.

COMMENTS: *Though for most VBAC women, going to the hospital early is not usually a good idea, being in the hospital early created a sense of safety for Barbara. There must have been times she wished she had been in he hospital sooner during her last labor, hoping that earlier hospitalization might have averted the death of Courtney. Barbara's sense of safety was not threatened by the presence of nurses, doctors, midwives, or technology; but was actually enhanced by this thorough attention that she had so sorely lacked during her first labor.*

BARBARA: The hospital's policies are pretty strict, but the midwives are very flexible. I was very comfortable with the midwives' attitudes toward birth, and I knew they wouldn't intervene unless they felt it was necessary.

DONNA: Although we use certain invasive procedures for a VBAC, such as IV and continuous internal monitoring, both Barbara and Pat understood that we would still attempt to give them the kind of experience they desired. They needed to understand every aspect of their care. And they needed to know that they would be making decisions along with us regarding their "management."

BARBARA: The midwives use a birthing room. It has a couch, rocker, and birthing bed. It felt homey. Pat and I just hung around. At 8 A.M. Ruth came on duty. I felt secure with her, too. By noon Tuesday I was 3 centimeters, but by 3:00 that afternoon, ketones were present in my urine.

COMMENTS: *When ketones are present, it indicates that the body is burning more energy than it is taking in. The body is turning its fat stores into energy. When these fat stores are burned, toxins are released into the body. These toxins can be dangerous to the unborn baby, and therefore a state of ketosis is to be avoided in pregnancy and especially in labor.*

BARBARA: Ruth suggested an IV to replace fluids and nutrients. (I was not eating, but could have ice). I agreed, because I knew I could still get around.

COMMENTS: *Clearly, some kind of fluid replacement and/or nutrition was indicated. If Barbara had been permitted to eat lightly in labor, or had been given honey or maple syrup in addition to her fluids by mouth, she may have prevented the ketosis, and thereby avoided the need for the IV. However, if these simpler solutions are not available or permitted, then the IV is the only recourse.*

BARBARA: I wasn't hooked to an external monitor, but every fifteen minutes, Ruth or one of the labor and delivery nurses would come in to listen with a fetascope and put me on the external monitor for a few contractions.

Labor was not progressing very quickly, and by 6 P.M. I was still 3 centimeters and 90% effaced. I was exhausted from lack of sleep and food. I was given some morphine to help me to sleep. I stayed on the monitor while I slept.

DONNA: Since I had expected that Barbara would stay at home longer in labor, I expected labor would be shorter at the hospital. Actually it was long and difficult.

COMMENTS: *Whenever progress is slow in early labor, resting the woman rather than stimulating the labor (with pitocin) is often a good choice in aiding further progress. In early labor a slight amount of sedation will often slow or halt the contractions long enough to allow the woman to sleep, helping her to regain her strength that she will need for the more demanding part of active labor. Often she wakes up in good active labor, and progresses rapidly because of her renewed energy.*

BARBARA: Ruth came and went during the day, and the labor and delivery nurses were almost always there. I felt comforted by their presence. Everyone helped me through contractions and kept a watch on the baby's reactions to contractions.

Dr. Amon, Ruth's backup, suggested that I could either have a cesarean or try pitocin for a while to get things going.

COMMENTS: *The doctor was treating her prodromal (prelude) labor as an arrest of labor. A slowdown during prodromal labor is not an indication for pitocin. Because of the history of a previous stillbirth, the doctor was probably feeling especially anxious about the outcome of this birth. He may have felt pressure to "get the show on the road," and left Barbara little choice.*

Had she stayed home longer and continued with labor-stimulating activities such as eating, walking, nipple stimulation, and orgasm, the prodromal (prelude) pattern might have resolved itself without intervention of any kind. However, since she was in the hospital early intervention was almost obligatory.

BARBARA: I knew that if they administered pit that they would have to break the waters to attach an internal monitor and a pressure catheter. I was frightened. I knew that when the amniotic barrier was broken that bacteria have pretty easy access to the baby. Vaginal cultures confirmed that I didn't have staph in my vagina. But I did have beta strep (another potentially dangerous strain of bacteria). Finally, Pat and I decided to try the pit before going to the more radical alternative of surgery.

At about 7:30 P.M. they broke the water and inserted the monitor and pressure catheter. Then they started the pit. The contractions got really hard, but I could handle them better because I was more rested. It also really helped me to see that the baby's heartbeat was responding well to the contractions.

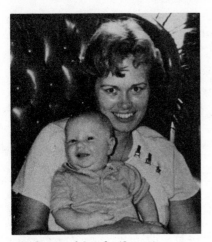

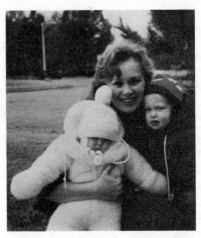

Barbara and Sparky (2 mos.)   *Pat, Cailan Aileen, and Sparky*

By about 3:00 A.M. I was 6 centimeters, and really tired. Pat was exhausted and scared, too. He thought a cesarean would be a good idea. I thought the idea of a few more hours of pain was lunacy. The night was just *so long.* Ruth had been with us the whole night, and she said she thought it would help if I got some rest by getting an epidural. I felt horrified by this notion. I didn't want an anesthetized baby. But I also didn't feel I could go on much longer. Pat said he felt he knew my limits, and that I was quickly approaching it. So about 4 A.M. I was given an epidural. Oh, sleep, glorious sleep!! It felt wonderful to sleep.

COMMENTS: *When a woman's labor appears to have been arrested later in labor, and especially after all else to stimulate the labor has been tried, often an epidural is "just what the doctor ordered." An epidural can change what appears to be an indication for a cesarean (CPD or failure to progress), into a rapidly progressing labor.*

Conscious or unconscious fear can result in the tightening of the pelvic floor. This tightening prevents descent of the presenting part and good application of the presenting part on the cervix, thereby preventing further progress. This situation often appears when the baby begins to descend, and a great deal of pelvic pressure is felt even between contractions. If the woman cannot find a way to release into the pressure rather than pulling up to stop the pressure, the epidural may be necessary to complete the dilatation.

The epidural takes away the sensation, and thereby takes away the fear and the fight against the process. The ligaments and muscles of the pelvic floor release, and progress continues.

BARBARA: Ruth and Dr. Amon said that if progress was not made soon, that they would recommend a cesarean. Luckily, another laboring woman came in and kept Ruth and Dr. Amon busy. So I just went to sleep for a while.

At about 6 A.M. Ruth checked me again, and I was 9 centimeters! I was so happy!! We let the epidural wear off, and Ruth told me to start pushing. I never felt the urge to push, only incredible pains.

Pat was really great. He tried to give me just what I needed—sometimes to be quiet and "stop touching me, for God's sake!!" I was getting really cold and asking for blankets. This really scared me because I got chills when the fever started when I was in labor with Courtney.

COMMENTS: *These chills were the normal chills of transition, that often result from hypoglycemia due to lack of food in labor, or overuse of refined sugar as in glucose water in the IV. However, to Barbara they were part of the tragedy of Courtney's death. Though intellectually she might have known the difference between these experiences, the association created tremendous fear for her.*

BARBARA: I was grunting and screaming with each contraction. God, it hurt so much that when Ruth said to look at the baby's head, I didn't even care. I just wanted to end the pain by getting him out *alive*, and *out now!* I kept on asking Ruth how much longer, and she said she didn't know. She said she could make it slightly shorter by cutting. But Pat said he thought I could handle it, and advised me to just let nature take its course.

COMMENTS: *It is possible that had Barbara not been told to push, but simply allowed to follow her own body (breathing through contractions, unless her body was telling her to push), that the pushing might not have hurt so much. Some people never get the urge to push, and simply breathe their babies out.*

However, it is also possible that the midwives wanted Barbara to actively push because they felt that Barbara was not releasing into the downward force of the contractions enough to permit her to simply breathe her baby out.

BARBARA: Pat and Donna helped me breathe and concentrate through the contractions. I tried various positions but found that sitting in bed with my knees up was the most comfortable. It also enabled me to keep the blankets on.

Sparky was finally born at 8:02 A.M. on Wednesday, April 10. He was 8 lbs. 3 oz., 22 inches long, and had a head circumfereence of 39.5 centimeters. He was limp and had swallowed meconium. A pediatric specialist from the intensive care nursery was rushed in. Since Sparky was so blue, Ruth just cut the cord quickly, suctioned him, and ran him over to the nursery table. They stuck a tube down his throat and nose, and got everything out.

COMMENTS: *Meconium is the baby's first bowel movement. It is dangerous for a baby to get meconium in his airways or lungs, so whenever a baby is born with meconium, a DeLee (a long tube with a suction device) is used to clear the airways before the baby takes his first breath.*

BARBARA: I was screaming inside with fright. I thought he was dead. I was so scared, my body was racked by sobs. Donna and Pat tried to comfort me, telling me Sparky was going to be fine.

COMMENTS: *In Barbara's mind, her worst nightmares were coming true. The fear of losing not only one baby at birth, but a second child as well must have been paramount in both her conscious and unconscious mind throughout her pregnancy and labor. Facing this fear was another hurdle in accepting Courtney's death, and realizing that she had a healthy son.*

Perhaps it would have been easier for Barbara if they had worked on Sparky immediately next to her, so that she could see that her baby was actually alive. Perhaps it would have been easier on Sparky if he had had his mother's loving touch along with the quick action of the medical personnel. Perhaps it would have even been easier on the medical staff if they had realized the power of the mother-child connection whenever life is threatened and resuscitation is needed. If this experience had been a shared one, perhaps the weight of it would have set more easily upon them all, but especially upon Barbara.

BARBARA: They let Pat cut the cord closer to his body, wrapped him up, and brought him to me. I was so numb, I couldn't believe he was all right. They gave him apgars of 8 and 10.

Ruth was really amazed that Sparky was healthy because there was a "true knot" in his cord. Pat and I really felt that somehow Courtney's spirit had protected Sparky through his development and birth.

COMMENTS: *Sparky must have responded quite quickly to the efforts of the medical personnel. An apgar of 8-10 is an excellent apgar for a baby who has swallowed meconium. He must have had a strong will to live.*

As for the knot in his cord, a true knot is quite rare. A knot, (as differentiated from a looped cord or a cord that is wrapped around the neck or body) has the potential of tightening during the descent of the baby and completely impairing the circulation of the cord blood to and from the baby. If the cord is long enough, the danger associated with the knot is averted.

BARBARA: We held Sparky for about three hours. I tried to nurse him, but he wasn't interested. Then he was taken to the nursery.

The nursery personnel wanted to start Sparky on prophylactic antibiotics because my temperature was 100.1 degrees at the time of the birth. I said, "No way!!" My temperature was so high (over 100 is said to be high) because I was without food and water for so long. Then they wanted to keep Sparky from me for 24 hours because of my temperature. It was going down gradually, and neither Sparky nor myself were showing any signs of infection, so we vetoed this, too. Then, they wanted to take blood from him to do a blood count because of my temperature at birth! Pat spoke to the chief pediatrician who said, "Let's wait, and see if he appears sick." Sparky never showed any signs of illness. I knew he wouldn't because I knew I didn't have staph this time. I just wasn't going to let them impose their arbitrary rules on me or our baby!

Pat and I took a shower together, and went up to our room. About three in the afternoon, I went down to the nursery. Sparky nursed like a barracuda! We all slept together in the same room that night, and the next day we went home.

VBAC was, and is, important to us. But always, always, a healthy live baby was paramount. I hated being drugged out and cut open for

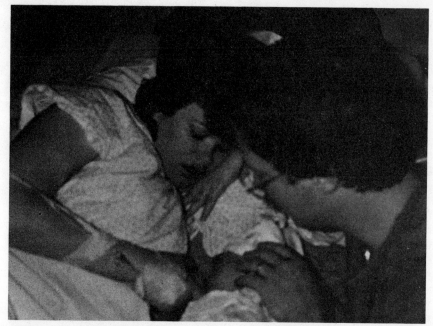

Barbara, Pat, and Sparky (15 mins.) Culligan, in the birthing room

Courtney's birth. Even a bad memory of her birth would have been better than no memory at all. But I would have certainly willingly had another cesarean if Sparky had been in trouble. Surely, it would not have been an optimal experience. But being in pain for 32 hours of labor is no cup of tea, either. The importance lies in priorities—BABY FIRST, EXPERIENCE SECOND.

I get angry when I hear women wallowing about their doctors. I know there exists in the obstetricial community a real interventionist atmosphere. But it hurt so much to go to a cesarean convention last year and hear the anger and resentment against these practices from women holding their *healthy* babies. *I had a cesarean, and no baby!* I wanted to yell to them, "Be happy with that kid! Sure, heal the pain, the jealousy and the disappointment of your birth experience, but also thank your lucky stars. Be joyful about your baby, no matter how she was born."

Birth was not the "look into each other's eyes meaningfully, and out pops a baby" experience that is often depicted. It was hard work! I believe in birth as a natural process, an opening of body and mind to a new soul. Looking back at it, I'm sure fright and anxiety added to the length of my labor. But I also feel that for his own reasons Sparky needed a long time to enter the world.

When Sparky arrived, I didn't feel overjoyed. I felt overwhelmed and exhausted—thankful that we both didn't die, thankful that it was all over and nothing major had gone wrong. The euphoria came later— the elation of knowing he was coming home with us!

If I could have changed anything, I would have liked to deliver Sparky at home. I would have been frightened, but it would have completed, somehow, the circle of conception and birth in our own bed. The hospital itself and the birth room weren't bad. It just would have been nicer at home.

The Birth of Cailan Aileen

On August 5, 1986, we had another baby, Cailan Aileen. She weighed 7 lbs. and was born vaginally and naturally, without any drugs. The labor lasted only *5 hours,* a record for me! She is beautiful—a delicate creature of strength and beauty. We just love her!

Sparky is now 19 months old and getting more fun every day. Those terrible twos have not yet arrived for he is a happy, joyful baby. He makes our lives exciting by doing the conventional things like flushing toys down the loo, not eating anything for what seems like days, hiding the cordless phone with the ringer off, and throwing the morning orange juice at the dog. The little things that make a house a home. . . .

Our lives have changed so very much. Our children are a joy, and we are elated to have them in our lives. Courtney's death hurts more now sometimes, though, because we really understand fully what we have lost.

Sparky and Cailan Aileen

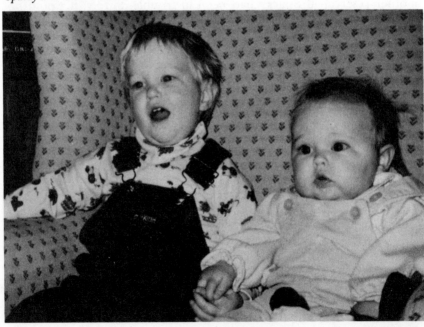

We've learned a lot these last few years—how strong we are, how much tragedy love can bear, how to communicate more effectively, how humor can get you through the worst of it all. But most of all, we learned about the love we continue to share. We've brought three lives into the world through that love. Cailan and Sparky are still with us. Courtney isn't on earth now. Hopefully, she's wherever her spirit needs to be. We've come to understand and to accept her death.

All VBAC couples face fear and have courage. It takes plenty of both to try a VBAC. Try it. You've got nothing to lose, and a new experience to gain. You are beautifully capable. Your body is wonderfully physically finely tuned to the process of giving birth. *You can do it!*

24

"*I Came Up and Up to Your Head, and I Touched You*"

JUDY GARVEY

The Birth of Matthew

J UDY: My first labor lasted two and a half days, ending in excruciating frustration—a cesarean due to cephalo-pelvic disproportion. I felt that the cesarean could have been avoided if I had had a coach and if I knew-what-I-know-now, then. But I didn't. Medical paranoia and technology took over. My baby was monitored, stuck in the head, removed of his water pillow, removed from his mommy, and left to wonder what had happened for 10 hours before we retrieved him. Never again, we swore. Three years of education and soul-searching later, we found no roads clear in New York City except our own bedroom.

My Cousin's Birth

JUDY: Two weeks before the birth of my second baby I learned that my cousin's pregnancy had ended with their baby dying in utero at 8-1/2 months due to a short wrapped cord. This news was very unsettling to me. I seemed to dwell on it, as much as I tried to ignore it. My empathy for their sorrow was very great, and dampened my own expectant joy in those last few days.

The Birth of Daniel

JUDY: Daniel, my baby of light, my life-loving little boy, was a VBAC birth. We had a midwife assist us at home and were prepared to go to the hospital if troublesome signs showed up during labor, but they didn't—not until the very end.

As labor progressed (12 hours of the hardest work in my life), there was never a doubt in my mind that my baby would live. It was a beautiful birth. We were a strongly united team — baby, mother, father, and midwife. We believed that the baby could do it. We squatted for two hours to help him out. At the end of the pushing, minutes before he appeared, the heart tones became fainter, then inaudible.

COMMENTS: *Inaudible heart tones at the end of the second stage is quite common. Usually this is simply due to the relative position of the baby as it passes through the mother's pelvis. As the shoulders begin to pass behind the pubic bone, the heart tones often become inaudible because a fetascope does not conduct the sound of the heart tones through the pubic bone. Therefore, we should not presume that the baby is in trouble because we can no longer hear heart tones. Usually, it simply means that the baby will be born momentarily.*

As the head crowned, however, its color was dark, not pink. This was my first real clue that the baby might be in trouble. However, to have transferred to a hospital at this time would only have served to increase the risk for this baby. The baby needed to be born as fast as possible, with the most positive energy possible.

JUDY: We all believed in the spiritual messages that go to the baby during labor. We *believed* that he would be born—that I could encourage him through my calling, my hope, my life-giving pain. Our midwife Lynn hoped and waited.

Daniel was born with a short cord wrapped firmly around his neck. Our midwife was ready for the cord as his head appeared. The force of the cut splashed blood on the bedroom wall. I knew at that precise moment he was in trouble, not a second before. I pushed without stopping, knowing that my baby must come out so that he could be saved.

I knew, even in my birthing trance, that others were worried — that Jim (my husband) was afraid, that my midwife was poised and ready. Matthew was quiet and curious.

Daniel was not breathing when he was born. He was grabbed up and suctioned, and suctioned again. "Come on baby," I remember hearing Lynn say over and over again.

COMMENTS: *Daniel was born lifeless by all scientific measure. But as I began to work on him, he looked at me. It was then that I knew that his spirit was with us—that there was hope for this life.*

JUDY: I was not alarmed. I felt alienated from everyone else's anxiety. I disassociated myself from the trauma. I remember thinking that perhaps after all of this, he wouldn't be alive after all. But at the time this thought did not make me sad or hysterical. I didn't really believe it could happen. I still had my ecstasy of birth. I stepped aside from the whole procedure, perhaps meeting his soul above us all somewhere, waiting to breathe, to be born. I felt out of my body, watching them all working, pleading.

The next thing that I remember is that he was sputtering, wheezing, sneezing, and there were happy sounds and crying. Lynn put him on me, and we rubbed and massaged him.

Even then, I was still removed. I refused to entertain the thought that there was still danger. I had to be reminded to rub him and massage him, preferring to let him lie on me, to watch and touch. "Rub him, rub him. He needs to be made to feel warm, to feel you—rub him." The midwife coached me into providing his still precarious body temperature with the necessary touches. Within minutes he was nursing and getting pinker and pinker. When he was born he was grey, not even blue, and at least thirty minutes passed before he was truly pink. We all kept massaging him. He was with us. He was happy.

We have a picture of him two hours later—a beautiful pink little baby. What a beautiful way to be brought to life! For him, it was the way of shared energies and spirituality, not the respirator and incubator. It was his choice to stay with us.

COMMENTS: *Technically, of course, resuscitation of an infant born in such condition is imperative. To rely solely upon the calling of the spirit to bring forth life that is on the brink of death would be foolish and irresponsible.*

Daniel, less than 1 hour after birth

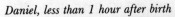

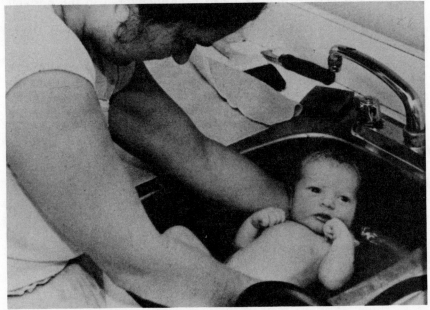

However, life is truly a choice—a choice of the spirit as to whether to stay or leave. In reality, at every birth (even with apgar 10/10 babies) every baby makes that choice. If we look carefully into the baby's eyes, we may see the moment of choosing—of choosing to breathe, of choosing life. Whenever we as parents, practitioners, friends, and family sense the significance of that moment and connect with the spirit of the child (even as we perform the necessary technical resuscitation), we may provide the necessary spiritual resuscitation as well.

It is my deep-felt belief that resuscitation of an infant should always be done at the side of the mother and father. Regardless of the circumstances, a baby should never be separated from its parents, especially if that baby is on the brink of choice.

JUDY: Those who have experienced the death of their baby should know that their baby did not die from their lack of belief. That soul was simply on the other side of life. Daniel was nearer to us, and made the choice to breathe.

I remember thinking of my cousin during those life-and-death moments, just after Daniel's birth. It *did* happen to me . . . I knew it would.

COMMENTS: *Judy experienced an empathetic premonition. Through her own empathy with her cousin, she realized the pain of the death of a baby—her own baby. She moved into this birth prepared for the possibility of her baby's death. Intuition and premonition are always powerful sources of knowledge, and a pregnant woman's intuition and premonition regarding her baby are often overwhelmingly clear and accurate. It is therefore imperative that we acknowledge these sources within ourselves, and follow our most deep-felt guidance regarding our choices in birthing.*

JUDY: Later the thought occurred to me, "If I had been in the hospital like everyone said I should have, this never would have happened." Perhaps, and perhaps not. If I had been monitored in the hospital, perhaps my recumbent position would have been even more stressful to Daniel's beautiful, sunny brain. My squatting position allowed Daniel the maximum nourishment.

COMMENTS: *Whenever a pregnant woman lies on her back, the weight of the pregnant uterus places pressure on the major vessels, infringing upon the placental circulation, and thereby compromising the oxygenation of the fetus. Maintaining an upright position such as squatting aids in improved circulation and therefore oxygenation to the fetus. In addition, squatting provides the greatest pelvic dimensions, and thereby allows the fastest descent.*

We often presume that with the use of the monitor a wrapped cord could be detected early in labor. However, a wrapped cord only becomes a problem when the cord is short, and tightens with the descent of the baby. It is only when the cord tightens that a change in the oxygenation to the baby will occur, thus changing the heart rate. Therefore, it is possible that even with the latest technological equipment the problem with Daniel's cord might not have been detected any sooner in the hospital than it was at home.

Had this apgar 1/8 baby been born in the hospital, he most certainly would have been whisked away from his parents—from the spiritual tie with his mother, who was perhaps the person most responsible for his choice to breathe, to choose life.

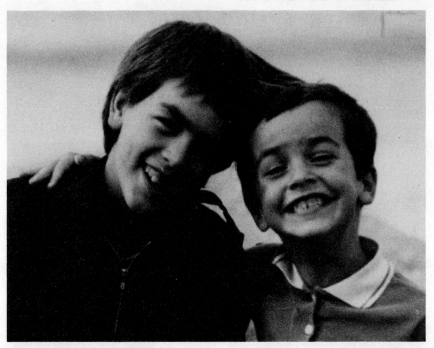

Matthew and Daniel now

JUDY: We believe strongly in the parallels of birth and death. My baby elected to live. My Daniel hovered momentarily and chose to breathe. He was greatly assisted by the quick actions of our midwife, Lynn. But in the end, he took that breath.

My beautiful, thoughtful Daniel—he has never known separation, trauma from technology, or undue medications. He responds in kind—happy and giving.

From Matthew's cesarean to Daniel's VBAC was a leap. I shall always share something special with Daniel. At birth, for a few brief moments, I contemplated his death. I met his energy during labor, still hopeful, and helped to bring him through. I watched him struggling for life in those brief seconds, and didn't feel emotion. I was also displaced. I was also in-between. We came back together.

We had never told Daniel that he wasn't breathing when he was born. Yet, on his third birthday, he began to talk about his own birth, saying, "And I didn't get dead—and I came up and up to your head, and I touched you!"

OPENING
A Photographic Birth Story
JUDY AND BOB

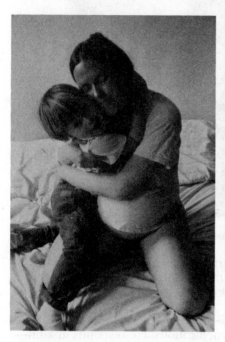 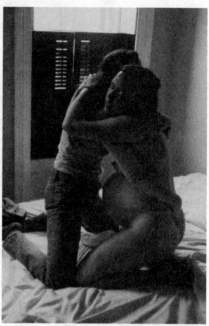

JUDY: Everyone is supporting me during my labor. They each have an important role, and I am glad they are all here. My son Brien's hugs are a very special kind of support. Just knowing he is nearby feels good. Between contractions I look out the window and watch him playing in the backyard.

BOB: Are we doing everything we can do for Judy? Are we doing what is best for her? It's hard to know how to help.

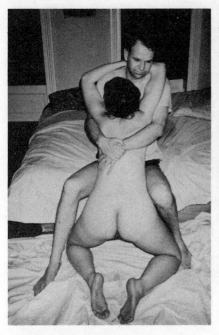

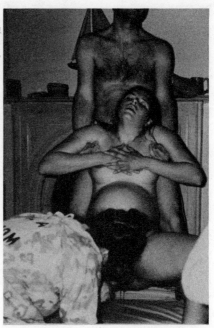

JUDY: I am totally focused on pushing. Feeling very inward . . . just going inside myself . . . thinking about the baby moving out of my body . . . as if nobody else is here. I am trying to draw on all the energy that I can.

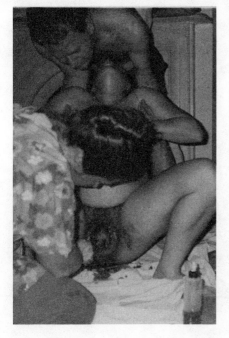

BOB: Feeling a pull on my energy. Psychological support becomes physical support. We all are drawn into the process as if we are attached to exactly what is happening. We are all pushing. Judy's sense of wanting the baby to move down — we are all feeling all the energy it takes to do that.

BOB: Relief! The baby is going to be born at home. I just want to see the baby come out. To prepare for this I should have meditated, jogged, and lifted weights every day of the pregnancy!

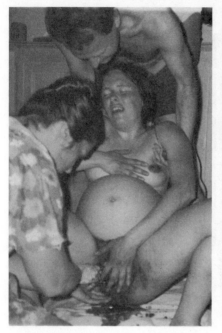

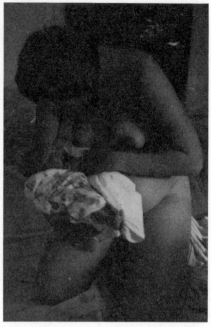

JUDY: Excited! When I touch the head I know it is really happening! My baby is really coming out. Now, at this very moment, I *know* that my baby will be born at home.

LYNN: A slow crowning. "Keep it coming, Judy . . . a little more . . . you're doing great!" The head is born to the eyebrows. Another push. The head is out. Push again. The shoulders are held up. "Stand up, Judy." Another push. Still no baby. I will have to assist. "Hands and knees, Judy." I reach in and hook my finger under the baby's armpit. I pull, and Judy pushes one last time. And WHOOSH! The baby is in my lap. A quick suction and a gasp. I pass the baby between Judy's legs and lay her face down in front of Judy. "Here she is! Here's your baby!"

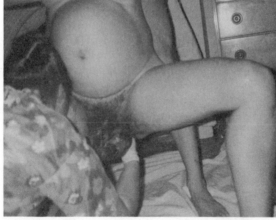

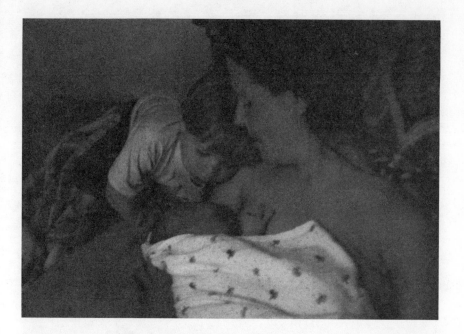

BOB: It's a girl! It's Dana. She's OK. She's alive! Tremendous feeling of happiness that the whole thing went well. I can sit down and relax for a while. Everybody's looking and feeling good. Some thoughts about how Judy's doing and a reassessment of Dana. Wonder what they'll need next. We're now a family of four.

JUDY: Looking at Dana for the first time. Marvelling at this new person who has just come into the world.

LYNN: To witness the moment of first meeting . . . such sweetness . . . the most precious moment of a lifetime . . . is my reward for all the work I have done.

JUDY: Very happy that Brien is here! It feels right. Being at home in my own bed with my two kids is just the way I wanted it to be. I know I made the right decision.

POSTSCRIPT: We named her Dana April because April means "opening" in Latin. Opening is what I needed to do to birth her.

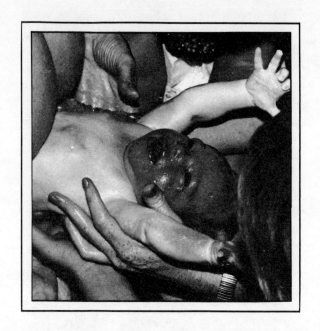

Out of the Hands of Practitioners

25

Defining Complication

KAY MATTHEWS
Family Nurse Practitioner, Nurse-Midwife, Domicilary Midwife

C OMMENTS: *I believe Kay Matthews was the first midwife in this country to attend home VBACs.*

KAY: In America anything other than a baby that falls out in the emergency room is considered a complication. According to my training in the British system, breeches, twins, and VBACs were simply variations, not complications. I began doing these so called "high-risk" births at home for the same reason that I did any birth at home—women wanted to have natural births, and truly natural births generally don't happen in American hospitals. In many situations where there have been variations in the birth process women are not even allowed to attempt a natural birth let alone be supported in such an endeavor.

Every birth requires a maximal level of attention by the attendant, a VBAC does not require more. If an intervention is indicated then the fact that there has been a previous cesarean should in no way influence the attendant's and mother's decision-making. Only when one can approach the birth process in an objective manner can the attendant really provide the laboring woman with the enthusiastic, confident support that she is entitled to.

26

VBAC Training 1947–1950

IRWIN KAISER, *OB/GYN*

I trained in obstetrics at Sinai Hospital in Baltimore from 1947 to 1950. It was a private hospital, and we had a fair number of practitioners working there, among them some pretty scholarly people whom I respected. A couple of them took for granted that they didn't have to do repeat sections, provided that the indication for the first section was no longer present. However, there were also a couple of staff members who were just as adamant against VBAC.

One of the "anti" practitioners had done a cesarean on a woman for a breech, on the basis of an incorrect pelvimetry report. The secretary had made an error in typing the report. Then, when they did the section, they discovered the baby wasn't a breech, but a vertex. Therefore, we knew from the chart that this woman had had a totally unnecessary cesarean section. The question was, "Would she have a repeat section?" A tremendous argument ensued between the staff members, particularly because the original doctor had done a classical section, and we were very leery of doing normal deliveries following a classical section.

The woman went into labor, and all the other staff members left, leaving me alone with her. She had a very rapid labor, and delivered a 9-pound baby with absolutely no trouble at all. The baby was just fine, and I was dumbfounded when I stuck my hand in to explore her uterus, and found that the entire length of the scar was defective. I reported this finding to the senior staff, and they decided that she should be sterilized.

This was *not a rupture*. The womb had simply come apart. Neither the baby nor the placenta had come out through a hole in the uterus. The baby was born quite safely through the vagina. The woman was not hemorrhaging.

I was pretty upset by the outcome of this woman's birth. It seemed to me that she had had rotten care in the first place (when she had the cesarean), and even though we had had the best of intentions, we had run a substantial risk around this woman's uterus. I decided that I had to seriously review the literature, after which I concluded that clearly vaginal delivery following a cervical cesarean section is probably perfectly safe.

The literature was clear in the 1940s, and it has remained clear. There have never really been any serious disagreements with this, and that is the way I have practiced ever since. It was never a big deal for me. The real question was, "Had the patient had a cervical section? Was the indication for the previous section still present?" And if the indication for the previous section was not still present, she was simply a pregnant woman, and that is the way she is treated.

27

Classical VBAC

MITCH LEVINE, *OB/GYN*

I have attended a few women who have had previous classical incisions. As with any other decision that has to be made, I explain to them that there may be an increased risk with a classical incision. But we also discuss the benefits of vaginal delivery. If people decide that they still want to to have a vaginal birth, then that is their option.

It's my job to explain the risks and benefits to people, not to decide for them. All the women who have decided to have a VBAC with a previous classical incision have had fine births, without a rupture or any other medical problems.

28

Mandatory Labor After Previous Cesarean

KENNETH MCKINNEY, *OB/GYN*

KEN: Barbara came to me for a VBAC after having had a cesarean with her first baby for a contracted pelvis. According to the history, she had been in early labor and wasn't progressing. So the doctor did a pelvimetry. He found her inner spinous diameter to be 8.8 or 8.9 centimeters.

COMMENTS: *The inner spinous diameter is the smallest transverse (side to side) diameter of the pelvis. An inner spinous diameter of less than 9.5 centimeters is considered by most obstetricians to be "inadequate."*

KEN: The doctor then presented Barbara with that information, and told her, "You will definitely need to have a cesarean. It's 5:00. Let's do it now and get it over with."

Upon review of the case, it seemed to me that Barbara might not have had an adequate trial of labor with that first baby, and that even though statistical probability indicated she might not deliver this second baby vaginally, I felt a VBAC was still a possibility.

I do not feel that previous CPD, failure to progress, or "contracted pelvis" as evidenced by x-ray pelvimetry are indications to do a repeat cesarean. One of the things that people lose track of is that the number values on x-ray pelvimetry that delineated an adequate pelvis versus an inadequate pelvis were really intended to indicate who was a candidate for pitocin.

COMMENTS: *It would be dangerous to give pitocin to a woman who had a truly impacted labor. If the baby could not be born because of gross physical disproportion between the size of the mother's pelvis and the size of the baby's head, then forcing the labor with pitocin could risk the life of both the mother and the baby. Use of pitocin with a truly impacted labor could cause uterine rupture. In fact, it has been documented that misuse of pitocin is the single greatest factor in causing uterine rupture. Therefore, pelvimetry was developed to risk out the use of pitocin on a woman whose pelvimetry indicated that pitocin might be dangerous for her and her baby.*

KEN: According to the first publication of those values (prior to 1963), 85% of the women whose inner spinous diameter was greater than 9 and a half centimeters would deliver vaginally. It really said nothing about whether or not the baby **could** come out vaginally, it was only an indication of the statistical probability of vaginal delivery. However, people made a quantum leap from that evidence of statistical probability of vaginal birth to using those measurements to label a contracted pelvis vs. adequate pelvis.

COMMENTS: *In other words, having CPD or even a "contracted pelvis" as evidenced by pelvimetry does not indicate that a woman cannot deliver her baby vaginally.* Even a woman with a "contracted pelvis" can overcome this label, and deliver her own baby herself—vaginally.

KEN: One day near term of this second pregnancy Barbara called me at the office to say that she was having this awful pain. This was early in my experience with VBAC, and I thought, "Oh, shit. This lady's ruptured her uterus."

COMMENTS: *"Unusual pain" with a woman who has a uterine scar may mean "uterine rupture."*

KEN: So I told her to come in to the hospital immediately. She came in, and was having contractions every 4 or 5 minutes. The "awful pain" she was experiencing was labor!

Clearly, she had never really been in labor with her first baby, which explained why her previous "labor" had been "unprogressive." She subsequently delivered vaginally a baby that weighed over 8 lbs.

Since I started doing VBACs in 1978, I have felt that unless there was an indication for cesarean in the current pregnancy (like placenta previa), then the woman was a candidate to deliver vaginally. Now that further data is available which supports trial of labor and vaginal delivery for women who have had previous cesareans for "CPD, failure to progress, or contracted pelvis," a case could almost be made for making a trial of labor following a previous cesarean mandatory. It probably represents the best obstetrical care for mother and baby.

29

A Perfectly Round Head

KAY MATTHEWS

KAY: On Friday of the fourth of July weekend, the doctor was planning to go away on vacation. He told Candice that she was past her due date, and that she could deliver a post-mature baby, which would be quite dangerous.

Candice went into the hospital for an induction. They started the pitocin, but that didn't work. So they ruptured her membranes and gave her more pit. The induction failed, so they did a cesarean for CPD. Her baby weighed 7-1/2 lbs. and was not in the least bit post-mature.

A couple of years later Candice came to me wanting to have a home VBAC. She had been to see several obstetricians all of whom said, "No way are you going to get a baby through that pelvis." She did have relatively narrow spines (the side-to-side measurement of her pelvis was small), but she had a very deep pelvis. Her diagonal conjugate measured greater than 12 centimeters. (The front to back measurement was very large.) I told her what I tell everyone who is worried about whether or not they really have CPD. "Nothing but labor will tell you whether this baby will fit through this pelvis at this time."

Candice went into labor, and from our phone conversations, she appeared to be puttering. Because the induction had failed the first time, I treated her labor as if it were her first labor, expecting a long inactive phase.

A few hours later she called back saying that the labor had picked up. I left immediately for her house which is less than a half-hour away. When I arrived, there in the middle of the floor sat Candice, her husband, and a 8 1/2 lb. baby with an absolutely round head.

COMMENTS: *If a baby has had any difficulty whatsoever in negotiating the pelvis, the baby's head molds, and develops what is called a caput. If a baby is born with a perfectly round head, there is absolutely no disproportion.*

KAY: I thought to myself immediately, "There's no way you can get a baby through that pelvis—Ha!"

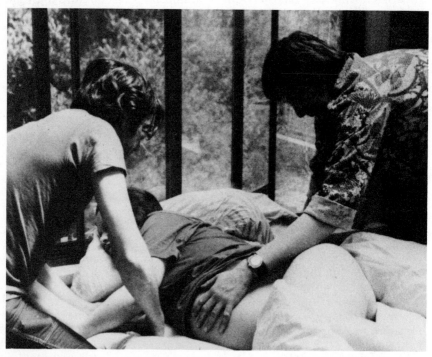

Kay Matthew, family nurse practitioner, nurse-midwife, and domiciliary midwife, uses her "eyes on the tips of her fingers" as a "natural monitor" to assess the strength of a laboring woman's contractions.

30

Once a Cesarean, Never a Cesarean

I R W I N   K A I S E R, *OB/GYN*

When I was chief resident we had a patient who had had a section for her first delivery. She was very upset about having had a section, and very much wanted to deliver from below. I took her through a three day labor, because we had decided to comply with her request not to have a section. After three days, she finally delivered, and we all heaved a sigh of relief.

This labor and delivery was the talk of the whole obstetrics department in this hospital. One of my teachers who was a fellow with a pretty good sense of humor met me in the elevator. He put his arm around my shoulder and said, "Well, Irwin, once a section, never a section."

31

Expert Witness

K A Y   M A T T H E W S

I have recently been called to testify in a malpractice case. The woman had had a previous cesarean for a rather nebulous reason. A routine repeat cesarean was planned for her next birth. A couple of sonagrams were done during the pregnancy, but not at the dates when accuracy of gestational age is most easily determined.

At approximately 36 weeks gestation the doctor popped in to measure her belly with a tape, and said, "How about Thursday?" There were no further tests for gestational age performed—no L/S ratio, nothing.

A cesarean was performed on the scheduled date, and a baby weighing less than 5 pounds measuring only 17 inches in length was delivered. The lungs were immature, and the baby soon died. Had this woman gone into labor and delivered her baby vaginally when the baby was ready, the lungs would have been mature, and the baby would probably be living today! This woman should have had a VBAC!

32

Talking Women into VBAC

KENNETH MCKINNEY,
OB/GYN

KEN: Whenever women come to me after having had a previous cesarean, I ask the question, "How is this baby going to come out?" And most people today say, "I want to have it vaginally."

Talking about VBAC today is a little like talking about breastfeeding. I don't have to tell people anymore that breastfeeding is going to be better for them and their babies. People know that. It's available in the lay literature. In people's constellation of friends, it's just the norm, not the unusual. Since 1978 when I first began to attend VBACs, I have seen attitudes towards VBAC change radically. It is quickly becoming the norm.

Today, if a woman has any question about the safety of VBAC, we sit and discuss the matter. I talk about what makes labor start—that the fetus probably plays a significant role in that determination. Therefore, it makes sense to let the baby say when it's ready rather than depend upon a laboratory to say when a baby is ready to be born. Next we talk about going into labor, anticipating that the baby will probably come out vaginally. Then I give the woman the statistics to support a VBAC. Usually, at that point folks are comfortable.

After much discussion of safety of VBAC vs. repeat cesarean, one woman, Sally, decided to try to have a VBAC. She came in to the hospital in active labor, and was progressing slightly slower than Friedman's curve of a centimeter a hour. I don't feel compelled to interfere with or interrupt a labor that doesn't follow that curve exactly. Therefore, since it was in the middle of the night and she and her husband were really doing fine, I went to sleep.

Perhaps an hour or an hour and a half later, one of the nurses came and woke me up saying, "This couple wants to see you right away. The lady doesn't want to do this anymore." When I walked into her room, she said, "I don't know how I ever let you talk me into this. This is just awful!" And her husband said, "Oh, honey, you're doing a great job!" And she said, "You're full of shit!" And I said, "Sounds to me like you're in transition!" When I checked her she had only a rim of cervix left. She delivered vaginally about twenty or thirty minutes later.

I see this phenomenon happen all the time. Women say: "I want to go home." "I can't do this." "I want to take a break and have supper and then I'll have a few more contractions." When a woman is in a lot of pain and voicing her frustration with her labor, it would be very easy to say, "You're absolutely right, let's go right to the operating room."

However, it's very important to remember that a woman in labor is a woman in labor. If she's had a scar from a cesarean section, that shouldn't influence you in your management. You should treat her like you would anybody else.

33

A Five-Hour, Second-Stage VBAC

THERESE DONDERO, *C.N.M.* and GERRIANNE BODD, *R.N.C.*

THERESE: Laurel wanted a midwife-attended hospital VBAC and couldn't find anyone in the area where she lived who was willing to do this. She came to our practice because we had somewhat of a reputation for delivering women who had previous cesarean sections. Laurel was quite comfortable with us. However, it took quite a while for her husband to develop some confidence in our noninterventive position. We not only had to work through all of her anger, but we also had to work through their decision to be taken care of by a midwife. His lack of confidence in us caused Laurel a great deal of interference during her VBAC labor.

Her first labor was arrested at the second stage, the baby was posterior, and she was sectioned. From a strict medical point of view, the appropriate thing was done. However, perhaps if she had been in a different environment, she might not have needed the cesarean. Laurel delivered her first baby in the same institution where her husband was a practicing physician. It seemed to me that there was physician-to-physician communication going on that perhaps could have created the decision to do a section.

COMMENTS: *Doctors' wives have the highest cesarean rate. Perhaps one of the factors is this physician-to-physician communication which Therese describes.*

THERESE: Laurel needed to feel that she could trust me. She needed to know that we weren't going to place a time limit upon her labor. We talked about how distrust could interfere with her birth and I was glad I could rely on a good childbirth educator to enhance this feeling of trust. I believe that the most important factor in positive birthing is the woman's ability to trust herself and have confidence in her body.

GERRI: Laurel and Stan came to me for a full series of childbirth classes. In class it seemed Stan needed the information more than Laurel did. My overall trepidations for this birth really were focused on him. I felt there was no physiological or psychological reason that Laurel could not have a VBAC, but that Stan was a strong deterrent. While taking classes, Stan was always very negative about Laurel having a VBAC, and was very supportive of all medical intervention, which he described as "labor enhancements." I had the feeling that he truly believed that the baby would be safer if born by cesarean. Clearly, he was going along with Laurel only because of his love for her, not because of any belief on his part. I wondered if Laurel would be strong enough to birth this baby despite his negativity.

Laurel needed emotional reassurance. She had lost confidence in her body's ability to function well. She had a rather passive personality and needed constant reassurance that things were going well and that her body was working fine. In addition to regular classes, in several private sessions, we "rebirthed" her cesarean baby, and went on to do birth visualizations of vaginal birth.

COMMENTS: *Rebirthing the cesarean baby is a visualization process by which the mother visualizes the past birth experience, changing it as she would have liked it to have progressed. This experience can be very healing, permitting the woman to move from the previous birth memories into the forthcoming birth with more freedom and openness.*

THERESE: During prenatals we talked about Laurel's feelings about labor. I suggested that she try to get rid of her anxiety about the baby's position. She was very much afraid that if she knew the baby was posterior again that this was going to interfere with her pushing. We agreed that we wouldn't tell her the position of the baby.

GERRI: Laurel called me several times the day of February 1, 1982, reporting the early signs of labor. Finally, she called and said she thought the contractions were getting quite close together. I drove over to her house and checked her vitals. I estimated that she was in middle-to-late active labor and that it was time to go to the hospital. She wanted to stay home as long as possible and did not want to leave her two-year-old son. She seemed unwilling to hurry in any way.

Laurel got dressed, and we headed with Stan to the hospital. He seemed somewhat nervous. He had a fear that the baby would be born in the car. I brought emergency equipment just in case, but did not have the sense that she was that close to giving birth.

Laurel and I were deliberately slow in transferring from the car to the hospital, urging Stan to go ahead and park—that we could all slowly walk in together and up to maternity. We had to do a little "doublespeak" maneuver to get both Stan and me upstairs with Laurel, as the hospital didn't want two labor support people. We explained that I was to be labor support; and Stan was there to view the birth of his baby, bond, and be a moral support for his wife.

An obnoxious female resident examined Laurel and found her close to full dilitation. But the baby was quite high (-3 station). The resident put pressure on Laurel to have the monitor attached (external), and we had to fight. Laurel was very uncomfortable with this woman, who was rough and nervous. She kept stating that Laurel was "high-risk" because of her previous cesarean, and therefore must be monitored. I was able to speak to the resident outside Laurel's room. I calmly told her that I understood her anxiety, but that she was transferring it to the patient. Perhaps she could call the midwife right away. Hurray! Done, no monitor, and midwife on the way.

Once Therese arrived, everything went very well. Laurel and I spent a great deal of time walking to the bathroom. She sat on the toilet. We tried a lot of labor positions, including semi-squatting, but that baby was still very high, and Laurel was still not completely dilated. There seemed to be very slow progress at this point.

THERESE: Stan just didn't trust what I was saying or what my exams were indicating, which created a great deal of tension.

GERRI: Upon Stan's insistence, the backup physician was brought in.

THERESE: Stan seemed to be attempting to create that same physician-physician communication, which had apparently undermined Laurel's first labor. So, I took my backup aside and told him to cool it, that I was managing the case.

GERRI: The presence of this physician agitated Laurel. She thought they were preparing for another cesarean. I was able to calm her and convinced her that he was there only out of protocol, and because Stan had insisted upon his presence. After Therese spoke with the backup, he was kind enough to be as inconspicuous as possible, coming in and out infrequently and remaining in the background.

THERESE: Laurel really did as most women do that I've taken care of with previous sections. It really comes down to trusting their bodies to go ahead and do what it can do. She ended up, basically ignoring her husband's anxiety about the whole thing and just went ahead doing what she felt she needed to do. We all ended up ignoring him.

GERRI: Therese and I discussed over coffee the possible psychological barriers that might be causing this labor to take so long. But as both Laurel and the baby's heart tones were doing well, Therese was unconcerned.

Against the strong advice of the obstetrical nurse on duty, Laurel was drinking "Third Wind" (an electrolyte-balanced juice) and water frequently, moving about and breathing slowly and deeply. When she experienced the urge to push, it was mild, but she was encouraged to go with it. With a few light pushes. . .

THERESE: Laurel got to full dilatation. But the next two or three hours of pushing were a waste of energy. She was pushing, but it was inef-

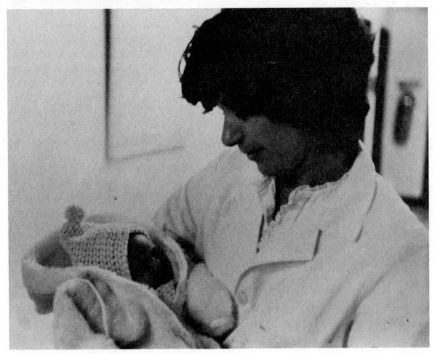

Therese Dondero, holding Laurel's baby

fective. Since the station was good, however—down to +1 or +2 station—and the head was in a good position, I had every confidence that
she could deliver her baby herself. The backup checked her, too, and
realized she could deliver—that it was just a matter of some good effective pushing. But Laurel was blocking it.

After about 2 or 3 hours of pushing, I felt that the fetal monitor
was indicated, as exhaustion could become a factor for mother or baby.
But we used it only intermittently. Had we seen evidence of fetal distress,
she could have been delivered immediately with forceps.

GERRI: But the baby never had an episode of distress. I think the combination of total relaxation and nutrition, and slow deep breathing allowed Laurel's body to recover from each contraction well, preventing
distress.

THERESE: She just needed time to get it together to push effectively. All
she needed was a real good push, and the baby would have come out.

We got her pushing on a mat, and that didn't work too well. Then
she went back into the bathroom and pushed on the bowl. And that's
when after 4 hours of pushing, it happened. Her contractions had been
good all along, but whether the baby's head turned a little bit or she
decided that she could do it, that's when it happened.

Things moved quickly. Stan got involved, and ended up being very
helpful and supportive.

GERRI: Laurel pushed for a total of a little over 5 hours! Finally, the baby was crowning! Laurel's labia were very swollen from the extended pushing, so Therese did an episiotomy. Then, we understood what had taken so long—this baby was born with her hands in a prayer position along the side of her head. Her head, arms, and hands were born all at once! The head had molded around the hands. Therese was concerned about getting the baby out and breathing, as she was somewhat blue.

Laurel nursed and Stan bonded with the baby, as her episiotomy was repaired. She was exhilarated and hungry, and I felt both relief and triumph for Laurel. After a while the baby was brought to the nursery, Laurel was cleaned up and given fresh fruit to eat. Stan and I went home.

THERESE: The next day I received a lot of flak about having a woman with a previous cesarean section push for five hours. I think they're still talking about it. We must give people their own time and space to give birth.

* * *

I regret to add that Therese Dondero, one of the finest most dedicated midwives I know, has recently died. We all miss her and appreciate all that she gave to women and their babies.

34

Saving the Doctor's Wife

STEVEN MELTZER, *OB/GYN*

STEVE: A woman who is married to a doctor was in labor, and was having a very hard time with her contractions. She was screaming for someone to do something for her. I knew she had a good-sized baby in there, and perhaps there was a slight degree of disproportion. Most of my colleagues would have done a cesarean. But I was tired of doctor's wives always being cut open. I mean, you never hear of a doctor's wife that doesn't get cut.

So when she reached full dilatation I just made her keep pushing. We set up the vacuum extractor. . . .

COMMENTS: *A vacuum extractor is a machine that creates a powerful yet controllable vacuum. A big rubberized cup rather like a plunger is placed on the head of the baby. When the cup is in place, during each contraction, the vacuum is turned on just enough to allow the woman's pushing effort to become more effective, but not enough to damage the baby's head.*

STEVE: The woman delivered a 9-pound baby from below. This kid had such a caput (the part of the head the molds to allow the baby to pass through the pelvis) that when the pediatrician came in to check the baby, he said, "Somebody put a hat on that kid, will you?"

But at least I know one doctor's wife who didn't have a cesarean!

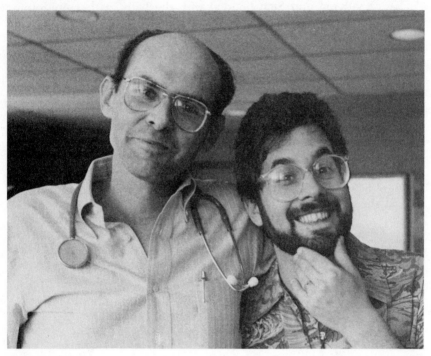

Dr. Steve Meltzer, Ob/Gyn, and Dr. Harlan Sparer, chiropractor, lighten the load through love and laughter.

35

The Effect of Malpresentation on Vaginal Birth

KENNETH MCKINNEY,
OB/GYN

KEN: Joan came to me when she was pregnant with her first baby. During that labor she had become fully dilated, but the head was stuck in the inlet of her pelvis. None of the maneuvers we tried were successful in altering that situation, so after more than two hours of pushing with no progress, she had a cesarean.

When she got pregnant again, she came in to talk about the next birth. We agreed that she would go into labor, and we would see what would happen. So Joan went into labor, and when she arrived at the hospital she was fully dilated. The head was coming through her pelvis a little bit further than it had the first time.

So, I said to her, "Why don't you just bear down and see if you can't just bring that head down a little bit." And she really got mad!

"I don't want to do this!"

"Well, come on try."

"No, I don't want to do this. I want to have another cesarean section."

"The head's way up there, so try."

"No, I don't want to. You set up for another section."

"I'll tell you what, I'll get it set up and you push."

So she did, and I did and she pushed the baby out. This baby weighed a few ounces more than the first one. Clearly, something was different in terms of how the head oriented through her pelvis.

Since I've been doing VBACs I have learned to have an appreciation of the effect of the presentation of the head upon the outcome of labor. Having watched women in labor after they've had a cesarean section (especially those who had cesareans for CPD), I've come to realize that much of the cause of abnormal labor must be due to malpresentation. A head that's a little deflexed (tilted backwards), or more asynclitic (tilted to the side) than you may be aware of may be playing a significant role in whatever the woman's problem is in labor.

That realization has indirectly affected my practice as a whole. When a woman is having a problem with her labor, I tend not to presume that the problem is CPD. I often approach those labors with the thought that perhaps with some positional or manual maneuvers the problem might be resolved, making a vaginal delivery a possibility.

36

Breech VBAC Without Pelvimetry

LEO SORGER, *OB/GYN*

L EO: When Brenda and George came to me their baby was due in about a week. Their first baby who weighed 6 lbs. 10 oz. had been born by cesarean because of a breech presentation. Even though their doctor had told them that their second baby was presenting as a vertex, he still wanted to do another cesarean.

When I examined her, I discovered that this baby was another breech. We attempted an external version in the office without drugs and without success. Then we tried another version in the hospital using medication (terbutaline 1.5 mg. and valium 10 mg.) to help to relax her uterus and make the version easier. But the frank breech was too deeply engaged in her pelvis and would not turn.

Meanwhile, she was due and said she definitely wanted to attempt to give birth to her breech baby vaginally. So we planned that she would go into labor and try to have a vaginal birth.

Unless a woman is adverse to a vaginal delivery, in my practice all women with breeches go into labor. I don't believe in the use of pelvimetry, although I do a very careful clinical evaluation of the pelvis. Whether the baby is footling or frank breech does not make too much difference as long as the baby is guarded against cord prolapse in the footling presentation. I'm very careful to avoid a cord prolapse with a footling, by checking often and carefully before the membranes rupture. Often if a cord is forelying, it can be palpated while the membranes are still intact. I now have a 70% success rate for vaginal breeches. In other words, 70% of the women who attempt vaginal delivery with a breech presentation actually give birth vaginally.

A few days later Gloria's labor started and she came to the hospital for her breech VBAC. She had a relatively short labor with good progress, did most of her pushing in a deep squatting position, and stood up a bit for delivery. With no episiotomy, and no problems whatsoever, she gave birth to a healthy (good apgar) 7 lb. 5 oz. baby (larger than her cesarean-born baby). The next day she took her baby home.

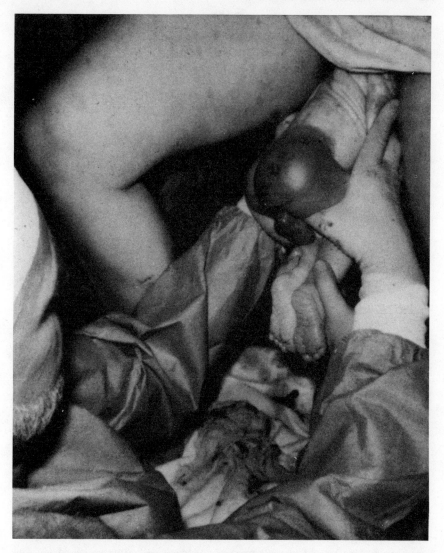

Dr. Leo Sorger assisting with the delivery of the head of a frank breech presentation. Dr. Sorger is on the floor, below, while the woman is standing. This posture encourages the head to flex, allowing for a smooth completion of the birth. The intense color of the baby's buttocks is o.k. with a frank breech and will return to normal soon.

37

Natural Protocol for Breech Birth

MICHEL ODENT, *OB/GYN*

In his book, *Birth Reborn* Dr. Odent writes the following about breech delivery:

From our experience with breech babies, we have found that by observing the natural progression of first-stage labor, we will get the best indication of what to expect at the last moment. This means we do nothing that will interfere with first-stage labor—no pitocin, no bathing in the pool, no mention of the word "breech." If all goes smoothly we have reason to believe the second stage of labor will not pose any problems. Our only intervention will be to insist on the supported squatting position for delivery, since it is the most mechanically efficient. It reduces the likelihood of our having to pull the baby out, and is the best way to minimize the delay between the delivery of the baby's umbilicus and the baby's head, which could result in the compression of the cord, and deprive the infant of oxygen. We would never risk a breech delivery with the mother in a dorsal or semi-seated position.

If on the other hand, contractions in the first-stage labor are painful and inefficient and dilation does not progress, we must quickly dispense with the idea of vaginal delivery. Otherwise we face the danger of a last minute "point of no return" when, after the emergence of the baby's buttocks, it is too late to switch strategies and decide on a cesarean. However, although we always perform cesareans when first-stage labor is difficult and the situation is not improving, most breech births in our clinic do end up as vaginal deliveries.

COMMENTS: *Unfortunately, most practitioners trained in this country have not been trained to do vaginal breech deliveries. Those who have, have been trained to do breech extractions, not vaginal breech births. A breech extraction involves much manipulation of the baby, with a large episiotomy, forceps, and sometimes even anesthesia, keeping the woman in the lithotomy position (flat on her back). Often much damage is done to the baby or the mother through all of these interventions. If more practitioners adopted or were trained with Dr. Udent's management, certainly the cesarean rate for breech presentation would be decreased with perhaps improvement in the statistics for breech outcomes.*

38

Obstetrical Training for Breech Delivery

IRWIN KAISER, *OB/GYN*

I have never in my life had trouble with a breech. And I rarely section for a breech.

Now, of course there are some skills involved in delivering breeches. And, many doctors trained today aren't learning them. However, if doctors don't have the skills, maybe they ought to be doing something else—perhaps administrative medicine.

39

Prophylactic Cesarean for Herpes Disputed

(from *OB/GYN News* 16(15):14.)

D r. Debauchez, from the Hospital for Sick Children in Paris, France, describes the following case:

The pregnancy proceeded normally until the 34th week when the mother developed an "unexplained" fever, which went away spontaneously and did not recur. Four days later, a male infant was born vaginally.

The infant arrived covered with fluid-filled blisters and blisters that had already broken and were scarring over. The newborn was otherwise normal.

The infection had obviously been contracted in utero. Herpes was not the first diagnosis to be considered, but subsequent tests showed unmistakable evidence of herpes.

The infant's skin lesions receded after four weeks. The baby is now 5 months old and there has been no sign of neurologic or any other sort of visceral involvement. (OB/GYN News 16 [15]:14)

COMMENTS: *Recent studies done by the Disease Control Center in Altanta have shown that neonatal herpes is not necessarily prevented by cesarean delivery. Thus, the use of prophylactic (preventative) cesareans for women who have a history of herpes is suspect.*

Since herpes is a stress-related disease, perhaps the effects of stress during labor and birth should be studied. In order to prevent neonatal herpes perhaps we should be looking for methods of giving both mothers and babies low-stress births.

40

Repeating Indications??

LEO SORGER, *OB/GYN*

LEO: Gloria had had her first baby with another doctor. The labor had been a prolonged prodromal (slow-onset-type) labor. After the first day she was admitted to the hospital and the doctor did a cesarean.

Gloria came to me for a VBAC with the next pregnancy. I assured her that a long latent-phase labor would not necessarily lead to a cesarean. And it did not.

Labor began, and once again, she had the same pattern as she had had with the first labor. She labored with contractions every 8–10 minutes for 3 days. She came to the hospital during her first day of labor, and I said, "You're not really in labor. Go home. I'll even give you a sleeping pill." Gloria slept. The next day the same thing happened. I checked her and said, "No, you're not doing anything. Go home. Take your sleeping pill." The third day she came back, and this time she was really in labor—about 5–6 centimeters dilated. She made fine progress, had the baby vaginally, and was very happy that she had a natural childbirth.

41

My Favorite Story

MITCH LEVINE, *OB/GYN*

A couple came to me who I especially liked. They had their first baby with another doctor at Beth Israel Hospital. She had a long labor. The doctor did an x-ray, and said, "Absolutely, no way could a baby ever fit through your pelvis." She had a cesarean.

She came to me early in the next pregnancy. She was due in the middle of July, and I told her I was going to be away for the whole month. I told her she should look for another doctor who would not be away in July. However, she said she really wanted to work with me for her prenatal care, and would accept my backup doctor for the delivery.

At the end of the pregnancy I left for my trip, and came back just for half a day in the middle of the month. I was curious to see if she had delivered. I called her and she said she hadn't had her baby yet.

She and her husband were avid windsurfers, and they invited me to come to the lake with them that day, to teach me to windsurf. When I got to the lake, she was already out windsurfing. And when she came into shore she told me her labor had begun while she was out on the lake.

I never learned to windsurf that day because we immediately left for the hospital. Two hours later she delivered a 9-pound baby, a pound and a half bigger than her first baby.

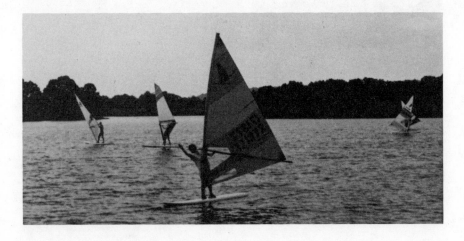

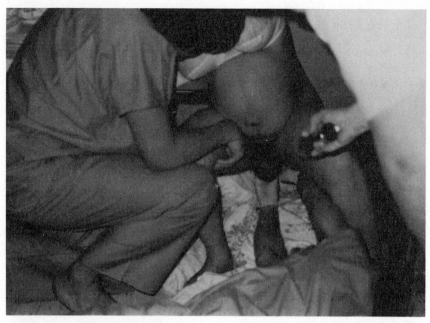

Dr. Mitch Levine, lying on the hospital floor to assist with the birth. The flashlight enables the doctor to see while the other lights are dimmed.

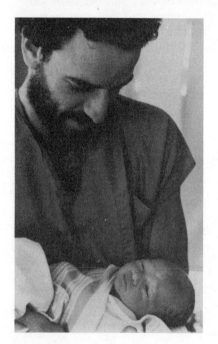

Dr. Mitch Levine, holding newborn

42

Two Out of Three Ain't Bad!

PIXIE WILLIAMS, M.D.

I can't remember when I first heard about VBAC—I just knew intuitively that it had to be right. My guiding motto in my practice of medicine has always been: "Above All, Do No Harm," which I take to mean: "Nature (usually) knows best, and you had better have a darned good reason for going against her."

It's bad enough for a woman to undergo major surgery (even if truly necessary) for the birth of her baby. How much worse to have that immediately foretell a future of major surgeries with each subsequent child! I dimly remembered hearing of women who had beat the odds by having their VBAC babies unintentionally by simply laboring and birthing before the surgery could be done. What an incredible natural force there is behind normal birthing! Surely, I reasoned, nature would not have those labors ensue without a very good reason—or at least *the burden of the proof is on us,* her relatively ignorant assistants, to prove beyond a doubt that VBAC is wrong and dangerous (if that is what we believe to be true).

I'm in the unusual position of being better informed and more progressive than most of my patients. (Probably those consumers in the forefront of change generally seek out midwives, and alternative health-care providers rather than a doctor at a community health center.) Betsy was my first patient who had had a previous cesarean. When I asked, "Have you thought about having your next child vaginally?" her eyes widened a little as she said, "No . . . is that really a possibility?" I thought to myself, "She probably thinks I'm crazy . . ." But Betsy was to become my most ardent supporter of VBAC.

By some quirk of fate I found myself with three VBAC patients early that summer, all due in the fall. To assuage my own anxiety I did copious literature searches on the topic but was still afraid to bring it up with any colleagues. When I heard that Lynn was doing workshops on VBAC for potential clients, I jumped at the chance.

I knew that in suggesting a VBAC to my patients, we were venturing into controversial territory, so I felt that it was of the utmost importance to me that my patients be well informed, prepared, and aware of any potential risks, and *most of all, aware that the responsibility and choice of VBAC was theirs, not mine.*

Unfortunately, our society has been programmed to "give up" responsibility for health choices to their doctors. I've never been comfortable with being responsible for other people's choices—in fact, I think it's a matter of denial (on all sides) of the fact that *one cannot give over responsibility* for one's choices to the "experts." The attempt itself to give over that responsibility is a choice—a choice which presumes that "modern medical technology" has the answers for the "right way" to handle things. However, just the opposite is true. In most instances, medicine does NOT know what is "right"—the answers are not to be found etched in stone. One must struggle to determine for oneself what is right. It's much easier, of course, to deny that uncertainty, and give the responsibility to the experts.

At the end of the VBAC workshop weekend my head was spinning with doubts. The workshop was over, and only my first patient, Betsy, seemed certain that VBAC was what she wanted and COULD HAVE. Bernice wanted a VBAC badly, but was full of self-doubt about whether she could do it. Evelyn was unconvinced. To her, it sounded unpleasant to go through a labor again, and what for? She felt "fine" about her cesarean. I felt discouraged. It seemed like only Betsy had a chance of doing it because of her positive attitude. I had hoped for more transformation in the others. After talking it over with Lynn, I tried to satisfy myself with having at least raised their consciousness about the issue of *responsibility*, even if they weren't ready to deal with it in a positive way. I sensed, too, that there was still some personal growth ahead for each of them in the last few months of their pregnancies.

Betsy was due first, much to my relief, since I felt she was practically a sure bet to succeed. Her first section had been for breech, her second a routine repeat. She had less feeling of failure to reckon with and had already faced up to the fact that she had unquestioningly bowed to her obstetrician's expertise when it came to her repeat section. She was excited and determined. Because of her previous passivity, and her positive attitude now, I figured she would have to come out ahead from the whole experience, even if for some reason her VBAC "failed." She had made tremendous personal growth during her pregnancy.

Betsy's labor started around 10:00 P.M., two weeks after her due date. We excitedly went to the hospital. She would have liked to have tried a home VBAC, but I was not yet attending home births at the time. By 2:00 A.M. she was 5–6 centimeters, but by 4:00 A.M. she was only 6 centimeters with vertex at 0 to +1 station. She was tired, and I chose (with her consent) to rupture her bulging membranes in the hope that the head would work better against the cervix to dilate it.

The head never came down well against the cervix, and it remained a loose 6, in spite of uncomfortable contractions every 2 to 5 minutes from then on. We tried everything but standing on her head—squatting, knee-chest, bearing down, etc. At noon I suggested an IV with glucose in the hope that it would give her contractions some extra strength (she wasn't able to drink because of vomiting); she refused the IV. To her the IV represented hospital technology and I think would have meant defeat.

Betsy was still determined. At 4:00 P.M. (she had been at 6 centimeters for 12 hours) I gently voiced my feeling that she had given it her best try, but that it wasn't going to work. She and her husband dealt with that realization. They discussed as well the possibility of her having a tubal, and decided against it because to her that would mean even more violation of her body. We all prepared for her cesarean. At about 6:30 P.M. (20 hours after her labor began) she had her third section, and *for the first time,* her husband was present, she was awake, and she was allowed to see and touch her daughter immediately. For all that she was happy—at least this section had met her needs more than the others.

I was exhausted and drained. I had been pleasantly surprised by the reasonably supportive attitudes of the general surgeons who do cesareans at our small community hospital. They seemed to feel, as I do, that VBAC is a choice we can offer in spite of the fact that we are not a university hospital with the ability to do a STAT (immediate) section in 15 minutes. A STAT section in 15 minutes is a MYTH. I had trained in several of the best hospitals in Boston and New York, and had *never* seen a STAT section pulled off in less than 30 minutes.

After Betsy's birth was over, I wondered if I had the strength to go through two more of these VBAC labors. At least the other two had been through labors before, and might go faster, or might even give up much sooner. I was worried about the effect Betsy's "failure" would have on the other two. Bernice was initially discouraged, while Evelyn was her usual noncommittal self. Soon, though, I realized that Betsy's outcome was in one sense positive for the other two—it gave them permission to *fail,* which they probably needed in order to *try.*

Twelve days after her due date, Bernice called me in the middle of the night to tell me that her waters had broken and that she was having contractions. I had been away studying with some midwives. I raced to the hospital from 2-1/2 hours away.

BERNICE: We arrived at the hospital about 4:00 A.M. and the doctor covering for Pixie said I was 3 centimeters and zero station. I thought to myself, "I'm farther along now than I'd been with Ben after 28 hours, and there's no stopping me!" That totally relaxed me—so much so that I slept between contractions, and was still sleepy during contractions. The nurses left us alone, except to check on us once in a while.

Looking back, I was so tense during labor with Benjamin that I didn't allow myself to be aware of the progress of his labor. I was so concerned with the breathing techniques from Lamaze classes, I wasn't paying attention to what my body was telling me. With Molly's labor, just tuning into my contractions, and letting events happen was so much easier for me. During transition, the urge to push was so strong, but Dick kept telling me to relax and let the baby come. I did just what he said, and found the contractions seemed harder, but at the same time, they were easier to deal with.

COMMENTS: *Transition is that part of labor where the sensation of dilatation of the cervix is coupled with the sensation of descent of the baby. The woman is working with two sensations at once. She is still feeling the intensity of the contracting uterus to complete dilatation. However, in addition to that sensation, she begins to experience the deep and ever-mounting pressure of the baby moving down and out of her pelvis. She may or may not be experiencing an actual urge to push. She may simply feel that her bottom is "splitting open." Relaxing into transition contractions increases the pressure of the baby moving down through the pelvis. This downward pressure (soon to become the urge to push) is often the sensation that women resist. They unconsciously tense their pelvic floor muscles and ligaments (that hold the pelvic organs in place) thereby holding the baby up from below. Thus the baby is prevented from moving down, and progress is impeded. Releasing into this downward pressure causes the pressure to increase, but with the release comes the inner connection of moving into the sensation, and letting go, thus facilitating an efficient and progressive labor.*

PIXIE: By the time I got to the hospital, Bernice was 9 centimeters, and totally involved in her experience.

BERNICE: Pixie checked me and said, "I almost missed the delivery! Would you like to give birth in bed, or use a birthing chair?" I sat in that chair, and thought, "Why couldn't I have sat here earlier, instead of sitting on the toilet seat?" It took so much pressure off!

PIXIE: Bernice's second stage was less than an hour.

BERNICE: Before I had a chance to think about what happened, Molly was in my arms. All I could do was look at her, touch her, talk to her. I didn't even know what was going on around me. I couldn't get over how Molly and I seemed to already know what we each wanted or needed.

PIXIE: The whole thing was so quick and smooth, that we all (Bernice, her husband, and myself) could hardly believe it was over—the force and wisdom of nature!

As time passed I wasn't quite as discouraged as I had been about the outcome of Evelyn's impending labor. She had offhandedly said during one of our office visits, "Oh, of course I'll try a VBAC, and I'll probably do it." I figured she might do it in spite of herself—in spite of her attempt to distance herself from the whole thing.

Evelyn went into labor one morning about two weeks later. Her labor was one of the easiest I have ever seen—about 5 hours of regular contractions during which she chatted and watched soap operas. She was fully dilated but remained unconvinced—"Last time the labor was easy, too, but it was the pushing that didn't work."

The indication for Evelyn's first section had been "soft tissue dystocia" (unyielding non-bony soft tissue was preventing the birth from occurring). She had adequate room in her pelvis. The baby's head was at +2 station when they did the cesarean. It had already passed through the most narrow transverse (side to side) axis of the pelvis, and technically it should have been able to be born vaginally. However, apparently her pelvic floor muscles were so tense that pushing was totally unsuccessful.

With Evelyn's VBAC labor, I saw an amazing transition as she began to push. She changed from being relaxed and chatty, to being tense and

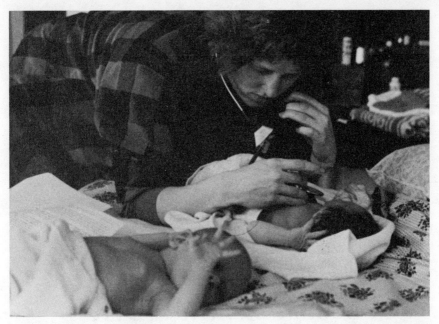

Dr. Pixie Williams, examining a newborn after a home birth, accompanied by her 2-week-old son, Ethan

almost panic stricken. As she let herself really push and felt the head come down, she seemed overwhelmed by the force within her. The feeling of "letting go" clearly terrified her. It was easy to see what had gone wrong the first time. I tried to deal with that fear, to help her to relax, to calm her, and she gave birth to her child.

I had cut an episiotomy because I didn't feel that we could work together to ease the head out, and ended up with the worst extension I'd ever had—to (but not through) the rectal sphincter, and a small tear through the floor of the vagina.

The episiotomy repaired quite smoothly, but she later claimed that having those stitches and having sore buttocks from sitting in a hospital bed for three days (her choice of how long to stay) were as bad as her section had been. I chuckled to myself, "Sometimes you just can't win . . .".

COMMENTS: *Not until we confront the fact that a good birth is not necessarily a painless birth will we absorb the full richness of the experience of birthing our babies naturally.*

PIXIE: Betsy and I are still dealing with her "failure." We've analyzed it from every angle. Did the previous uterine scars interfere? Should I not have ruptured her membranes? Would the IV have mattered? Would she have done better at home? Was her nutritional state less than perfect? Should she have tried to sleep for a night during the labor, rather than trying so hard to give birth?

The answers to these questions are nowhere to be found, so I am left back with my fundamental belief that *sometimes we cannot know why things turn out as they do, and often we must live with that mystery.*

Betsy is still asking the questions, though, and I feel the need to help her sort it out. I recently suggested she get in touch with another woman in our area who had a very similar experience and outcome. That woman said to me, "I think maybe I copped out . . . that I knew I had a way out through a section all along, and I just didn't give it my all . . . But I feel okay about it now. I've forgiven myself." I think Betsy *did* give it her all, but I think she has NOT yet forgiven herself. I think she expects much more of herself now than before this pregnancy, but I think she needs to be able to forgive herself for being less than perfect as well.

43

Commitment to VBAC

KENNETH MCKINNEY,
OB/GYN

Back in 1978 when I first started attending VBAC women, VBAC wasn't something that patients were talking about. It was hard to get information on VBAC and it was hard to find a woman who had had a VBAC.

At that time we gave everybody who was interested in VBAC a packet of journal articles which supported VBAC, and the names and phone numbers of the women in the local VBAC support group. For most women knowing there was literature and a support group available was all they needed to feel good about having a VBAC. They would take this information readily saying, "Oh, thank you very much. I'm really happy to have this information."

However, one woman, Nancy, came to our practice because she was good friends with the nurse that was working in my office at that time. When I gave her the VBAC information, this woman said, "Oh, no thank you, that's fine." I hate to prejudge people by way they carry themselves and the way they talk, but this was a woman who never had a hair out of place, and never really talked about "Gee, I hope this baby will come out vaginally. . . ."

Something just didn't sit right, at least by the tenor of the times and the way most women were approaching it. Nancy never had any fears about it . . . Never had any qualms or questions . . . At that time almost But this woman never talked about any fears or concerns.

When Nancy came in in labor, she was all duded up, wearing a real pretty nightgown. She just sat in bed with the head of the bed up, made 5 centimeters, and said, "I've had my trial of labor. I want a repeat cesarean section." She had just begun to get into the active phase of labor, and she just didn't want to have to be bothered with the pain. You truly have to be committed to having a VBAC, and I don't think she was!

As I look back over my years of VBAC experience, I realize that a number of women whose trials of labors had ended with repeat cesareans did not have cesareans because of physiology. They had cesareans not because they were physically unable to deliver their babies vaginally. They had repeat cesareans because they chose to have repeat cesareans.

* * *

It is with deep regret that I report Ken McKinney's death. He committed himself and his life to mothers and babies. He never placed himself on a pedestal, but most of those who knew him would have placed him there. The world has truly lost a special being.

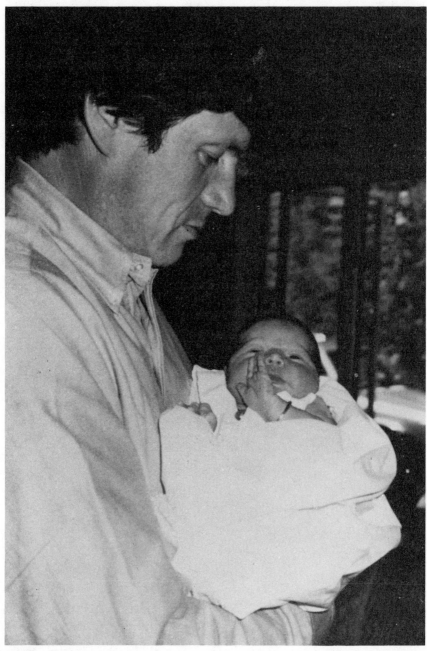

Ken McKinney, with his niece, Morgan Leonard. "Morgan's parents, who live in California, came to New Hampshire to have Morgan, their first child. On July 20, 1986 at 1:20 A.M., Morgan (8 lb., 10 oz.) was born in the guest room of Ken's home," writes Carol Leonard, midwife and wife of Ken McKinney.

44

By the Skin of Her Teeth

ALEXANDRA PAYTON, *Midwife* and
BARRY GOLDIN, *OB/GYN*

ALEXANDRA: Deva had been planning a hospital birth with the two local obstetricians. Here in Oregon obstetricians are rather relaxed about hospital routines, but most of the new-age women in this small community have home births. So I think Deva felt a good deal of pressure to perform from her peers. Late in the pregnancy she came to see me about doing a home birth.

However, not only did her husband, Rama, not want a home birth, he didn't want to be at the labor. He didn't want to see her in great suffering and agony.

I don't think she ever pictured herself giving birth at home with Rama at her side, or even holding her baby after the birth.

I also sensed that she didn't do too well with discomfort or pain. Whenever the baby's head would pivot and turn a little bit on her cervix at the end of her pregnancy, she would call me up really late at night to tell me it hurt. It almost seemed as if her feelings were hurt—as if the baby were hurting her, doing something wrong to her. It brought her to tears.

When Deva went into labor, I went to her house. She appeared to be in transition. She was barely breathing—holding her breath to hold everything up to avoid the pain. She didn't want to let her breath go because then the baby would come down and the pain increased.

I didn't examine her. She didn't want to be touched. I think she didn't want to be touched because she would relax into those touching hands. As she would relax she would let the baby down, and she she didn't like that. She coped with her labor similarly to the type of meditation where instead of contemplating something and moving into it, you push things away. She seemed to spend a lot of time pushing things away perhaps because she didn't know what she could move towards. Perhaps if I had examined her that night and had told her that she was perhaps two centimeters, I could have said, "You know, we really can't go on like this." But I didn't. So, that first night I just tried to help her let out her breath.

I examined her that morning and she was four centimeters. But her cervix was very stretchy. Her uterus was working very well, but the head hadn't come down onto the cervix. I asked if I could keep my fingers in during the contraction, and with the next contraction, I stretched her cervix to eight centimeters. But as soon as she went to eight, she planted her heels and pulled way up, and of course pulled the baby back up. It was "back to the drawing board."

I asked her if we could try it again. I had just begun to edge the cervix back, and she yelled. Rama was really furious. He said, "You're hurting her."

Deva and Rama also had a friend, Krishna, whose wife had just had a cesarean. He kept calling Rama during the labor. He belongs to the same spiritual group that Deva and Rama belong to, and Rama somehow bows his head to him. Rama would come back after talking to him and say, "Well, Krishna said this, Deva . . ." and "Krishna said that. . . ."

Rama was really pushing for transport after he talked to his friend. However, there was no medical indication for transport. The baby sounded all right. There was no problem. But I decided to transfer because Deva didn't seem to believe anything else would ever happen at home. I decided to go to a physician in Eugene (almost two hours away) who I knew would be very patient, and try to help Deva have a decent birth. I also didn't want to wait too long at home and be forced later on into a transport to the nearest hospital.

Just the year before I had called the local hospital to report that I wanted to transfer a woman who had thick meconium staining. They said, "Oh, thick meconium is no big deal." I said, "Well, we also have tachycardia (fast heart tones)." And they said, "We don't worry about that." I listened to one more contraction after I talked to them, and the baby's heart was just racing. The fluid was thick like clay. So we went in to the hospital. The woman labored there for five more hours, and they finally did a forceps delivery. The baby was born pink, but covered with meconium. The baby's pink tone told us that he was born in good condition.

But the baby was not suctioned well on the perineum. He gasped and inhaled meconium, and from there his condition worsened. His breaths were labored, and his color quickly changed to grey.

The oxygen at the hospital didn't work. They couldn't get their suction going. The pediatrician went crazy. The respiratory therapist attempted to assist in setting up the ambu bag (an instrument used for newborn resuscitation), but the pediatrician thought he was sending the oxygen out the wrong end, so she tore the extendor off the ambu bag and threw it across the room. She made the nurses crazy. She was screaming so that the nurses were dropping things on the floor. It was a bad movie! The baby was flown to the ICU in Portland, and finally died there two weeks later from meconium aspiration pneumonia.

As midwives we usually decide to transport to the hospital because we believe that the people there have more equipment and experience with newborn intubation and resuscitation. However, after witnessing the hospital's mismanagement, I realized that we might have had a better outcome had we stayed at home, monitored the woman vigilantly, and suctioned the baby properly on the perineum.

I had been exceedingly frightened by this experience. Although Deva's labor was not yet characterized by the same physical symptoms of meconium and mild distress, psychologically Deva's labor was extremely reminiscent of the other woman's labor. Inside of myself I felt that I would do anything to prevent that from happening again.

I decided to bring Deva to Barry Goldin, OB/GYN, in Eugene. I was glad to be able to transfer to a hospital and doctor I really trusted.

After we had made the decision to transport, I went into the bathroom to gather some of Deva's personal items to pack for the hospital. I noticed large brown apothecary-sized bottles of tylenol, codeine, and percaset (a codeine derivative). And suddenly I thought to myself that perhaps she had been taking these drugs all through her labor without my knowledge. She had looked strange, and I realized now that I was very naive because I just never thought that a woman who was planning a home birth would take drugs.

When we arrived at the hospital, Deva was seven centimeters. I had been hoping that during the transfer that all that moving around might help the baby down. But Deva moved as little as she possibly could. She waited in the parking lot for a wheel chair to come. I was very disappointed that the nurses spotted us where I had parked the car. I thought we'd have to at least walk all around the hospital to get in. But some very kindly nurse came out with a wheel chair for Deva.

Deva actually got worse when we got to the hospital, because she didn't like the walking or having to continue to relax and deal with her labor. She thought going to the hospital would mean that she would get medication. A couple of times she asked Barry for pain medication and when she asked the second time he said, "As your servant and doctor, I wouldn't withhold from you something that you wanted just because I had the key. But I would discourage you in any way that I could from taking medication. You might not feel too proud of yourself afterwards." She never asked for the pain medication again.

Though of course I know that Deva truly wanted to give birth herself, I almost felt like we were tricking her by forcing her along.

BARRY: As long as we were never dishonest with them, it's not trickery. Sometimes you have to do things to push people—like confronting her about her relationship with her husband, or making her walk to the hospital. That's pushing her, not really tricking her.

When I first walked into the labor room, Deva just looked totally withdrawn, she was like a shell. She was really weak and tired, sort of huddled up in the bed, cowering. Terrible. Throughout the labor I noticed that there was almost no interaction between her and her husband, no eye contact, no physical contact.

ALEXANDRA: He had slept during most of the labor at home.

BARRY: He would start talking to me about totally inappropriate things. He started talking to me about business right in the middle of her contractions.

ALEXANDRA: Once we got to the hospital Rama spent most of his time in the father's lounge, looking for other men to talk to, and seeming very much surprised that there weren't any other men in the waiting room. The other men were in the labor rooms with their wives. But Rama very much avoided supporting Deva in her labor.

Deva needed to get up to pee once in a while. In order to do that she would have to get up off the hospital bed and take two steps to the bathroom. We (myself and the nurses) would offer to help her to do this, by moving a stool over to the bed, and she would say, "No, no. I don't want to go to the bathroom yet."

However, when Rama would occasionally walk into the labor room suddenly she would declare that she needed to get up. She would almost loll off the bed, as if someone should catch her, looking towards Rama to fill that role. She wouldn't drink for me, so I would ask him to offer it to her. I think she did so much want him to help her that it was hard for her to do anything to help herself. But I think that he was uncomfortable with the idea of support and help.

Towards the very end, she sort of laid back into his arms. He would come and sit next to her, only because there wasn't any place else to sit in the room. He must have finally gotten tired enough to really relax into being there with her. She would lean against him and start to melt. Things would look better. But then he would start to resent it for some reason, and he would get up and do something else. I almost thought that if I had taught him some kind of Lamaze technique where you stand there and go, "one, two, three," that he would have liked that a lot better. But I don't think that kind of "support" would have worked for Deva. If Rama could have done something to control the labor. . .

BARRY: I think it's really difficult for men because it's more scary to a man. They have no connection to labor physically or emotionally. So they revert to what they know, which is control. I'm sure there's a lot of despair. When a man sees his wife going through this intense thing, out of his love for her, he feels helpless. Most men have a hard time perceiving themselves as helpless.

ALEXANDRA: Interestingly, Rama is pretty helpless in their relationship, although he acts like he's the one in control. He had a hard time with her becoming a mother and having the baby because he really is the baby.

COMMENTS: *It is often the case that women have cesareans because they need their husband's love and attention; and fathers often encourage cesareans because they don't want to lose their status as the baby. They really aren't ready for their wife to have a baby.*

ALEXANDRA: I don't think Rama was ever uncomfortable with the idea of having a cesarean. But he was very uncomfortable with birth.

BARRY: With a cesarean, perhaps the father feels more equal to the mother in the birth.

ALEXANDRA: In fact, the man often gets more from the cesarean.

BARRY: Because the woman's knocked out.

ALEXANDRA: The man gets to hold the baby first. He gets to stay with the baby while she is in recovery, so he's the one who gets to bond with the baby, and the mother does not.

During the actual birth he is upright and she is strapped down. The gesture in the birth of the woman bringing forth the child is significant. Rather than the mother GIVING birth and the father receiving the child, when it's a cesarean the father is posed upright across from the doctor with the woman strapped down lying flat between them. She gives them nothing. They only *take* from her.

And, in fact, women will often refer to their cesareans with the phrase "They had to take my baby." They do not say, "I lay on the table and gave the baby to the doctor and my husband." So, even though it may be on an unconscious level, women are aware that their babies have been taken from them.

Rama had a hard time with anything that was physical in a feminine sort of way. He was really afraid of anything blossoming. After the birth Deva disclosed that Rama and she had a very difficult sexual relationship. She rarely got the physical and sexual attention that she needed and wanted. Perhaps giving himself sexually and physically did not blend with his beliefs that men need to be in control of themselves at all times.

When we confronted Deva about her relationship with her husband, at first she denied there was any problem. But then on further confrontation, she actually got angry. But that anger, in and of itself, seemed to help her labor. She seemed to become a little bit more energetic and lively, which was useful.

BARRY: She had been in the hospital about nine hours, and in labor at home for about 12 hours before that. She had had what seemed to be reasonable, frequent, regular strong contractions. Yet apparently she remained at the same place. During a contraction she would dilate to 9 centimeters. But between contractions, she would pull the baby back up, and go back to 7 centimeters.

ALEXANDRA: She would begin to breath deeply as the contraction began and then as it got stronger, she would breath more and more shallowly, so that her breathing was almost imperceptible at the end of the contraction. She was holding her breath up.

BARRY: Generally, I don't like to intervene because I like people to work out what's blocking them for themselves. I very rarely believe in the possibility that the baby doesn't fit. It's usually that there is some kind of block physically or emotionally or spiritually that's preventing the progress. I think it's very valuable for people to work that out for themselves, rather than for us to intervene somehow to push past the point. But I felt in her case we had made numerous attempts to try to get at some kind of emotional issue, to get her to move around more, to do many different things to try to help her to get her labor to progress. But she was really totally unresponsive. Also, we were a little concerned because the baby's heart variability was quite flat.

Therefore, after about nine hours without progress, not having figured out any other thing to do, and not seeing any end in sight, I felt that we should push her along by giving her pitocin. When I use pitocin, (particularly in the face of meconium, which she had) I usually like to use an internal monitor. I feel that as long as things are happening naturally, you remain sort of well protected. But when you start artificially intervening and augmenting the labor with pitocin, then it's very important to do that in the safest way possible. So, we put a monitor in and we started pitocin.

The pitocin was on, I would say not more than five to ten minutes, when what had been just marginally flat heart tones turned into multiple decelerations. So we turned the pitocin off. However, I still was not convinced that the only alternative was cesarean, as it seemed that even that five or ten minutes of pitocin had caused her labor to pick up somewhat.

I don't like to make decisions for people unless it's an extreme emergency where I have to say, "Look, you have to trust me. I have to do this." So usually even if I'm contemplating cesarean, I like the couple to make the decision themselves. They decide for whatever reason, because I think that when they're behind the decision, then they feel better about it afterwards. I want the couple to feel that they're just *using me to perform* the operation, not that I'm doing an operation to them. I think the surgery itself goes better because it's their energy and spirit that's behind it. They don't have the anguish of thinking maybe something else could have been done, or at least they feel they're in control of a situation and it was their choice. I've operated on people who have literally never needed any pain medication and gone home the following day, because they had made the decision to have done whatever was done.

Therefore, I was trying to find out how Deva and Rama felt about the possibility of having a cesarean. As soon as the subject was broached, Rama very clearly asked for a cesarean. Then I said, "Okay, Deva, what do you think?" And her husband said, "She wants a cesarean." I said, "No, no, Deva, what do you think?" Her husband said, "She wants a cesarean." And then I finally turned to him and I said, "You know, I really appreciate your wisdom in this, but what I would like to hear is Deva's thoughts on this because I feel it's very important for both of you to make the decision." He said, "I agree with you. Deva wants a cesarean." He even wanted her to have general anesthesia. When I said to Deva that perhaps right now she'd be happy with general, but that it may be a very disturbing to her for a long time afterwards, he said, "We don't care about later."

ALEXANDRA: Then we left the two of them alone together. Rama was really angry at us. As we were leaving I said to them, "It's possible that while we are gone that Deva could suddenly dilate again." Rama put his hand on her head, and said in a hypnotic monotone, "No, what Deva wants. . . ."

BARRY: We made preparations to do a cesarean. I had told her that if she continued to have no progress, I didn't see any other option. But when I was out talking with the nurses during that hour, they said, "Well, are you going to do one?" And I said, "Well, let's have everything ready in case we develop fetal distress, but I'm really not convinced yet that we need to do that."

ALEXANDRA: Actually, I wanted to have the cesarean done more than Barry did. When I saw the late decelerations coupled with early meconium I really felt scared. I had that hospital transport last year after which the baby had died from meconium aspiration, and I think the labor was just too similar for me.

BARRY: It's probably a different feeling being the midwife or being the doctor in that place, because as a physician you feel that you have that under control. You have a monitor on, and if at any point the baby started showing signs of distress that did not recover right away, you have the cesarean. You can take out the baby in a few minutes.

ALEXANDRA: That should be the advantage of a hospital birth. Since all the equipment is there you can actually let things go further than you could if you're at home. Instead of hospital births being intervened faster, they should be able to wait even longer to intervene.

BARRY: After a short time Deva and Rama decided (maybe he decided, maybe she did) that they wanted a cesarean. They said, "Check us now, because we want a cesarean." I said, "Let's wait 40 minutes." Then after only about 20 *minutes,* they called me back again and said, "No, we want the cesarean now, can you check us now?"

ALEXANDRA: Barry came back in to check Deva. She was much more relaxed now, and she leaned back against Rama as Barry began his exam. Without a word, Barry braced his arm against her left knee, and gently pushed the cervix back over the head.

Midwives generally don't try to intervene without first asking a woman's permission, but had Barry asked Deva first for her permission to try to push her cervix back, she probably would have tightened up and screamed just as she had done at home with me. However, as she was relaxed because she felt that this was just the last exam before her cesarean, it worked. When Barry took his hand out, he said, "Well, you've got nothing in your way now. You're fully dilated. You can push your baby out." Actually, Rama looked very angry. Even Deva looked a little aggravated at this new turn of events.

I think we could have stayed home for a week, and she still wouldn't have had her baby. I think that I really wasn't medical enough for her, in that if I had done more things like frequent exams, it would have been better for her. I usually don't use a doppler, unless I really can't hear the baby. I think that disturbed her. I think she would have felt safer if I had used a doppler. There are people who feel better if you keep all of your instruments and equipment out of visibility (but close by in case you need it). And there are other people who feel safer if you put IV bottles on their dressers. I think Deva would have liked it if all the equipment had been hanging around her.

BARRY: She wanted a hospital birth at home.

ALEXANDRA: I had hoped that in suggesting transport that she would feel safe enough let go and to have her baby. But I think that it wasn't until she had already planned her cesarean, and Rama told her, "It's all over now," that she allowed herself to let go.

Although we usually have a woman wait for the urge to push, in this case we instructed her to push. Within four or five contractions her own urges to push took over and she was actually into her labor for the first time. As a new contraction would start to build, Deva would lean up more and breathe gently but deeply (as she hadn't been breathing before), and intermittently bear down with her own body's rhythm making great progress. We were already seeing some of the baby at the peak of the contractions.

Rama had been silent during this time while the nurses and I were teaching her to push. But as soon as he saw her moving with the pushing with her own rhythm, he became very instructive. Even though we had by now backed off completely with our instructions, and were only offering comfort measures between contractions, he was being quite bossy about the way she was pushing. He would tell her to push as long and hard as she could. Even when it was apparent that the contraction had ended and she was leaning back into the pillows to relax, he would say, "You should push more with that contraction." Yet, at the peak of the contraction, he would tell her, "Now, don't push if you don't have a contraction." After watching this a few times and biting my lip, I finally worked actively with her by saying, "You've got it, just go with it, open up for your baby." And in between contractions, I would say, "When you feel the contraction has ended just lean back and relax."

Deva really loved pushing. She had color again. She was excited. She was totally involved with herself and the sensations of her body.

BARRY: At the end, with all the concerns about the baby and the cesarean, her husband got really involved. He was right there with her. He had not even been on the bed with her until that point. He had been on the other side of the room during the whole labor. But when she was pushing, he was right there with her, telling us what to do, telling her what to do. But he was right there, and I think that that was very crucial for her. Maybe the rest of the struggle with the labor was the only way she knew of getting him to be there for her.

ALEXANDRA: Deva was in a borning bed (a bed that can break down like a delivery table). The little seat part was laid back with the bottom still attached. As she gently birthed her baby, Barry laid the baby about 6 inches beneath her on a warm baby blanket. He did not put the baby on her belly. He just said, "Go ahead, pick up your baby." She picked him up, held him, and kissed him on his head. She really welcomed her baby.

Deva has had incredible closeness with Arjuna, her son, from the very first moment and has had confidence in herself as a mother. When I see her with her son now, I can't help but to think of when she just scooped him up like that, and held him. I do wonder if the birth had been a cesarean, if they would have had to reach across many barriers to find this kind of closeness that they naturally have now. It seems to me that in pushing her baby out, Deva burst through a barrier, and she was then clear on the other side of it to meet her baby.

45

The Spitting Image of His Father

ANASTASIA HOLMES, *Midwife*

Allison was pregnant with her first baby, but there was a question of paternity. The man who was most likely the father was Mike, with whom she had been living for a few years. However, it was also possible that the father of her baby was James, a man with whom she had been having an affair.

Allison and Mike had not had a very smooth relationship, and there were times when he had emotionally and physically abused her. She was under his power of authority, and as soon as the pregnancy was confirmed, Mike made it quite clear that she should have an abortion.

So, Allison made an appointment to have an abortion. James, out of his love for her, volunteered to go with her to the clinic to support her during this time. The abortion was scheduled for early afternoon. She and James met at his house in the morning. As they talked over lunch Allison expressed her reticence about having an abortion. She told him that she was getting older and had been thinking about having a baby even before she became pregnant. And now that she was pregnant, she felt she really wanted to have the baby.

As a total surprise to her, James offered to marry her, move away to Oregon with her, and have the baby together. It was shortly after their move to Oregon that I met Allison and James. Although at the time of our meeting Allison did disclose that she was not sure about the paternity of her baby, she did not want to talk about her feelings. In fact, in her mind it seemed that all her problems had already been resolved out of the kindness of her husband, James.

However, about a month before her due-date, Mike telephoned her. She felt very threatened, but still chose to keep her feelings to herself.

When Allison went into labor, she called me immediately. She wanted my assistant and me to come to help her. She was having a hard time dealing with her labor. When we arrived Allison appeared to be in transition, but she was only one centimeter dilated. Six hours later, she was still only 1 centimeter, and five hours after that she was 2 centimeters. She needed me to be there with her every minute. Everytime I went downstairs to have a nap, she would scream until I came back. The only way she would stop screaming was if I was touching her the whole time.

Finally, she got up to go the bathroom and said, "I don't think I want to do this. I don't think I want this baby." So I sent her husband into the bathroom with her, to be alone with her. A few minutes later he came out to talk to me. He asked, "Do you think this has anything to do with Allison feeling badly about the baby's father?" I said I thought it did. Many women in labor will say, "I don't think I want to do this," or "I don't want to be in labor," but I had never before heard a woman say that she didn't want the baby.

Usually I don't interfere because I believe that the woman needs to resolve her feelings internally. But Allison started saying that she wanted to go to the hospital and have a cesarean with general anesthesia. So, in order to buy time, I said to her, "No one's going to be at the hospital at this time of night to set up for a cesarean, so if you go to the hospital now you're only going to have to do this agonizing labor under the constraints of the hospital monitors, which will only make labor more painful. Perhaps we should wait a few hours until everyone will be there. Then you can just go in and have a cesarean." I wanted her to feel that she could relax and not worry that we were going to force her to birth this baby. She seemed to feel so strongly that birthing this baby was not something that she wanted to do.

My feeling was that she didn't want to see this baby be born. I asked her if she could have this baby with absolutely no pain whatsoever, would she want to see it born? Did she think this baby would look like this awful man with whom she had lived? Did she not want to see this baby who would look like him come out of her body?

There were times during this conversation that her friend would interject, "Oh, but you really love this baby, Allison." And I would motion to her to wait, because I felt that Allison really needed the space to release her negative feelings first, before she could uncover her real feelings that, of course, she loved her baby.

Then I told Allison a story of another woman in a similar circumstance whose birth I had attended. This woman had conceived a baby with a man she did not know very well. As time passed and she grew to know him better, she grew to dislike him more and more. When her baby was first born she loved and cuddled her baby for a short time. Then she put on her glasses, looked at the baby, and said in a rejecting tone moving a bit a way from the baby, "Oh, he looks just like Marvin (the father)." But then I noticed her wry face changing into a grin, and then into a loving smile as she looked into her baby, saying, "Oh, but if you look into his eyes, you can see who he really is. Of course his shape looks a little like Marvin, and of course he would have to I guess, but when you look into his eyes, you can really see him. Oh, just look at him, isn't he a wonderful boy!" I told Allison this story so that in case this baby did look like Mike, all she would have to do is look into the baby's eyes, and she would know just who he was.

Finally, Allison shared that she did not want to hurt James who had been so good to her, by birthing this other man's baby in front of him. She was so appalled by this situation that she felt she could not complete the act of birthing this baby.

Then I asked her, "When you decided to keep this baby and not have the abortion, did you feel like this at all?"

"During the pregnancy after you and James had married and planned for the coming of this baby, did you feel like this at all?"

And she answered quietly, "No, no . . ." as if she were very much in touch with that feeling of loving the baby and being loved by James.

And when I asked, "How did you feel when you first felt the baby move?" she just looked totally radiant.

Then her friend said, "All this baby needs is that word of love to come from you now." She cried and cried with her friend, and I left to wash my hands.

Over the sound of the running water, I heard a familiar sound. I could hardly believe my ears. Could she? So soon? I turned off the water and listened more carefully. My ears had not lied to me! What I had heard was the familiar catch in the throat, the sound of bearing down. Within a half-hour from the time we had started this discussion, Allison had moved from 2 centimeters to pushing!

Within another half-hour her baby was born.

Once Allison realized that her fears—that this baby was this man— were not reality, she was able to connect once again with her baby. She was able to realize that though she had had no conscious wish to conceive a child, that indeed unconsciously she had asked this child to come to her. Now she needed only to open the door for him. Once she realized that she did indeed love her baby, she was able to give birth quickly and easily.

I feel that it was very important for this woman not to have had a cesarean because I think it would have been very harmful to her relationship with her baby. Having a cesarean would have allowed Allison to turn her back to her baby. It would have allowed this baby to be born without her participation and removed from her so she didn't have to deal with him. Though Allison and her baby might have been able to reweave a connection later, I feel there would always have been a soul-rift, some kind of tear, between the baby and the mother.

46

Knockout

PHYLLIS MALONEY,
R.N., C.C.E.

A young black couple, Glen and Linda, were actually still single, but considered themselves married in the eyes of God. She was 17 and he was 19, and they had been sexually active since she was

14. They never used birth control. They believed that when she got pregnant that this was what God wanted. They were very happy during the course of the pregnancy. When they came for childbirth classes, they listened very intensely, and had lots of questions.

When she went into labor, they went to the hospital. She was laboring slowly but surely. However, the doctor didn't think she was progessing fast enough. There were no other complications—no fetal distress, no increasing blood pressure, just slow progress.

After 14 hours, she was 6 centimeters. The doctor determined that she had "failure to progress," which he told them might lead to fetal distress. He told her they were going to do a cesarean. He didn't ask her, he told her. The couple conferred between themselves and decided to refuse the cesarean.

However, the doctor ignored the couple's refusal to have the cesarean. Even though to Glen and Linda this was an important decision made from their deep convictions, the hospital saw them as young crazy kids, and presumed they were ignorant because of their minority status. The hospital was surprised at this couple's assertiveness, and actual refusal to follow what the hospital was attempting to force upon them.

So instead of acknowledging their refusal for surgery, the hospital personnel proceeded to roll her gurney down to the OR. Glen followed them down the hall, keeping in the background. No one noticed that he was there. The OR had a little window that he watched through. He watched the doctor pick up an instrument, which he thought was a scalpel. In a state of panic, he burst into the operating room. He punched the doctor. The doctor was on the floor. Everyone rushed to help the doctor.

Meanwhile, Linda was screaming, "The baby's coming!" Glen rushed to Linda and caught the baby. Within seconds there were security guards in the operating room, pressing charges against Glen for assault. He replied that if they were going to press charges against him, then he would press charges against the doctor and the hospital for their attempted surgery without consent.

He spent the night at the hospital security office, and was later released. They did not want to be liable for surgery without informed consent.

Afterwards Glen called me to tell me what happened, and said, "I done good, right?"

47

Everything You Didn't Do

CINDY DUNLEAVY, *Midwife*

Christine came to me seeking labor support for a VBAC which she was planning in the hospital with Dr. Sorger. She had had five previous cesareans—three low-segment transverse incisions, and two vertical incisions. The first cesarean was done for a frank breech presentation, and a vertical incision was used. The second was an attempted VBAC with an English doctor, but she had fetal distress. In retrospect Christine felt that the fetal distress had occurred because she was so nervous. For although the doctor supported her efforts to have a VBAC, she felt that perhaps "Once a cesarean, always a cesarean" was in the back of HER mind. The next three cesareans were simply scheduled routine repeat cesareans.

Pregnant now with her sixth baby, Christine lived an hour and a half from Dr. Sorger. But she chose to have him attend her birth, despite the travel involved, because of his noninterventive reputation with VBAC.

Christine had several false labors during which she drove all the distance to the hospital, only to return home still pregnant. Finally after the third false start, she and her husband and her good friend who she referred to as "her sister in the Lord" arrived at the hospital. Dr. Sorger checked her and told her she was 5 centimeters. She remained 5 centimeters for some time.

Then Dr. Sorger came in to check her again, and even though he had found no cervical change, he said, "There is absolutely nothing in the way, nothing stopping this birth." Placing one of his fingers next to his lips, he added, "You're just so soft and loose, just like this." Then he left to go down to the hospital library to work on his charts.

Within a half-hour Dr. Sorger was called to delivery. When he walked in he found his patient cuddling her moments-old baby with tears rolling down her cheeks. He apologized profusely for not having been there for the delivery. She replied with a smile on her face, "Doctor Sorger, I paid you for what you *didn't* do to me."

48

Completely Unscathed

LEO SORGER, *OB/GYN*

LEO: Joan came to me during her second pregnancy. She had seen another doctor for her first baby. During that first labor her dilatation had been "arrested" (delayed) for 2 hours at 6 centimeters. The labor was evidently pretty poor (contracting only mildly and infrequently) at the time, so maybe all she needed to do was to walk around. But the doctor never gave her a chance. He did an immediate cesarean in the absence of maternal or fetal distress.

When she came to me for the second birth she had never heard about VBAC, and was not interested in VBAC classes. I persuaded her to attempt the VBAC.

When she was in labor, she screamed, "I want my C-section now!" But I said, "No way. You're making nice progress and you're having your baby just the right way, and that's it." Then I left and went down to the office. She screamed and hollered, and the nurses called me. So, I said, "OK. Give her 25 mg. of visterol," a small amount of medication, just to help her relax. Two hours later, without further medication or anesthesia, the baby was born naturally. She and her family were so happy and grateful about the birth that they invited me to the christening of the baby.

She had a second VBAC since then, two years ago. With the first VBAC she had a small episiotomy with a few stitches. But the second time she had not one single stitch, and walked out of that hospital completely unscathed—not even a track mark of the baby. This time after the birth she was so happy that she sent me an expensive bottle of German wine, and she's a poor woman, on medicaid. Perhaps we should have put an announcement in the local paper that a woman who had had a previous cesarean could come away from a birth so completely intact. That was so nice, so beautiful.

49

Dispelling the Final Naivete

ISABEL ANDREWS, *Midwife*

Nina first came to me for counseling about VBAC. She was expecting me to give her a pep-talk about why she should have a VBAC, and was surprised when our session together divulged no pat methods to VBAC preparation. As we talked about her needs for this birth (which was coming within a few short weeks), she found herself deeply moved emotionally and spiritually. A few tears flowed gently over her cheeks. A chord had been struck in her, and she wanted to come back for more.

As time passed Nina dealt with many issues which had related to her past cesarean—her fear of becoming a mother and losing her own identity, her past abortion, her relationships with men . . . She worked hard both in our sessions and at home on her own to seek out the growth she needed in order to give birth to this baby naturally. I was deeply impressed with her commitment to her personal growth, and surprised myself by agreeing to attend her planned hospital birth as a labor coach.

Upon my request, at our next meeting Nina brought her husband Nick and mother with her, so that we could meet and discuss our various roles with her labor. Nick was clearly worried about when we would move to the hospital. He did not want to have this baby born at home or in the car, or any place but in the "right" place—the hospital. Nina's mother, however, was quite supportive of staying at home for the labor. She had had four children and understood the value of being up and walking around in labor.

Nina planned that Nick would not be coming to the hospital with us—that he would be out working on their newly started family owned business. I was to call him at the last moment when she began to push, and he would come to the hospital to be there for the birth. I felt that plan was a good one, in that he clearly felt the most anxiety about this labor and birth.

The next visit was the home visit, and Nina and I were alone in her dark quiet house. We did a healing visualization about her abortion, and afterwards she disclosed that she really wanted to have her baby at home with me. She was now a week away from her due date, and her husband was nowhere close to being able to make the transition from hospital-do-anything-the-doctor-says birth to home-take-the-responsibility-yourself birth. So I did not advise her to confront her husband with changing their plans about the place of birth. I suggested that she should talk to her husband about her feelings of safety and comfort, hoping that he might sense her needs and follow them. Then I planted the seed that it was possible that she might have this baby so quickly that there would be no time to make the trip to the hospital.

As we talked there was a strong feeling of closeness, of sisterhood between us. Nina seemed to relax deeply, spoke quietly and moved softly. She talked of her belly—how it had been tightening and relaxing the entire time I had been there. She had the look of labor and, had I stayed with her that evening without interruption, I believe she might have had her baby then and there. But my own family needed me, and as she was not actually in labor, I left.

During the next week or so, Nina had several episodes of contractions during the day, which then stopped when she went to bed. Although these contractions did not progress into active labor, they did do a great deal of work. Prior to these episodes of contractions, her baby's head was still floating and her cervix was only 1 centimeter dilated. The next time I checked her she was 4 centimeters and the head was down to −2. I expected this labor to go very quickly once it became active. Perhaps she really would precipitate this baby at home.

Nina called me a few days past her due date in the middle of the night, saying she was having contractions that felt different and stronger than the others. As her pattern had been contractions during the day which stopped at night, I felt that contractions starting in her sleep was a sign of true labor. I left for her house immediately, as she said she wanted me to come to be with her.

When I arrived almost an hour later I expected to walk quietly into a dimly-lit room with a half-dressed woman having over-powering contractions. But she came to the door fully dressed and greeted me as if she were having a party and I was the first guest to arrive. She and her husband were tidying up the house and planning their next business day.

Nina paused only momentarily at the peak of contractions to squat alone, unsupported. Her contractions passed Nick by completely. He gave her no acknowledgment whatsoever that she was in labor. He would talk to her continuously through contractions about everyday affairs, bustling about around her, as if she should really get this labor over with and get back to business.

It soon became apparent to me that it was difficult for Nina to actually allow the labor to become active because she was so distracted. I escorted her into the bedroom and closed the door with the excuse of examining her. The baby was posterior, about −2 station, and she was 6 centimeters. I was impressed with the progress she had made already considering the atmosphere of her labor, and felt that with focus to bring upon truly active labor, she could progress quickly. She did some posterior-turning exercises on her hands and knees, which she really enjoyed, and then she moved back to the bed to lie on her right side to rest and to continue to encourage rotation of the baby. During these contractions she began to breathe deeply and moan lightly. The pace began to quicken. I felt encouraged.

But every time the contractions would begin to overpower her, and she would begin to release through sounding, Nick would appear in the room to unconsciously interrupt her focus. I didn't want to remove him from the labor because Nina kept trying to get him to become involved. So I tried to find a way to involve him in actual labor support. This was difficult because my attempts at instructing him as to how to support her actually interrupted her energy focus as well. Soon he gave up, and it wasn't long before the haven of her bedroom had been totally invaded by long, involved discussions of complications in plans for the day which were clearly labor-induced.

Nina's parents arrived about 7 A.M. which was quite relieving because her mother could act as a buffer zone between Nick and the privacy of Nina's bedroom. Nina began to regain her focus on the labor, and I checked her again. She was about 7 centimeters, and the baby's head had moved down somewhat. However, it was still not rotated and not yet at 0 station. Since the last cesarean had been done for CPD at full dilatation because of lack of descent, I wanted to stay home with Nina until the baby had at least reached 0 station.

However, I made the devastating tactical error of announcing to Nick what wonderful progress Nina had been making. Much to my surprise, he strode angrily to her bedside, moving close within her space and glared at her demanding, "I thought we discussed this! I thought you told me you would go to the hospital at 6 centimeters!"

Nina cringed into her pillow like a scared puppy. "But the head isn't down yet. I want to stay home until the head comes down," she whimpered as Nick turned his back on her and strode back into the kitchen.

I tried to explain to Nick that Nina needed to be the one to decide when to go to the hospital—not him or me—Nina. But within a few short minutes, Nina conceded that she was ready to go to the hospital, and that she wanted Nick to drive. I suggested that we all go out and take a walk first, just before we leave for the hospital to get the contractions coming stronger and faster. But Nina was afraid to have strong contractions in the car, so she passed on the walk.

In the car the contractions slowed to about 20 minutes apart, and I feared that she would have regressed in dilatation as well. After the usual hospital red tape, Nina was settled in her labor room, (about the size of a large walk-in closet) and the doctor examined her. He told her she was 7 centimeters but that the head was floating. She blurted out, "My midwife checked me at home and the head wasn't floating. It was coming down."

The doctor responded by saying to me, "Since Nina has engaged the professional services of a midwife, it would be confusing to her if we gave her different opinions. Perhaps when it is time to do the next exam that both of us should do the exam together to see if we both agree on our assessment." Since doctors generally do not ascribe to the belief that babies can move back up once they have descended into the pelvis, the doctor's inference was that my skills were of course lacking (since I had assessed her station "wrongly") and therefore he would use this opportunity to "teach me a lesson" and overpower me in the eyes of Nina.

The doctor felt threatened by a midwife who might question his decisions or his authority, or act as a legal malpractice witness if anything were to "go wrong." I knew it would be to Nina's advantage if I could dissipate the threat the doctor felt with my presence. He would be less likely to try to be authoritative with Nina, less likely to rush into an unnecessary cesarean. Therefore, I chose to concede my power to him.

In addition, Nina's disclosure of my role as a midwife placed me in a difficult position. In this state lay midwives are illegal practitioners. If I had accepted the doctor's challenge and done a vaginal exam in his presence, it would have been legal suicide. I had no choice but to turn the power of assessment over to the doctor.

The nurses then came in to attach the external monitor and the IV, neither of which were negotiable. Nina was wired, both physically and emotionally. Then Nick appeared at the door, and I had to leave as only one support person could be present at any one time. I left them alone to talk privately.

Nick left at about 10:00 A.M. saying that he would be back about 3:00 P.M. and to call him if *anything* happened before that (meaning a cesarean), as he didn't really believe that she could have this baby vaginally.

At the next vaginal exam, Nina was 8 centimeters. The doctor shook his head as if she was wasting her time by attempting to labor, not failing to remind her that the baby's head was still floating.

After he left, Nina asked me to check her. I found her to be 8 centimeters with the station at −2 to −3. The head had moved back up from all the tension, but it was certainly *not floating!* It angered me greatly that the doctor defined this station as floating. The baby was still working on rotation. As I examined her, I could feel the baby's head twisting and wiggling (not floating) against my fingers.

Nina was tired and wanted to lie on her side to rest rather than be in an upright position. She hadn't slept all night, and the side-lying position would help to rotate the baby. In addition, it was while she had been lying on her side that her labor had become active at home, so I concurred. Using reflex points and the Logan Basic Contact (a chiropractic technique which lifts the ligaments and relaxes the muscles of the pelvic floor), I tried to help her to release her bottom to let the baby come down—the issue which seemed to be the focus of the doctor's attention.

At noon, an hour after the previous exam, the doctor authoritatively entered the room. Without consideration for whether Nina was having a contraction or whether she was prepared for the exam, he jammed his hand roughly in and out of her vagina and announced, "No change." I found it quite amazing that in literally two seconds he claimed to assess dilatation, descent, rotation, and application of the presenting part!

Nina looked defeated. "Just how long do you want to be 8 centimeters?" he challenged her. She just stared across the room at him.

"Nina, I asked you a question . . . How long do you want to be 8 centimeters?" he demanded.

"I can't answer that question."

"Well, I can't go on without a plan for managing your labor. If you can't tell me how long you plan to be at 8 centimeters, then I'm going to tell you that if you don't consent to having a cesarean by 1:00 P.M. (one hour from then), then you will have to get another doctor."

Tears began to well in Nina's eyes, and I quietly said to the doctor, "Well, Nina will have to think about that," hoping that the doctor would then stop harrassing her and leave us alone.

The doctor strode out, but the nurse began to lecture Nina on the dangers of a protracted labor. I wanted so much to argue with both the doctor and the nurse, but I couldn't because of my position as a lay midwife. All I could do was wait until they had finished with their scare tactics to instill Nina with the truth about her actually impressively progressive labor, given the negative surroundings.

I told Nina that we could easily change doctors if she wanted to, that I knew doctors who would manage her labor differently. She said, "You do? Here, in this hospital?"

"No, not in this hospital. We would have to go to another hospital, but . . ." Then I looked at her fearful eyes. "What are you afraid of, Nina?"

"I promised Nick that I wouldn't go against anything that the doctor said." My hands were tied. What real alternative could I offer her if she couldn't do anything except what the doctor said? I began to wonder why I was there.

Nina called her sister who is a medical student to get her opinion. Her sister was appalled by the doctor's behavior, which gave support to Nina's ability to continue her labor. Then she called Nick, who much to my surprise also supported her laboring at least until 3:00 P.M. when he was planning to return. I hoped that with the support from her family, she might really let go and finish her dilatation.

I got her up, and started belly-dancing and nipple stimulation. We were both dancing together with our eyes closed to music of primal body rhythms. Whenever she would open her eyes and try to come back to the physical reality of the hospital setting, I would quietly remind her to stay in that special labor place. "Let the labor take you away . . . carry you away . . . feel the feelings . . . see the visions. . . ."

"Oh, the colors, I see beautiful colors," she murmured, as she continued to move her body with the breath of her labor.

The contractions got closer together, stronger, longer . . . down to 2 minutes apart. Then the door burst open and we both jumped about a foot off the ground.

"Nipple stimulation is dangerous," the doctor admonished. He went on to explain how nipple stimulation creates waves of hormone imbalance which could cause uterine rupture. I tried to explain to Nina that nipple stimulation was certainly not dangerous, that if she were pregnant and nursing her toddler her breasts would be having constant stimulation. She asked me if I thought that her uterus would rupture, and I tried to assure her that if the doctor were really worried about uterine rupture the nurses would be taking her vital signs every few minutes, whereas in fact, no one had taken her pulse or pressure since the initial exam at 8:00 A.M. However, regardless of my attempted reassurances, it seemed Nina was afraid of trying nipple stimulation again.

All Nina needed was really active labor even for just an hour or two, and she would have been fully dilated. I wanted to take her for a walk to try to stimulate contractions, so I told the nurse she needed to go to the bathroom. But instead of letting her off the monitor to go to the bathroom, the nurse brought in a bedpan. It was absurd because whenever Nina would move even slightly, the belt would slip and the monitor would no longer be recording accurate tracings of the fetal heart.

Finally, it was 1:30 and I asked the nurse for a half-hour of privacy. Nina got on her hands and knees, and I massaged her cervix for that half hour. The baby was attempting to rotate the entire time. I could literally feel the baby slowly making the rotation and moving downward. By the end of the half hour, Nina had progressed to almost nine centimeters, the head had rotated considerably, and descended slightly.

At 2:00 P.M. the doctor burst into the door (not one person ever knocked before entering), put on a glove and once again jammed his hand into and out of her vagina in two seconds. "No progress," he gloated, as if he knew he were winning a battle.

I thought to myself, "Well, the progress had been slight. Perhaps he just hadn't noticed such slight progress."

"Can I talk to your husband?" he asked. "What's your husband's phone number?"

Before I could catch Nina's eye to let her know that I didn't feel that this would be a wise maneuver, Nina began telling him her husband's phone number. I knew that the doctor would try to use her husband as a power-play to get Nina to concede to another cesarean. The doctor continued to badger Nina until she finally said that if there were still no progress when her husband arrived at 3:00 P.M., that she would consent to having a cesarean.

When her husband arrived, once again I had to leave. I stood out in the hall wondering if there was anything I could do to alter the course and prevent Nina from having what I considered an unnecessary cesarean. Finally at about 3:30 I returned to the labor room. Nina was being prepped for the cesarean, and the nurse asked her to sign the consent.

"I don't want to sign it. Nick can sign it," she said through repressed tears. Subtly, Nina was saying that she didn't want a cesarean, that she didn't consent to a cesarean of her own free will —that it was Nick who wanted the cesarean, and she was having a cesarean to please him. How powerful and gentle Nina had always been when she and I were alone together, yet whenever she was in the presence of men (especially her husband) she became a scared puppy. I wished that there were magic words I could have said to empower her to stand up for her own needs, despite her husband's wishes. But Nina had given her power to birth her baby to her husband. She was having a cesarean to prove her love for her husband.

Nina asked me to examine her because she said that although her contractions were still 6–8 minutes apart, they were very strong. She was making strong gutteral sounds, almost as if she were pushing at the peaks of the contractions. When I checked her she was fully dilated except for a slight lip on one side. Had I had the time to keep my hand inside her, I probably could have pushed the cervix back within a few contractions. "Lie on your side and push during the contractions. Then, just before they are ready to do the surgery, ask the doctor to check you. You'll probably be fully dilated, and they'll have to let you continue your labor."

I felt hopeful. Twenty minutes later, after the nurses had finished their prep for the cesarean, Nina asked for the doctor to examine her again.

"No change," he announced, knowing he was victor in the struggle for power over the outcome of this birth. I wanted to scream, "Liar! She's fully dilated. I checked her myself." But I couldn't. Never had silence been so painful.

Tears began to roll from Nina's large eyes. I put my head next to hers and rubbed her back. "I'm so confused," she whispered.

"You must be," I said. I wanted to say, "He's lying to you. Why don't you just stand up and refuse to have another cesarean? We can go to another doctor, to another hospital . . ." But somehow I felt that pressuring her to avoid a cesarean would be as wrong as the doctor's insistence on doing a cesarean. I had already offered those options to her, and she refused them. I couldn't push a vaginal birth on her.

So, instead I said, "Follow your feelings. Do what you feel is best . . ." The nurses released the lock on her gurney, and began to roll her down the hall to the OR. "Have a nice birth, and a healthy baby."

An hour later I saw her in recovery. Her whole body was shaking, and she was in tremendous pain. She would open her eyes slightly to see who was with her, but she could barely talk. Nick was standing next to her holding her baby, who kept wrenching his neck, looking around for someone.

I asked Nina if she had held the baby yet. She said she was afraid to, her arms were shaking so much. I asked Nick to put the baby next to her. He tried, but he didn't understand what she needed. He put the baby's feet by her face, and all she could do was stroke them with her cheeks.

Then the doctor came in to give Nina his final instructions for the evening. He was no longer wearing his hospital greens. Nina's cesarean had put an end to his required attendance for this VBAC labor, and now he was going home. According to ACOG's (American College of Obstetricians and Gynecologists) guidelines for VBAC the obstetrician must be in the hospital during the entire labor. With other vaginal births the doctor is notified that the woman is in labor, but is not expected to appear in the hospital until she has begun to push. With other cesareans the doctor can schedule the surgery at his convenience, and leave as soon as the patient is stable. No wonder he wanted to do a cesarean by 1:00 P.M.!

Nick was too busy getting pictures taken by the nurses, and feeling proud of his 9 pound 13 ounce son to notice Nina's pain. But I soaked it up like a sponge. Suddenly I saw myself ten years ago after my first child was born by cesarean. All the pain I thought I had forgotten came back as if it were yesterday. I wanted to offer some words of comfort to her. I wanted to take away her pain. But once again I was powerless. I kissed her goodbye, and let her know that she could always call to talk anytime of the day or night.

I was numb for days afterwards. How could anybody do that to anyone—lie to a woman to force her consent to have a cesarean? I wanted to cry, but there were no tears, only emptiness.

I was a failure.

For ten years I had been working to help women to avoid cesareans. I knew all the power plays, all the scare tactics, but I was still powerless to change what I knew was a totally unnecessary and unjust cesarean.

I had always believed that even though the doctors often made misjudgments, that even though their education was lacking in alternatives to cesareans, that deep down inside they were doing only what they believed was best for the woman. Somehow this belief had kept me sane. Now, my sanity was being pressed to its limits.

Nina's birth had forced me to question my beliefs. How can a woman know if her practitioner is telling her the truth? A woman must seek out a relationship of equal trust with her practitioner—the practitioner must show evidence of giving his/her trust to the mother, as well as expecting trust from the mother. Perhaps this can be the only true test of whether or not a practitioner can be trusted. Trust between mother and practitioner is of great significance, for without trust we have nothing.

However, now more than ever, I realize that the basis of real trust between individuals is the ability to first trust oneself. A woman must look inside herself, and trust herself above all others, especially when she is in the process of giving birth. To give away her trust of herself is not only to give away the power to give birth to her baby, but to give away her power to give birth to her own power, her own essence, her own self. Had Nina been able to trust herself above all others, perhaps she would not have been led down the road to an unnecessary cesarean, despite what the doctor or her husband or anyone else were saying to her.

However, although Nina might have been able to stand up to this doctor had she had a greater belief in herself, the unethical conduct, the malpractice of this doctor ate through me like acid from the inside out. I wanted to expose him to his colleagues, to the nurses in that hospital who believed he was so right and just in his diagnosis that a cesarean was really necessary. I wanted to expose him to the women who, like Nina, are won by his smooth-talking authoritative manner. But who would listen to me? Even if it could be brought to court, I couldn't get up on a witness stand and testify that I, the unlicensed midwife, had checked this woman and know for a fact that she was progressing, that at the time of the cesarean she was fully dilated! At best I would be laughed out of court, and at the worst I'd be brought up on charges of practicing medicine without a license.

So I did what I thought would be the next best maneuver. I called my friendly doctor, Karl, to tell him of this doctor's practices, hoping that he would have a suggestion as to how to stop this injustice. When I told him the story, he said, "It happens all the time."

"All the time??" I asked, as I couldn't believe my ears.

"All the time," he repeated.

Aghast and appalled, my naivete now fully destroyed, I sat in silence.

"By the way," Karl went on, "I have a terrifying article for you from the *New England Journal of Medicine* that has all the statistics to support prophylactic cesarean sections at 39 weeks for everyone . . ."

Soon women may have the choice of staying at home to have a vaginal birth or going to the hospital for a cesarean.

50

Failure

THREE MIDWIVES

CATHERINE: Whenever I have to transfer a woman to the hospital and the woman has a cesarean, I feel I've failed. Just as the woman feels she has failed, and that her body has failed, I feel that I have failed the woman. I'm embarrassed to see the woman. I usually get depressed and cry over it.

JEAN: I usually feel more depressed than the mothers do.

CATHERINE: Usually the women help me get through the postpartum period. But I don't think I ever come to terms with it. I'm always looking for the answer to the question, "How else could I have done it differently?"

Half-way through one woman's labor, she asked me in tears, "Would you still love me if I had a cesarean?" She was a close friend, as well as a client. Of course, I said yes, that I would still love her. I hugged her, and held her, and told her how wonderful she was. But when her birth actually did end in a cesarean, I had a hard time keeping it together.

I find it very difficult to have a good relationship with a woman after we've worked through a labor together that has ended in a cesarean. In the years following the cesarean I find that I'm always trying to avoid these women.

JEAN: I find that I want to contact these women more. I'm very worried about how they feel about me. I feel guilty, that if only we had done . . . then we could have avoided a cesarean. I just want to be magically absolved of my tremendous feeling of responsibility. Of course, I realize that no matter how much reassurance I receive from that woman that she feels at peace with what has happened, her words could never absolve me. I must work through the feelings and learn what I can from the experience for future births.

SABRINA: I don't necessarily feel less close to the women who've had a cesarean. In fact, a couple of them are very close friends. One of these women went on to have a VBAC with her next birth, and I felt just as excited as she did. I felt the sense of completion.

I've noticed that women whose births have ended in cesareans, call me on the phone quite often afterwards. It is almost as if they're looking for what they've lost. After I've been to a cesarean, I find myself just sort of wandering around, crying, looking for something, but I don't know what it is. Then I have a talk with myself and say "As midwives, we don't have control over what happens to women." Yet, I still keep asking myself if there is anything I did wrong or should have done differently.

Out of all the births I've gone to (about 200), I've only been to about 5 cesareans. Of course, I don't attend all the births of all the couples I teach in classes, and a greater percentage of those women whose births I have not attended have had cesareans. However, interestingly, I'm usually better able to help the women whose births I had not attended deal with their grieving than I am able to help the women whose births I've been to. I'm too close to them, I'm still feeling the cesarean. I'm still grieving, too.

JEAN: It seems to me that the really good practitioners are the ones who take each and every birth to heart. They are the ones who really care about the women, really feel with the women. And when one of those women has a cesarean, or even just a highly complicated birth, it's almost as if that experience is happening to the midwife.

In some ways this is a marvelously rare closeness between a woman and her midwife, which should be treasured. However, it is the major cause of burn-out for practitioners. It seems that the practitioner can only feel so much, and then they have to choose to either shut down their feelings (become more calloused and removed from the women who come to them), or quit because they can't take the pressure and the pain. I'm still searching for that middle ground of balance between the two choices.

I have always believed that a good practitioner needs to have a great deal of humility, that he/she needs to examine his/her role after each and every birth, after each and every visit, with great scrutiny. To me, this is the process through which a practitioner grows. I know that I have been called to midwifery because it has forced me to grow in so many ways as a woman. I want to keep practicing midwifery. I want to continue to grow. But I don't want to end up in an asylum because the amount and depth of feeling was just too much for me. I'm still searching for the balance.

When a birth ends in a cesarean, I feel most out of balance. I have trouble leaving the emotional space of the birth. I have to talk about it over and over with my husband, friends, other midwives. Sometimes I come home saying, "I'm going to quit. This is just too much for me." But somehow I regain my balance, and keep on practicing and feeling.

SABRINA: I don't know how much longer I would continue to practice if I had to attend a lot of cesareans. It takes me about 20 times longer to recuperate from a cesarean than from a vaginal birth.

I haven't been with that many women who've had cesareans. In the early years of my practice if a woman had a cesarean, I would come home feeling so frustrated that I wanted to punch walls. Then I began to change the way I practiced. I realized that there were certain hospitals and situations in which I just couldn't help anyone. I can't be effective if from the minute I walk in I have to fight.

I realized that in agreeing to go with a woman to a place where the cesarean rates were high and women were treated abusively, I was subtly contributing to this abuse. So I refused to go to those places. I made a decision to attend only those women who I felt had made careful choices about their doctors and about their place of birth.

Since making that decision only a couple of births I went to have ended with a cesarean. In all those cases women were not separated from their husbands and got their wishes as far as having a cesarean was concerned. And in all except one, I was there for the actual cesarean, as well.

I'll never get used to watching someone's uterus be cut open. If I saw a million cesareans, I'd never get used to it. It's a feeling of invasion. I feel that women all over the world are screaming.

When I watch the baby's face as it is delivered from the uterus, I am always saddened by the child's look of painful surprise, as if it had been horribly interrupted from a primal process. Their journey has been abruptly ended, and they don't know why. To help the baby with this transition I began to spend a moment together with the parents prior to the surgery explaining to the baby what was going to happen. And during the surgery I always talk in my mind to the baby, and I let the baby know what's happening when it's time to come out.

Once the baby is born, then there's some joy in the birth if the mother is participating. I'm always happy to see the baby, and even happier when the mother gets to be with the baby. There's a lot of joy there. I always make sure that the mother and father get to spend time with the baby alone. Then I go home and cry. Even if I'm not really certain that there could have been a different outcome, I still feel really sad. The women themselves often feel somehow peaceful about their cesareans. Sometimes that peacefulness is denial, but some seem to really be at peace.

Everyone has the right and responsibility to work through their own lives. It's my job to be supportive. I can't base everything on how many births end in cesareans. I can only be a person who is really there for the mother and the baby. That is the hardest thing to deal with as a midwife—to realize that it's the woman's responsibility, but yet at the same time we must always be watchful and mindful of not being part of the co-option of a woman's rights to give birth.

I've changed over the years that I've practiced. I've come to accept that it seems OK for some people to have cesareans, and I realize I can't impose my own values on them. One of the most important things about being a midwife and a labor coach is to let go and realize that it's not your birth. It's just as important for midwives to let go as it is for women in labor to let go.

I don't feel that a cesarean is a failure, and I work very hard to help women to feel that they did the very best job that they could. But sometimes it's difficult to sit down next to someone whose birth I've been at, hold her hand, look her in the eye, and hear her say, "Do you think it could have been different?"

Out of all the births I've been to, even though I just couldn't understand at the time why women made the choices they made, afterwards I always felt close to them. Even if I didn't agree with them, I really felt close to them in some way. I consider it a privilege to be at births—whether it's a cesarean or a vaginal birth.

51

From Marshmallow to Monster

KATHERINE HUGHES
VBAC Educator, Labor Coach, Midwife

With her first birth Alice had a very interventive vaginal birth and was very disappointed with the experience. When she was pregnant the second time, she prepared herself very well. She searched for a noninterventive practitioner, and found an old family doctor to attend her labor in a small country hospital near her home just outside of Waupakka. "Old Doc Hawkins" as she was commonly referred to by the locals was a grandmotherly woman, who still made housecalls for sick children and the elderly. She had a wonderful way of making her patients feel at ease. They could always call Doc Hawkins whenever they needed to ask questions or to get medical help. Alice's birth with Doc Hawkins was a totally natural event. She had absolutely no interventions, not even an IV. Alice really loved the whole experience of giving birth to her second baby. She especially loved that she, not her doctor, had made the decisions about her birth.

By the time Alice was pregnant again, Doc Hawkins had retired from practice, and Alice and her husband, John, had moved to Madison so she was forced to seek another doctor to attend the birth of her baby. She went to a doctor whom her friends had recommended at their community hospital. However, she never felt she had the communication that she had with the old doctor she had loved.

She interviewed 3 other doctors, hoping to find someone she could really trust. But the other doctors were worse than the first. Her husband pressured her about interviewing so many doctors, so she stayed with the first doctor. The other ones seemed worse because they were working in the major medical center. She decided to stay with small hospital thinking she would have more control.

She went into labor at term, and went to the hospital when her contractions were 4 minutes apart. She would have stayed home longer but her husband John was terribly nervous about not getting to the hospital in time, even though it was only a 10-minute drive. He was annoying her so much that she felt he was interfering with her labor. So they left for the hospital.

Alice and John got to hospital, and waited about 20 minutes for the doctor to arrive. The doctor examined her and said, "This baby is breech, and we're doing a cesarean." There was nothing else wrong, no fetal distress, no failure to progress. In fact, her labor was moving along quickly—she was 7 centimeters after only 2 hours of labor. It was just a routine cesarean for breech.

Even though Alice had talked about cesarean with her doctor prenatally, she had never thought to ask about breech. She had presumed that since she had two previous vaginal births, that even if the baby was a breech, she could still deliver vaginally. She had such easy births with her first two babies that she completely trusted that her body knew how to give birth.

Alice felt overwhelmed by her doctor's demands to do a cesarean. He told her the baby would have brain damage if he didn't do the cesarean. When she tried to refuse the surgery the doctor told her that if she refused the cesarean then she would have to leave this hospital. He would no longer take care of her.

Then the doctor took John out to the hallway. Through the doorway Alice could see the doctor put his arm around her husband. The doctor was talking to him, but Alice couldn't hear what he was saying.

Alice's contractions were even stronger now than they were when she arrived at the hospital. A few minutes later the two men, husband and doctor, came into the labor room like a coalition and began talking to her. John said that he refused to take her to another hospital.

Alice would have to look elsewhere for support in avoiding this cesarean. She called her mother to ask if she would drive her to another hospital. Her mother said, "Do what the doctor says," and hung up.

Alice cried hysterically, as the nurses began prepping her for a cesarean. She told them she didn't want general anesthesia, so they agreed to give her a spinal (not an epidural). They wheeled her into the OR alone, as her husband was not permitted to be with her. Actually he appeared to be relieved because he didn't want to see surgery. Alice was crying on the table, saying that she knew that she could give birth, that nothing was going to go wrong . . . and the next thing she knew she awakened in the recovery room.

She said to the nurse, "I was supposed to have a spinal. What happened?"

The nurse said, "The spinal must not have worked, so they gave you general." (Though epidurals at times do not work, for a spinal not to work is almost completely impossible, unless it has been administered improperly.)

Later the obstetrician told Alice that they gave her general anesthesia because she was crying.

Alice was separated from her baby, Sandra, for two days, even though she screamed and cried for the nurses to bring Sandra to her. She wasn't able to get out of bed because of post-surgical complications, so she couldn't get down to the nursery on her own power. Every time her husband came to visit she would ask him to fight for her right to have her baby, but he wouldn't do it. He was a marshmallow. By the time she finally got to see Sandra, the baby wouldn't nurse. Alice was very upset, as she had never had trouble with nursing before. It seemed like everything was going wrong.

Alice left the hospital on the fourth day and came home. Her mother was there to help. Alice was so depressed that she was crying every day. She didn't want to see anyone. People would say, "At least you had a healthy baby." Her own sister, Suzie, who had had all her babies by cesarean, offered no support to Alice. Suzie had a hard time dealing with Alice because she thought Alice was lucky, and said, "At least you had vaginal births before." Alice had no one who understood her pain.

After her mother went home, Alice started taking care of the baby on her own. She noticed that she really didn't have the same interest in the baby that she had with her other babies, and she felt very guilty. She recognized that the baby was very good, but she just didn't feel the same kind of connection that she had felt after her other babies were born, even though she and Sandra finally did establish nursing. These feelings interfered with her mothering. She still took care of her baby, and never abused her, but she just didn't have the same feeling in her gut that tied her to her baby. She especially remembered the time when her baby fell, and she just didn't feel that really sinking feeling in her stomach. When she realized that there seemed to be nothing she could do to change this void in her relationship with her baby, not only did she feel she had failed because she had had a cesarean, but she felt she had failed because she just wasn't a caring mother.

When Sandra was two years old, Alice and John moved back to the country again, this time rural northern Illinois. Alice was glad to be going back to the country, as she had hoped that the country would bring her the peace she had when her two boys were little. She hoped that in the country her motherly feelings toward Sandra might blossom. However, although certainly Alice did feel more at ease with the slower country pace, she still noticed the gnawing emptiness in her relationship with her daughter.

Alice's realization about the effect of her birth on her mothering forced her to decide that she would not go through that experience again. Even though she desperately wanted to have more children, she felt she could not have any other children unless she could have a vaginal birth. No one around her really understood why she should be so concerned about having more children. Since her last baby was a girl and her first two were boys, everyone told her her family was complete. But she always wanted more children.

This conflict between wanting more children yet fearing another cesarean brought her to seek out VBAC counseling and classes with me. Alice came to classes before she was pregnant and dragged her husband along. He managed to be sick for at least three quarters of them, but she came to every class, even if she had to come without him. She loved the classes, loved being with the women, and wanted to keep coming to classes until she gave birth to her next baby. Before Alice was even pregnant she asked me to be her labor coach for her next birth. We had a close relationship long before her pregnancy, which allowed us to flow more easily into the pregnancy and birth.

John wasn't interested in the classes. He made it quite clear that he didn't want to have another baby. For a long time it appeared that he was simply against having more children. But later he disclosed that he didn't want Alice to have another baby because Alice's post-partum depression had been so difficult for him to cope with, that he feared what would happen if she had another cesarean. He didn't feel that he could cope with another depression. He wanted to avoid the possibility of another depression by simply not having another baby.

During class we always discuss the importance of being assertive about getting your needs met in the hospital. John was completely frustrated by this concept. He wanted to be able to find a doctor Alice could completely trust. But Alice felt that she could never ever give her trust to a doctor again, no matter how wonderful or agreeable the doctor seemed. She wanted the final word herself.

Alice interviewed probably 20 doctors, both locally and in the Chicago teaching hospitals, and finally reluctantly picked a doctor who was associated with one of the teaching hospitals. Dr. Dworkin's wife had a VBAC, which seemed encouraging to Alice. In addition, Dr. Dworkin was paid on a salary basis by the hospital. He received no extra compensation if he did a cesarean instead of a vaginal birth. Therefore, Alice reasoned, Dr. Dworkin had nothing to gain by doing a cesarean, and therefore she felt her chances were better of having a VBAC with this doctor than with a doctor who receives extra remuneration for cesareans. But Alice never really felt that she was as connected with Dr. Dworkin as she had felt with "Old Doc Hawkins."

Alice went to Dr. Dworkin for her prenatals and to Dr. Silverberg, too. He was Dr. Dworkin's backup, and was considered the "breech expert" in the Chicago area. Alice wanted to know that if she had another breech, that she would still have a vaginal birth.

We talked about why people had breeches. I asked her why she felt she needed to protect her baby. Why did her baby need to be held up close to her heart? She realized that during the last pregnancy she hadn't felt that the birthing situation at the hospital was very safe, and wanted to protect her baby because of it.

In addition, Alice had always had a sense that her third baby was a girl. When she was a child she and her father had a very difficult relationship. Although he never physically abused her, he was totally insensitive to her feelings. He somehow expected that she should be just like her brothers. To him, there was no difference between girls and boys, and whenever she got cramps with her period as a teenager, he would never let her stay home from school, or lie down to rest. She was expected to push through the pain like a soldier. As the time grew closer to the birth of her third baby, she became more and more fearful for the little girl she knew she was carrying. Even though she didn't consciously think her husband would ever be as insensitive to their daughter as her father had been to her, subconsciously her fear for her baby and her need to protect her baby grew and grew. Acknowledging these feelings was very painful for Alice, but she felt greatly relieved having begun to explore the significance of her baby's breech presentation. This discovery allowed her greater freedom to move into the next birth.

John, on the other hand, could not relate to the concept of physical manifestations of emotional fears. He gave Alice no support whatsoever for her emotional explorations, and he would never talk about or deal with his fears. He never once admitted that he had had any fears whatsoever during the last pregnancy or birth. Whenever I would ask him how he would feel or what he would do if a particular complication happened, he would always say, "I'm just not going to think about it. It's not going to happen, and you (meaning me, the labor coach) are going to be there."

"What if I'm not there? Other people are due at the same time. Maybe I'll be at someone else's birth. What are you going to do then?" I asked. I always try to help people to realize that the birth can be whole and complete whether or not their doctor, midwife, or labor coach would be there. But John refused to accept that he needed to take any of these responsibilities.

As time went on Alice wanted to have a home birth more and more. She took out lots of my books. John just froze everytime she brought up the issue, and wouldn't talk about it. Finally, Alice just told John, "I'm going to plan a hospital birth, but I want to know that you will support me if during the labor I decide I want to have a home birth." I gave her the list of supplies to get to have the baby at home, and told her she should get people to help her.

Alice called her mother telling her she might want to have her baby at home. She asked her if she would come to help. This time her mom said she would back her up no matter what she decided to do. And her sister, Suzie, who had been so unsupportive previously, also agreed to help.

John remained very noncommittal. Finally, a week before Alice was due he told her, "I'm really afraid. I don't want you to have the baby at home. I would just be too nervous." Having already experienced the effect of John's nervousness upon her in labor, Alice felt that labor might go smoother if she planned to have the baby in the hospital with me there as the labor coach. If she were in the hospital she knew that John would be more relaxed; and since she really wanted him to be there for her, his being relaxed was very important to her.

I asked her, "Aside from having a healthy baby and a noninterventive vaginal birth, what's most important to you about this birth?"

And she said, "Having him with me supporting me is the most important thing." So, since John felt very safe in hospitals, Alice gave up her home birth so that he could feel safe and spend his energy supporting her.

A week before Alice went into labor, she and I had similar dreams. In the dreams her labor had gone very quickly, and she had the baby at home. She seemed very happy with the dream. But when she told John about the dream, he was a nervous wreck.

A week later I got a phone call from Alice. She said, "I'm in labor, but it's no rush."

I replied, "Well, I'm going to get dressed anyway, and you call me when you need me to come."

Ten minutes later she called back saying, "The contractions seem a little stronger, so I'm going to take a shower."

I said, "I'm going to come down to visit you, see how you're doing, and I'll come back home again, if you really don't need me yet. How do you feel about that?"

"That's fine."

I grabbed my birthbag, packed a bag for my son, and took him to the baby sitter immediately. I was glad we had no new winter storms in the last few days, so I could speed along the back road. From the dream I had I knew that it was important for me to get there fast.

Fifteen minutes later I arrived at Alice's. An older woman was running down the middle of the road screaming at me. Alice had told me that the old woman who lived in the farm down the road was rather strange, that although she was usually reclusive, from time to time she would wander around bothering people. I presumed this screaming lady was that elderly seemingly confused woman, and I didn't pay any attention to her. I directed my focus and started walking into the house.

Then this woman came right up to me and asked me if I was looking for Alice. The woman was Alice's mother, and as she dragged me to the car where Alice was sitting, she kept screaming hysterically at me about how Alice had to get to the hospital. When I got to the car, I asked Alice, "Is this what you want—to go to the hospital now?"

Alice's contractions were now 5 minutes apart and strong. "I have to get out of here, they're driving me crazy," she said. Her sister, her mother, and husband were there, and although they had all promised that they would support her, when she went into labor they were all screaming at her to get to the hospital.

We drove a mile down the road, and her contractions went from 5 minutes apart to 3 minutes apart. After another mile, Alice said with great certainty, "The baby's head is moving down. I can feel it. The baby's head is coming down."

I said, "Let's go home." But John refused emphatically.

Then I said, "Let's go to my house," as by this time we were very close to my house.

John said, "No way! We're going to the hospital."

I said, "There's no one home at my house. It'll be private."

"I'm having the baby in a few minutes. I've pushed before and I know I'm getting close." So I said again that we could go to my house, but John was already headed for the Tollroad. "I just want to go somewhere and have my baby in peace."

I leaned forward from the backseat where Alice and I were sitting, and said right into John's ear, "We're not going to make it to the hospital. The hospital is an hour and a half away, and we're not going to make it."

Finally, Alice said, "Just pick a good hospital, Kathy, because he'll never be happy if we don't go to a hospital." I thought we could make it to one of the western suburban hospitals where they have a birthing room, and are known to be supportive of VBACs, although not as liberal as the hospital she had chosen. I started to give John directions. But once it sunk in that we weren't making it to the planned hospital, John just wanted to take Alice to the nearest hospital. I suggested that we could just pull over and do the birth in the car, but John just kept heading for the local hospital.

The thought of going to this hospital was excruciating. This hospital had absolutely no experience with birth alternatives. As John drove into the hospital parking lot I suggested that we could still have the baby here in the car, and afterwards go into the hospital to have her checked. But John just started bugging Alice again, so she decided to go into the hospital.

We entered through the emergency room, hoping to be able to skip the usual hospital red tape, but the nurses sent her to admitting anyway. When we got to admitting, Alice was pushing and told them, "I'm having this baby now!" Suddenly, the admitting clerk's face dropped and turned pale, and they took her up to delivery immediately. That clerk really didn't want to have to catch this baby!

As we were going up in the elevator, I explained to Alice and John that this hospital would certainly not permit Alice to have both of us with her in the delivery room. She would have to choose between us. Alice said that although she really wanted me to be with her, that it was extremely important to her that John be there. So I told John that he had to really fight for their rights, which of course was the very issue he had resisted learning about in class. I was secretly praying she would have the baby in the elevator.

When we got to the door of labor and delivery, the nurse wouldn't let John in. "Has he taken classes here?" the nurse asked.

"No, they hadn't planned on having their baby here. They took classes with me," I responded.

"But he didn't take classes HERE. He can't be admitted to the delivery room without classes," she went on as if she hadn't heard what I had said.

"I don't care what you say, I'm going in anyway," John said, as he walked toward the door. Suddenly a guard appeared from nowhere, and physically stopped John from passing. Another guard was called up.

"We're arresting you both (John and me) for trespassing and disturbing the peace."

"Is it illegal for a father to be at the birth of his child?" I asked facetiously.

"In this hospital it's illegal if he hasn't taken our classes."

John said, "I don't care. I'm going to see my child born."

"I don't see what the big deal is, I wasn't there to see my child born," said one of the guards.

Then they started screaming at us that they were definitely going to arrest us. "How do you know so much?" they asked me. "What do you really do? Don't you know that's illegal in this state?"

I was becoming very angry and worried that by the time we had resolved this, Alice would have had her baby alone. I had to find a way to create counter-pressure on the hospital, so that they would be forced to let John into the delivery room. "If you don't let him in, I'm going to call the TV station," I stated firmly. One minute later the hospital administrator appeared. I said to him, "This man has taken a class, if you don't let him in I'm going to call every TV station and newspaper in Chicago to tell them the story."

Meanwhile Alice was back in the delivery room trying not to push too hard to wait for John to get there before the baby would be born. The doctor was telling her she couldn't have a VBAC. "You can't do this. We don't allow it. You'll have to sign for a cesarean." Alice ignored the doctor as much as possible and tried to concentrate on holding back the birth.

In addition, the nurses were harrassing her for my name and address, so that they could press charges against me. But Alice put them off cleverly, and didn't reveal any important information.

Finally, the hospital administrator decided to let John in the delivery room, but on the condition that the guards would escort me to the lobby. I would have to wait there with the guards because the hospital was afraid that I would call the TV station. As the guards were walking me to the elevator, I yelled to John, "You don't have to do anything. They can't make you do anything you don't want to do." The guards escorted me downstairs to the lobby, and sat down and watched me. They wouldn't even let me go to the bathroom alone, and escorted me there.

While I was waiting downstairs I was nauseous and terrified that something would happen to Alice or the baby. I ran through the events of the entire night over and over again, wondering if I could have done something differently, or suggested something else. Finally, I realized it was out of my hands, and I had to sit back and wait. I realized completely what fathers of the fifties must have felt before they were allowed in the delivery room. Each time I paced the lobby it was under the watchful eye of the guards. I wondered what the guards would have done that night, what their normal job would have been, if I weren't there. I walked over to the phone on the wall and called another midwife for emotional support. The guards immediately came over to listen to my conversation. I felt like I was in a weird dream and I needed to tell another person outside of the hospital what was happening and what was going on. I also wasn't totally sure I wasn't going to jail.

John walked into the delivery room and immediately held Alice's hand. As soon as she felt his touch, Alice started to push. The doctor kept saying, "You can't do this, you can't do this!

And John said, "But she IS doing it!" In complete frustration, the doctor left the room to get the chief of obstetrics.

Alice said, "The baby's coming!" and John caught the baby. When the doctor returned, John turned around with the baby in his arms, and said with a smirk on his face, "She did it!"

About two hours later John came down to the lobby to tell me what had happened. "This is the last baby we're having," he said, as he was shaking from all the adrenalin rushing through his body.

John went to the phone to call Alice's mother to tell her of the news of the birth. Her mother asked, "Where are you?"

John said, "At the hospital."

"Good," she responded.

"Not good," he said.

He reviewed the details of the birth, and Alice's mother said, "Why did you make such a fuss?"

The next day he went into the hospital to see Alice. It was past visiting hours, but John just walked in anyway, and nobody tried to stop him. The whole hospital was afraid of John. In fact, the hospital was afraid of both of them. Alice had the baby with her the whole time she was in the hospital. The nurses were too afraid of her to come in and take the baby back to the nursery. She signed out AMA (Against Medical Advice), and while she was getting the baby dressed to go home, a nurse came in and said, "You are the bravest woman I've ever seen. I heard about you, and I just had to come in and shake your hand. I'm so proud of you. Don't tell anyone I said this to you."

The story of Alice and John's birth spread like wildfire around our small town. Neighbors said, "Was that you, John?" No one could believe that he would fight like that.

"When I went in there I kept remembering all the things that Kathy had said in class, and all these protective fatherly feelings took me over. A monster took me over. I was even afraid of myself," John described. When the hospital told John he couldn't be there for the birth, all his anger from not being able to be there for Sandra's birth came back.

When the hospital sent Alice and John the bill for their services, Alice wrote a letter describing the terrible treatment they had received. They got a letter back saying that their bill had been cancelled. The hospital was still afraid that John and Alice would bring suit against them.

When we got together again after the birth, Alice said to me that she felt very disappointed that her mother had let her down once again, and she would have liked to have had her other children present for the birth. "I wish it all could have been easier. I didn't want to have to fight, but I'm so proud of John for standing up for us. I hated being in the hospital, but John caught the baby, and he never would have caught it if we had been anywhere else."

And John said, "Maybe it wouldn't be so bad to have a home birth with the next baby. It would be a lot less stressful."

52

VBAC as Triumph

LEO SORGER, *OB/GYN*
and BARBARA BROWN-HILL,
VBAC Educator and Birth Attendant

LEO: A VBAC is extra triumph. It's exhilarating because you have this feeling of winning a battle. We know that we've accomplished something. We have won one person from the pool of routine repeat sections. Every time we get another turned away from routine repeat cesareans, she will convince someone else to have a VBAC instead of another repeat cesarean.

Doing VBACs has changed me, and it's changed my practice. It's made everything more interesting and pleasurable. It's not as boring as sitting in a small town outside of Boston, and seeing the regular people from the neighborhood coming into us, for interventions and cesareans. We get a lot of exciting people coming to our place. We have people coming from all sorts of backgrounds and social strata from all over America. We've made a lot of friends with patients. Some of them we continue to visit. It's changed our lifestyle, and it's made life more rewarding. I feel better because I know I'm doing something unique, working to prevent unnecessary interventions and cesareans.

I see other obstetricians still using anesthesia and interventions, and not letting women even get up to go to the bathroom in labor. Knowing that such practices still exist brings forth anger and sadness in me. It's nice to see obstetrics differently, and be a little in the forefront of a change for the better.

I love working with midwives. Midwives are the spice of birth, the essential ingredient to a good birth. With their gentleness much harm is avoided. The greatest honor of my life was when the Radical Midwives of London bestowed upon me the title of "honorary midwife," placing one of their pins on my shirt.

BARBARA: I remember after one birth I was riding home on the train, totally disheveled and exhausted from being up all night. I was just sitting there smiling and smiling. And as I looked around the train I

Barbara Brown-Hall, labor assistant, and Marsha Levy, VBAC mom, rest and laugh between Marsha's contractions, enjoying her very active VBAC labor.

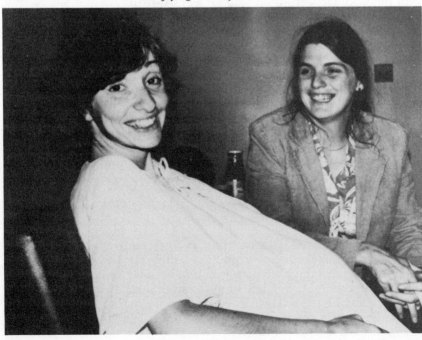

noticed that everybody was staring at me. They must have thought there was something wrong with me. After a VBAC I walk around for days elated. I just start thinking about the birth, and I get this big smile on my face.

Everyone at a VBAC gets excited. Even the stoggyish nurse ends up smiling. I've seen women say, "I did it, I did it, I did it" for ten minutes. After one birth as the father and I walked out of the hospital in the middle of the night, he screamed, *"We did it!!"* It's such a good feeling to watch women work through their cesarean experience and have a VBAC, and feel that they've really done it on their own. The entire room is filled with the feeling of triumph and so much love.

Being at all births is a privilege and a joy, but there seems to be something extra special about a VBAC. It connects us to the strength of all women.

I feel very connected to the people who have had VBACs. People call me on their baby's birthdays, and it's just like celebrating all over again.

If people knew what it's like to be at a VBAC, they would never want to do drugs. It's the most incredible high in the world.

Dr. Leo Sorger and midwife Cindy Dunleavy, with smiles of VBAC triumph

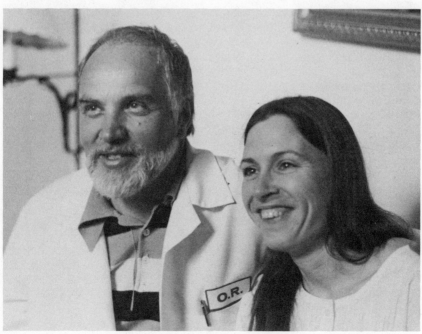

Glossary

Anatomy and Physiology

ACTIVE LABOR: Timeable consistent contractions, increasing in strength and frequency. The woman cannot walk or talk through the contractions. Active labor begins at 5-6 centimeters. If the woman is less than 5 centimeters dilated, even though contractions seem very strong, this is not yet active labor.

ANTERIOR LIE: The back of the baby is facing the front of the mother. Usually refers to a vertex presentation, but may refer to a breech or other presentation as well. An anterior vertex is the ideal presentation.

BONDING: The sensitive period of attachment betweeen parents and infant.

BRAXTON HICKS CONTRACTIONS: Prelabor "practice" contractions. Occurring throughout pregnancy, they become progressively stronger as the woman nears term. With each subsequent pregnancy, a woman will usually feel these contractions earlier in her pregnancy. These contractions are often mistaken for labor, but may be differentiated by their lack of consistency—not timeable, do not grow in intensity, and will cease when the activity level of the woman changes.

BREECH PRESENTATION: The buttocks and/or feet of the baby come out first. A variation of normal, not a complication. Should not necessitate routine cesarean. Should be attended by practitioner skilled and experienced with vaginal breech delivery.

CATECHOLAMINES: Hormones which prepare the body for fight or flight, and specifically prepare the fetus to survive outside the womb.

CERVIX: Neck of the uterus which opens and closes, through which the baby must first pass in order to be born.

DILATATION: The opening of the cervix, measured in centimeters, with full dilatation said to be 10 centimeters.

EFFACEMENT: The thinning of the cervix, measured in percentages. May occur prior to or during labor.

FIRST STAGE: Dilatation and effacement of the cervix.

FUNDUS: The top of the uterus.

INACTIVE LABOR: Timeable, infrequent, mild contractions, which do not require the mother's full attention. Usually, the longest phase of labor; 1-4 centimeters dilatation.

ISCHIAL SPINES: The internal knobs of the pelvis which can be felt by the practitioner when he/she does an internal exam. They are approximately 2/3 of the way between the top and bottom of the pelvis. The distance between the ischial spines is the smallest side-to-side internal diameter of the pelvis.

LOWER UTERINE SEGMENT: The less muscular lower part of the uterus, close to the cervix.

MECONIUM: The baby's first bowel movement.

MULTIPLE GESTATION: The presence of more than one fetus—twins, triplets, etc. Depending upon presentation of babies, should not necessitate routine cesarean.

OXYTOCIN: Hormone secreted during labor which causes uterine contractions.

PERINEUM: The muscle and tissue between the vagina and the rectum.

POSTERIOR LIE: A variation of normal. The back of the baby is against the mother's back. Usually refers to a vertex, but may refer to a breech or other presentation as well. Creates much low-back pressure. Though it does not preclude vaginal delivery, the birth can be made easier if baby rotates to an anterior presentation (back of the baby against the front of the mother).

PRODROMAL LABOR: The prelude to labor. Inconsistent contractions of variable length, strength, and frequency. May have timeable contractions for a few hours, then contractions stop or weaken, returning a few hours or days later.

RUPTURED MEMBRANES: The breaking of the sac which contains the amniotic fluid which surrounds and protects the fetus.

SECOND STAGE: Expulsive stage of labor, pushing the baby out.

STATIONS: A method of approximation of the descent of the baby through the mother's pelvis, measured in centimeters above or below the ischial spines. If the presenting part of the baby is at the level of the ischial spines (midway through the pelvis) it is said to be at 0 station. If the baby is still approximately 2 centimeters above the ischial spines, it is said to be at −2 station. If the baby has already passed through the spines and is now 3 centimeters below them, it is said to be +3 station. Minus 5 station is defined as a head not yet into the pelvic brim, and +5 station is crowning.

Since the ischial spines are said to be the most narrow part of the woman's pelvis, once the baby has passed through the spines, (past 0 station) the possibility of cephalo-pelvic disproportion is said to be dispelled.

THIRD STAGE: Expulsion of the placenta.

UPPER UTERINE SEGMENT: The muscular part of the uterus close to the fundus.

VERNIX: White creamy covering on the baby's skin which protects it from the watery environment prenatally. Most term babies are born with only a small amount of vernix; premature babies have a heavier covering; and post-mature babies are without vernix.

VERTEX PRESENTATION: The head of the baby is coming out first.

Skills and Equipment for Labor and Birth

AUSCULTATION: Listening to sounds within the body.

BACH FLOWER REMEDIES: Flower essences to assist in regaining spiritual and emotional balance. Designed to heal emotional difficulties and the emotional causes of physical difficulties.

CAULOPHYLLUM: Homeopathic blue cohosh. Contracts the upper uterine segment. May be used judiciously for induction or augmentation of labor, or hemorrhage control. Requires careful monitoring of the baby and mother.

CERTIFIED NURSE MIDWIFE: Midwife trained first as a nurse, then in a midwifery school in a hospital setting. May work at home or in the hospital.

EAR FORMATION: The degree of development of the ears is a significator of the actual gestational age of a baby.

EMPIRICAL, DIRECT-ENTRY, OR LAY MIDWIFE: Midwife trained by apprenticeship in a nonhospital setting. Knowledge and skills based primarily upon experience. Usually works in home environment.

FETASCOPE: Instrument used to listen to the heartbeat of a fetus.

GELSEMIUM: Homeopathic remedy which softens a rigid cervix.

KEGELS: Exercises to focus upon and develop control over pelvic floor muscles. Release of these muscles lets baby come down more easily. Tightening muscles returns pelvic organs to proper positions postpartum.

LEBOYER BATH: Leboyer was a doctor in France who, through his observations, became aware of the violent nature of birth as is common with obstetrical practices today. In his book, *Birth Without Violence*, he advocates the use of a body-temperature bath immediately following the birth of a baby, allowing him/her a quiet, unfolding transition from the world of the womb.

LOGAN BASIC CONTACT: Chiropractic technique to release ligaments of the pelvic floor.

OPTIMUM BIRTH LETTER: List of requests/demands for labor and birth presented during pregnancy to all those who may be involved in your care.

PERINEAL MASSAGE: Massage of the muscle and tissue between the vagina and the rectum. Done to prevent tears and/or the need for episiotomy.

ROLE-PLAYING: Pretending to take the part of another person to help facilitate better interpersonal relationships. Especially helpful for those who are fearful of confrontation with a practitioner.

TOILET TORTURE: Use of the toilet in labor to facilitate release and to stimulate and strengthen contractions.

VISUALIZATION: Positive guided visions to heal difficult or painful experiences, and create or reinforce positive experiences.

Complications and Emergencies

ABRUPTION: Breaking or tearing away of tissue (see specific types of abruptions)

ABRUPTION OF THE CORD: The tearing away of the cord from the placenta. May be partially or completely abrupted. Usually occurs only if the cord insertion is weak. May occur prior to birth which may cause fetal distress or death. Occurrences after the birth are often caused by too much traction on the cord during attempted delivery of the placenta, in which case manual removal of the placenta becomes necessary. (See UTERINE EXPLORATION).

ARREST OF LABOR: Cessation of contractions or progress after active labor has been established. Hormone levels which control labor are subject to environmental or psychospiritual disruption. Therefore, what appears to be "arrest of labor" can actually be "disruption of labor." Ameliorating the cause of the disruption should be attempted prior to use of medical intervention such as pitocin augmentation.

CEPHALO-PELVIC DISPROPORTION (CPD): The baby's head is supposedly too large for the mother's pelvis. Although in a few cases there is an overwhelming condition (such as pelvic deformity due to rickets), most of the time cephalo-pelvic disproportion (CPD) is relative to a particular baby in a particular position during a particular labor at a particular moment in time. Most of the time relative CPD can be overcome with great determination on the part of the mother and good skills and intuition on the part of the practitioner.

DEHISCENCE OF THE SCAR: A nonbleeding separation of the scar of the uterus. *Not a uterine rupture.* It is not symptomatic, with no evidence of shock, fetal death, or maternal complications.

DEHYDRATION: Excessive loss of body fluids. Risk of fetal distress, placental dysfunction or cardiovascular collapse.

DIABETES: A metabolic disorder affecting the ability of the body to use carbohydrates and fats. The pancreas fails to produce insulin, therefore blood sugar levels are high. Sugar spills into the urine, which can be detected with urine test sticks. Symptoms: increased thirst, hunger, and urine output. Diagnosis through blood work: serum glucose, or glycosylated hemoglobin, glucose tolerance test (GTT). Increased risks associated with diabetes in pregnancy: disproportionate fetus (cephalo-pelvic disproportion), rising blood pressure, placental dysfunction, kidney damage, growth retardation, fetal distress, intrauterine death, shoulder dystocia, stillbirth, neonatal hypoglycemic convulsions and/or shock, postpartum hemorrhage, increased chance of fetal anomalies.

ECLAMPSIA: (See TOXEMIA)

EDEMA: Swelling of tissue. A small amount of edema is common in late pregnancy to conserve fluid which will be needed following the blood loss associated with the birth of the placenta. Normal edema is characterized by a feeling of tightness in the ankles and/or hands which goes away after a short period of rest. Abnormal edema is characterized by obvious puffiness which, when touched by a finger, leaves a depression. It is a symptom of toxemia, although the presence of edema is not *diagnostic* of toxemia. (See TOXEMIA).

FETAL DISTRESS: Condition of the unborn baby which indicates that the baby's health is at risk.

GESTATIONAL DIABETES: Due to changes in metabolism in pregnancy, some women who were not diabetic prior to pregnancy become diabetic in pregnancy. Usually can be managed and/or prevented with diet alone.

HERPES: A viral infection of the mucous membranes, related to chicken pox, characterized by fluid-filled blisters. May infect skin, eyes, ears, nose, throat, mouth, genitals, or brain. Transmitted by direct contact of mucous membrane to mucous membrane, during a time of reduced immunity due to high physical or emotional stress. In pregnancy may be transmitted through the placenta. Recurrent outbreaks may be avoided through special diet and stress reduction. There is a direct risk of death or brain damage only if the infection travels to the brain.

HYALINE MEMBRANE DISEASE: Respiratory distress caused by lack of surfactant (a body fluid which allows the lungs to expand) in immature lungs of premature babies. Also referred to as Respiratory Distress Syndrome (RDS).

IATROGENIC COMPLICATION: Complication caused by the practitioner.

JAUNDICE: Yellowing condition of the skin and mucous membranes resulting from presence of bilirubin in the blood. Jaundice can be normal, a physiologic response due to lack of maturity of liver and increase in red blood cells. Or it can be abnormal, caused by infection or blood incompatibility. The abnormal condition requires active treatment. The normal condition requires only increased hydration and sunlight.

LARGE FOR GESTATIONAL AGE (LGA): Baby that is larger than normal range for its gestational age. May be a normal variation of fetal growth, or may be caused by abnormal physiology. Often associated with diabetes. (See DIABETES).

MECONIUM ASPIRATION: Inhaling meconium into the airways and/or into the lungs. Usually requires deep suctioning and possibly resuscitation. May cause aspiration pneumonia.

MECONIUM STAINING: When the baby's first bowel movement is passed prior to birth. Although the presence of meconium in and of itself is not a complication, it may be an indicator (not an absolute diagnosis) of possible past, present-time, or potential fetal distress.

PLACENTAL ABRUPTION: Separation of all or part of the placenta from the uterine wall prior to the birth of the baby. Symptoms: painful sustained contractions, persistent pain at site of placental implantation, enlargement of uterus. There may or may not be obvious bleeding or changes in the heart tones of baby. Risks: maternal hemorrhage and/or fetal death. However, if carefully monitored, if only a partial abruption, vaginal delivery may still be possible.

PLACENTA PREVIA: The placenta is either partially covering or fully covering the opening of the cervix. If the condition persists at the onset of labor, the result can be severe hemmorhage and possible death of baby and/or mother. In some cases a partial previa can be managed with a vaginal birth. However, a complete previa at the onset of labor is an indication for a cesarean delivery. However, diagnosis of placenta previa prenatally does not necessarily indicate a scheduled cesarean because the placenta can migrate (move). Thus, the condition may be totally eradicated by the onset of labor.

POLYHYDRAMNIOS: Too much amniotic fluid. Although often associated with diabetes, multiple gestation, and fetal anomalies, it may simply be a normal variation.

POSTMATURITY: An "over-cooked" baby caused by a placenta that is not working properly because it has begun to break down. It is characterized by lack of fetal growth, unresponsive fetal heart tones, abrupt decrease or cessation of fetal movement, calcified skull. Increased risk of fetal distress, failure of head to mold, placental abruption, stillbirth. May be prevented with good nutrition and positive emotional state. There are no absolute diagnostic tests for postmaturity.

POSTPARTUM INFECTION: Infection, usually of the uterus, which occurs shortly after the birth. Most common after cesareans because the uterus has been opened and exposed to bacteria. Can also occur following vaginal birth, due to introduction of bacteria through the vaginal canal. If not diagnosed and controlled, can cause sepsis (infection throughout the body), and possibly death.

PRE-ECLAMPSIA: An avoidable condition which if not arrested can lead to eclampsia or toxemia (See TOXEMIA).

PREMATURE RUPTURE OF MEMBRANES (PROM): Rupture of membranes as the first sign of labor without onset of contractions within 12 hours following rupture of membranes. Risk of infection substantially less if "hands-off" approach (nothing inside the mother's vagina, including fingers of practitioner) is taken. Precautions should be taken to avoid infection, and every effort should be made to stimulate contractions, beginning with the least interventive approach as possible.

PREMATURITY: Birth at gestational age of less than 37 weeks. Increased risks: fetal distress, lung immaturity (Respiratory Distress Syndrome), jaundice, poor sucking reflex, inability to regulate temperature, dehydration and weight loss, apnea (failure to breathe), brain damage, stillbirth, neonatal death. Often preventable with good nutrition.

PROM WITH PREMATURITY: Rupture of membranes prior to 37 weeks gestation. Rupture of membranes as first sign of labor may be beneficial to the maturation of the lungs. It appears that the longer the membranes have been ruptured prior to delivery, (taking infection-prevention precautions) the greater the chances are of fetal/neonatal lung maturity.

RESPIRATORY DISTRESS SYNDROME (RDS): (See HYALINE MEMBRANE DISEASE).

RETAINED PLACENTA: Placenta which is not expelled within 2 hours following the birth. Risk of obvious or concealed hemorrhage, shock, or death. May be resolved with change in maternal position, environment, use of oxytocin-containing herbs, remedies, or drugs, manual removal of placenta.

SHOULDER DYSTOCIA: The head has been born, but the shoulders are stuck. Unpredictable and not resolvable by cesarean, as baby is already partially born. Quick action necessary as intracranial pressure increases risk of brain damage and death.

SMALL FOR GESTATIONAL AGE (SGA): Baby that is smaller than normal range for its gestational age; usually associated with placental dysfunction. Complications: inability to breathe, low blood sugar causing brain damage, inability to regulate body temperature. May be confused prenatally with normal fetal size variations.

SPINA BIFIDA: Developmental anomaly. Defective closure of the encasement of the spinal cord. Cord and meninges may protrude from it.

TOXEMIA (METABOLIC TOXEMIA OF LATE PREGNANCY): A disease of malnutrition and/or high stress which results in poor absorption of food, thus effectively creating malnutrition. Findings associated with toxemia are profound edema (swelling), protein spilling in the urine, and a marked increase in blood pressure. In more advanced cases, blurred vision, headaches, and dizziness occur. Blood tests should be done to confirm diagnosis. Damage to the placenta (and thus to the baby), the liver, the kidneys, and brain may result. At its most advanced stage (commonly known as eclampsia), convulsions, coma, and fetal and/or maternal death may occur. These complications are preventable through good nutrition and stress reduction.

TRANSVERSE ARREST: The baby's head is stuck at the ischial spines and will not descend further until its position changes. The baby's head is facing sideways (transverse). The largest diameter of the head is trying to pass through the smallest transverse diameter of the pelvis (the ischial spines). In order to pass through the spines, the baby's head must rotate to either an anterior or posterior presentation. Rotation may be affected through change in mother's position, increase in quality of the contractions, and/or manual rotation by the practitioner.

TRANSVERSE LIE OR TRANSVERSE PRESENTATION: The baby is lying across the uterus. At onset of labor, often the lie of the baby changes to either a vertex or breech presentation. However, if the lie does not change spontaneously and labor is permitted for too long, the shoulder or arm is compressed into the pelvis. This presentation is not deliverable vaginally, but may be changed through version.

UTERINE RUPTURE: The forcible tearing of the uterus, causing bleeding or hemorrhage (as differentiated from dehiscence of the uterus). Incidence varies according to studies between 0.05–0.5% with previous cesarean scar. Possible causes: misuse of pitocin, malnutrition, mismanaged impacted labor with malpresentation or CPD, many pregnancies, placental abruption. Risks: hysterectomy, death of mother or fetus, although there have been no documented maternal deaths associated with low-segment scars. Outcome of rupture worse with an unscarred than with a scarred uterus.

VOMITING IN LABOR: Can be a normal physiologic response in labor. If vomiting is persistent, and fluid volume cannot be replaced, vomiting can be a complication. Risks: dehydration, fetal distress, low blood volume.

Tests and Interventions

AMNIOCENTESIS: Procedure during which a small amount of amniotic fluid is extracted from the uterus with large syringe. Tests which can be performed from this fluid are genetic anomalies, sex of the baby, Rh-sensitization, and L/S ratio. Risks associated with this procedure are trauma to fetus or placenta, infection, hemorrhage, rupture of membranes, premature labor.

ANESTHESIA: Controlled poisoning which renders patient without sensitivity/feeling and/or without consciousness. The greatest risks of any surgery are the risks of anesthesia.

ARTIFICIAL RUPTURE OF MEMBRANES (AROM): Intentionally breaking the amniotic sac which surrounds and protects the fetus. AROM increases risk of distress or infection to the baby. This situation often threatens the woman with a cesarean if she does not deliver within 12–24 hours.

BETAMETHASONE: A cortisone derivative which has been found to be somewhat effective in assisting the maturation of the fetal lungs, when given to the mother at least 12 hours prior to the birth of the premature fetus.

CERVICAL INCISION: When a low segment transverse cesarean is done late is labor, the incision is actually made through the cervix.

CLASSICAL INCISION: A vertical incision from the fundus (top) of the uterus to the cervix (bottom of the uterus). The presence of a vertical scar on the skin does not necessarily indicate that the uterine incision was classical.

DE LEE RESUSCITATION CATHETER: Suction tube which clears the upper airways.

DILATATION AND CURETTAGE (D & C): Mechanically dilating the cervix, then scraping the wall of the uterus and removing its contents. Often done routinely following miscarriage. Indicated with uncontrollable hemorrhage of the uterus. Risks: uterine perforation, uterine infection, sepsis (infection of whole body).

EPIDURAL ANESTHESIA: Anesthesia injected above the dura (tissue layer surrounding the spinal cord and the nerves). Contraindicated if mother is hypotensive (has extremely low blood pressure), or if a true emergency exists and great haste is required. Risks include drop in blood pressure (affecting the entire cardio-vascular system); total spinal (causing inability to breathe); long-term paralysis of the legs; depressed infant. Spinal headache does not result from epidural anesthesia.

FRIEDMAN'S CURVE: A bell-shaped curve which was the result of a study of the progress of many women's labors. The average progress of labor was determined to be 1 centimeter cervical dilatation per hour. Although the curve was never intended to define the average as being normal, it has been misused by standard obstetrical practice to define normal labor.

GENERAL ANESTHESIA: Rapid induction of unconsciousness using barbiturates and a drug causing total body paralysis. Breathing is done by the anesthesiologist through tube down the throat. Risks to mother: injury to teeth or eyes, swelling of vocal cords, difficulty in breathing long-term, inflammation from IV, allergic reactions to drugs, aspiration pneumonia, dangerously low blood pressure, cardiac arrest, brain damage, death. Risks to baby: respiratory depression, brain damage, death.

GLUCOSE TOLERANCE TEST (GTT): A diagnostic blood test for diabetes. Measures the body's ability to deal with a sugar load, following a fast. Requires fasting, then ingesting a large amount of sugar water. The safety of this test is questionable, as the test itself could actually cause diabetes.

GLYCOSYLATED HEMOGLOBIN: A diagnostic blood test for diabetes that measures the amount of sugar attached to the red blood cells. This test also requires fasting. However, since it does not require the high sugar load, it is safer than the GTT.

HALOTHANE: An anesthetic that is inhaled.

HERPES CULTURES: Cultures done from cervical or blister scrapings to diagnose presence of active herpes virus. Procedure may actually cause recurrent herpes outbreak, as it physically stresses already sensitive tissue.

HYSTEROGRAPHY: A graphic recording of the strength of uterine contractions during labor.

IATROGENIC COMPLICATION: A complication caused by the practitioner.

INDUCTION: Causing labor to begin. May be done with herbs, homeopathic preparations, rupture of membranes, or pitocin. Risks: prematurity, insufficient labor with subsequent cesarean, specific risks associated with herbs/drugs utilized.

ISOLATION: Forced separation of one patient from all other patients to prevent spread of infectious disease. Maternal-infant separation often done routinely in the face of fever or history of herpes. Condition should be diagnosed as currently contagious prior to enforcement of such isolation. May induce risks of decreased milk production, mastitis, increased neonatal jaundice, and decreased maternal-child attachment.

IV: Intravenous fluids. A catheter is fed into a vein with a needle. Through the catheter fluids such as saline solution (salt water) or dextrose (sugar water) are infiltrated directly into the cardio-vascular system. Indicated when patient is dehydrated or if a major blood loss has occurred. Often used routinely for women in labor. Could be avoided by eating and drinking in labor. Risks include: infection at the site of the catheter, damage to bladder or kidneys, hypervolemia (too much blood volume), high blood pressure, stroke, or heart attack.

LOW SEGMENT TRANSVERSE INCISION: An incision across the lower part of the uterus. Even if the external scar is vertical, the uterine incision may be low segment transverse.

L/S RATIO: A test for fetal lung maturity, done with amniocentesis. A ratio comparing the amounts of L (lecithin) and S (sphingomyelin) in the amniotic fluid. When the ratio is at least 2:1 then the fetal lungs are said to be mature. Risks are the same as the risks of amniocentesis.

METHERGINE: Long-acting synthetic hormone which contracts the uterus used to control hemorrhage. Contraindicated in the presence of high blood pressure.

PITOCIN: A chemical simulation of the hormone oxytocin which is secreted by the woman's body during labor.

PITOCIN AUGMENTATION: When a woman's labor has been arrested (without progress) for several hours in *active* labor, judicious use of pitocin can often stimulate contractions enough to complete the dilatation. Not usually effective if active labor has not yet been established. Contraindications to use of pitocin include: a floating fetus (not in pelvis), questionable fetal condition, evidence of true disproportion. Significant risks of misuse to mother and fetus include: placental abruption, uterine rupture, and fetal distress.

PITOCIN INDUCTION: Use of pitocin to begin labor. Often pitocin inductions fail because the mother's own hormones have not readied her cervix by softening and ripening it. Therefore, pitocin induction should be used only when absolutely medically indicated after all other more natural attempts at induction have been tried.

SCOPALOMINE: Hallucinogenic amnesiac used extensively in the 1950s–1960s, still occasionally used. It causes women to writhe in pain, completely disoriented and disassociated from the experience of giving birth.

SERUM GLUCOSE: A test of the amount of sugar in the blood following a fast. Usually used in conjunction with glycosylated hemoglobin as diagnostic tests for diabetes, and in differentiation between gestational and non-gestational diabetes.

SONAGRAM: Ultrasonic scanning that provides a two-dimensional picture by bouncing high frequency sound waves off tissues. Risks include changes in cellular replication, insufficiently studied to determine long-term effects.

SPINAL ANESTHESIA: Anesthesia injected directly into the dura (tissue layer surrounding the spinal cord and its nerves). Risks include abrupt drop in blood pressure (affecting cardio-vascular system); total spinal (paralysis from neck down, thus unable to breathe); spinal headache. Long-term paralysis of legs and depressed infant are less likely to occur with spinal than with epidural.

STRIPPING MEMBRANES: Weakening the membranes by sweeping the internal opening of the cervix with a finger. A method of induction. Increases likelihood that rupture of membranes will occur within 24 hours. Increased risk of infection and of having a cesarean for failure to progress.

SUPINE POSITION: Lying flat on back. When done for an extended period of time, not safe for mother or fetus in pregnancy or labor. Pressure of the pregnant uterus compresses the major vein returning blood to the heart, thus reducing oxygenation to the fetus. It is often enforced upon women in labor or delivery for convenience of practitioner.

SYNTOCIN: A chemical simulation of the hormone oxytocin which is secreted by the woman's body in labor.

TERBUTALINE: Smooth muscle relaxant.

TOTAL SPINAL: Complication of spinal and epidural anesthesia. Loss of sensation and paralysis from the neck down, instead of from the breasts down. Patient cannot breathe. Anesthesiologist must intubate (place a tube down the throat) and breathe for the patient.

UTERINE EXPLORATION: Checking the inside of the uterus manually. Indicated with unexplained or uncontrollable postpartum hemorrhage, to remove retained placenta and/or blood clots. Often done routinely following VBACs to check the scar. Risks include uterine infection, uterine perforation, and uterine rupture.

VACUUM EXTRACTOR: A machine that creates a powerful yet controllable vacuum. A big rubberized cup rather like a plunger is placed on the head of the baby. When the cup is in place, during each contraction, the vacuum is turned on just enough to allow the woman's pushing effort to become more effective, but not enough to damage the baby's head.

VERSION: Changing the baby's presentation. May be done non-interventively with visualization and anti-gravity exercises. If not successful may be done by practitioner either externally (external version) or internally (internal version). Risks of external or internal version include tightening a wrapped cord, placental abruption, and fetal distress.

X-RAY PELVIMETRY: Irradiation to determine the internal measurements of the pelvis. Often no more accurate than a good clinical evaluation of the pelvis. Accuracy is dependent upon the positioning of the patient. Cannot measure the amount of stretchability of the pelvis. If done during pregnancy, the fetus is exposed to full-body radiation, thus greatly increasing the risks of radiation to the baby.

Resources

Workshops

VBAC and Cesarean Prevention Workshops
with
Lynn Baptisti Richards

Workshop for parents includes learning from and taking responsibility for our births and our lives, choosing our practitioner and birth place, complications and intervention-prevention, hurdles of previous birth—repeating indications???, trusting your intuition, letting go, visualization, affirmations, color and sound, and special exercises designed to focus and strengthen from within in order to flow with the body.

Workshop for professionals includes understanding the cesarean experience, bridging the psychological gap between the needs of the VBAC mother and the needs of the VBAC practitioner, physical and psychospiritual tools for prenatal care, working through hurdles of previous birth—repeating indications???, improvement of outcomes for women with a previous cesarean, political considerations for VBAC professionals, case studies and sharing.

VBAC teacher training workshops include philosophies, theories, issues, knowledge, teaching techniques, counseling and labor support skills in an atmosphere of warmth and sharing to challenge you to meet your greatest potential.

Box 637, N. Bellmore, NY 11710
(516) 781-0785
M-F, 9:30 A.M.-2:30 P.M.

VBAC and Cesarean Prevention Workshops
with
Nancy Wainer Cohen

Includes experience of support, caring, enthusiasm, information, energy and safety that serves as a model for birthing. Primarily for parents, but professionals are welcome. To help women remember that they are capable of giving birth.

> 10 Great Plain Terrace
> Needham, MA 02192
> (617) 449-2490
> M-F, 9:00 A.M.-2:00 P.M.

Pediatrics for Parents Workshop
with
George Wootan, M.D., AAFP/ABFP

Includes physical examination of the child, treatment of certain common childhood conditions and illnesses (both routine and emergency), health maintenance techniques, disease prevention, selection of a health care provider that meets your needs.

> Box 101 K, RD7,
> Kingston, NY 12401
> (914) 331-4075

Professional VBAC Counselors

Lynn Baptisti Richards
Box 637, N. Bellmore, NY 11710
(516) 781-0785
M-F, 9:30 A.M.-2:30 P.M. Eastern Time
By appointment (phone or in person)

Nancy Wainer Cohen
10 Great Plain Terrace
Needham, MA 02192
(617) 449-2490
By appointment (phone or in person)

VBAC Practitioners

For information regarding supportive VBAC professionals in your area or to obtain a directory of midwives who attend VBAC births, contact Lynn Baptisti Richards at the above address, or your local Cesarean Prevention Movement chapter (see below)

Support Groups

C/SEC (Cesareans/Support, Education & Concern)
22 Forest Road
Framingham, MA 01701

ICEA (International Childbirth Education Association)
Box 20048
Minneapolis, MN 55420

La Leche League International
9616 Minneapolis Avenue
Franklin Park, IL 60631

NAPSAC (National Association of Parents and Professionals
   for Safe Alternatives in Childbirth)
Box 267
Marble Hill, MO 63764

Workshop for Special Needs
Kay Matthews
R.F.D. Windham Hill Road
Windham, VT
(802) 874-4165

Cesarean Prevention Movement Chapters:

NORTHEAST

CPM of Central New York
102 Bradley Street
Syracuse, NY 13204
Contact Person: Evelyn Gallagher
(315) 475-7101

CPM of Utica/Rome
326 Glen Rd. N.
Rome, NY 13440
(315) 332-8080

CPM of Northern N.Y.
129 Haney St.
Watertown, NY 13601
Contact Person: Sally Dear
(315) 788-2182

CPM of Mid-Hudson Valley
Julia Court Box 141
Campbell Hall, NY 10916
Contact Person: Bea Mooney
(914) 496-6163

CPM of Troy, N.Y.
42 Donegal Ave.
Troy, NY 12180
(518) 273-5421

CPM of Central Westchester
20 Willow St.
Irvington, NY 10533
Contact Person: Linda Nugent
(914) 591-7878

CPM of Northern Westchester
2673 Evergreen St.
Yorktown Heights, NY 10598
Contact Person: Joyce Gleason
(914) 962-4154

CPM of Suffolk, N.Y.
1063 Manor Lane
Bayshore, NY 11706
Contact Person: Terri Jaisle
(516) 666-2324

CPM of New Jersey I
11 DeBarry Place
Summitt, NJ 07901
Contact Person: Pat Kenny
(201) 273-3532

CPM of New Jersey II
20 Coville Drive
Browns Mills, NJ 08015
Contact Person: Lori Stetson
(609) 893-4783

CPM of New Jersey III
28 Serviss Ave.
North Brunswick, NJ 08902
Contact Person: Louise Rosenberg
(201) 545-9348

CPM of Fairfield County
1590 N. Benson Rd.
Fairfield, CT 06430
Contact Person: Nancy O'Sullivan
(203) 255-4043

CPM of Lehigh Valley, Pa.
RD1, Box 870
Alburtis, PA 18011
Contact Person: Debbi Donovan
(215) 682-4769

SOUTH

CPM of D. C./Suburban Maryland
8411 48th Ave.
College Park, MD 20740
Contact Person: Lily Werbos
(301) 474-2762

CPM of Greater Washington/North Virginia
5802 Norton Rd.
Alexandria, VA 22303
Contact Person: Ymelda Martinez-Allison
(703) 960-3899

CPM of Tampa
15611 Timberline Dr.
Tampa, FL 33624
Contact Person: Judy Zaritt
(813) 962-7238

MIDWEST

CPM of Greater Cleveland
PO Box 29011
Parma Heights, OH 44129
Contact Person: Michaelene Bratton
(216) 967-7207

CPM of Northwest Ohio
Rt. 1 S-236 Rd. 11
Napoleon, OH 43545
Contact Person: Sherry Oberhaus
(419) 592-7138

CPM of Kansas City, Mo.
RR1 Box 450 - 1AA
Liberty, MO 64068
Contact Person: Linda Nelson
(816) 781-4301

CPM of Austin
1307 Kinney Ave #130
Austin, TX 78704
Contact Person: Renee Potenze
(512) 447-0847

CPM of Dallas
13023 Jasoncrest Trail
Dallas, TX 75243
Contact Person: Mary Milner
(214) 690-4870

CPM of Houston
14618 Miranda
Houston, TX 77039
Contact Person: Vicki Huckabay
(713) 442-0327

CPM of Western Indiana
758 Edgemoor Rd.
Terre Haute, IN 47802
Contact Person: Karen Lukens
(812) 299-2507

CPM of Lafayette
4460 Douglas Dr.
W. Lafayette, IN 47906
Contact Person: Maureen Delp
(317) 743-4905

CPM of Southwestern Indiana
200 Roladn Dr.
Vincennes, IN 47591
Contact Person: Jane Hughes
(812) 882-6352

CPM of Southeast Minnesota
11718 50th Street
Albertville, MN 55301
Contact Person: Tessa Bridal
(612) 497-3511

CPM of Southeast Michigan
2405 N. Wilson
Royal Oak, MI 48073
Contact person: Jan Frasher McIntosh
(313) 548-8033

CPM of Ann Arbor
819 S. Seventh
Ann Arbor, MI 48103
Contact Person: Ann Sterling
(313) 996-2599

CPM of Mid-Michigan
1632 Four and 3/4 Mile Rd.
Midland, MI 48640
Contact Person: Sue Gaul
(517) 832-8287

CPM of Madison
1416 E. Dayton
Madison, WI 53703
Contact Person: Mary Jo Schiavoni
(608) 255-6931

CPM of Milwaukee
2428 N. 41st St.
Milwaukee, WI 53210
Contact Person: Jane Sullivan
(414) 873-2746

CPM of Baraboo
1036 Crestview Circle
Baraboo, WI 53913
Contact Person: Linda Mohar
(608) 356-6756

CPM of Fox Valley
1332 Traders Rd. #1
Menasha, WI 54952
Contact Person: Janine Romnek
(414) 725-8833

CPM of Wichita
716 S. Yale
Wichita, KS 67218
Contact Person: Jolene Brotton
(316) 684-6634

CPM of St. Louis
3871 Juniata St.
St. Louis, MO 63116
Contact Person: Anne Bader
(314) 773-1067

WEST

CPM of Los Angeles
12741 Evanston St.
Los Angeles, CA 90049
Contact Person: Deborah Hamza
(213) 395-4590

CPM of San Gabriel/San Bernardino
5618 Hawthorne
Montclair, CA 91763
Contact Person: Diana M. Peterson
(714) 988-8221

CPM of Solano
249 Cascade Dr.
Vacaville, CA 95688
Contact Person: Dale Flores
(707) 446-3438

CPM of San Francisco Bay Area
32455 Lake Barlee Lane
Fremont, CA 94536
Contact Person: Susan Huffman
(415) 471-1669

CPM of Las Vegas
6669 Gazelle Dr.
Las Vegas, NV 89108
Contact Person: Bekki Leier
(702) 646-5913

CPM of Sonoma County
4444 Alta Vista Ave.
Santa Rosa, CA 95404
Contact Person: Jennifer Gunderson
(707) 523-0919

CPM of Greater Phoenix
7885 E. Windrose
Scottsdale, AZ 85260
Contact Person: Jana Robb
(602) 483-2921

CPM of Northern Arizona
Box 22521
Flagstaff, AZ 86002
Contact Person: Kristie Pagel
(602) 774-2598

If contact person in your area has moved, or if no CPM chapter exists in your area, contact the main office of CPM:

Esther Booth Zorn
P.O. Box 152
Syracuse, NY 13210
(315) 424-1942

INDEXES

Birthing Terminology

Abortion, 45
Active labor, 5, 6, 12, 16, 23, 32, 43, 49
American College of Obstetricians and
    Gynecologists (ACOG)'s guidelines
    for VBAC, 1, 3, 12, 42
Amniocentesis, 19
Amniotomy, *See* Artificial rupture of
    membranes
Amphetamines, 22
Anesthesia: epidural, 21; general, 3, 10,
    11, 14, 17, 18, 23, 45, 51; regional, 3,
    10, 12, 13, 16, 42
Application of the head to the cervix, 21,
    44
Arrest of labor, *See* Disruption of labor, in
    Index of Environmental Factors
Artificial rupture of membranes (AROM),
    6, 10, 11, 13, 21, 23, 42
Asynclicism, 35

Bedrest to maintain pregnancy, 19
Bottle-feeding, 14
Breech, 11, 12, 16, 25, 36, 37, 38, 51; *See
    also* Version

Catheter, 9, 10
Cephalo-pelvic disproportion (CPD), 6, 9,
    14, 16, 18, 29, 33, 34, 35, 41
Cervical lip, 9
Chiropractic in labor and birth, 16
Chorio-amnionitis, *See* Infection
Congenital abnormalities, 19
Contracted pelvis, 18, 28, 41
Contractions, techniques to encourage, 21,
    44, 49

Numbers refer to chapters.

Corticosteroids, 11
Court-ordered cesarean, 9
Cross-matched blood, 10

Defective scar, *See* Dehisence
Deflexed head, 35
Dehisence, 26
Dehydration, 16, 23
Descent of the baby, 6, 7, 9, 12
Diabetes in pregnancy, 7, 19
Diarrhea in labor, 9
Dilatation and curettage (D & C), 11, 19

Epidural, *See* Anesthesia
Episiotomy and vaginal tears, 5, 6, 10, 42,
    48

Failure to progress, 5, 6, 7, 11, 13, 14, 21,
    24, 33
False labor, *See* Prelabor contractions
Fetal distress, 10, 23, 24, 33
Fetal lung maturity, 11
Fetal monitor, 3, 5, 7, 8, 10, 17
Fetal scalp sample, 10
Fetascope, 10
Forceps, 12, 22
Foreign guidelines for VBAC, 1, 2, 3, 17,
    18, 19

General anesthesia, *See* Anesthesia
Glucose tolerance test, *See* Diabetes
Glycosylated hemaglobin, *See* Diabetes

Heparin lock, 10
Herpes, 9
Home induction, 12, 14, 16

Induction of labor, *See* Home induction;
    Pitocin induction

Infection, 23; *See also* Postcesarean
   infection
Infertility, 19, 21
IVs, 3, 5, 6, 7, 8, 9, 10, 11, 12, 23, 42

Jaundice, 19

Ketosis, 23

Logan Basic Contact, 17
Loss of fetal heart tones, *See* Fetal distress
L/S Ratio, 19

Malpresentation, 6, 7, 11, 15, 17, 20, 35;
   See also Breech; Version
Manual dilatation, 44, 49
Meconium staining, 7, 14
Miscarriage, 11, 19
Mismanagement of labor, 4, 5, 6, 10, 13,
   14, 16
Multiple gestation, 11, 25

Nutrition in pregnancy, 4, 9, 17, 18, 22

Palpation of the fetus, 3, 13
Perineal massage, 16, 17
Pitocin induction, 6, 7, 10, 19, 29; and
   augmentation of labor, 6, 11, 21, 23;
   and fetal distress, 10; and placental
   abruption, 10
Placental abruption, 10
Placenta previa, 3, 17
Postcesarean infection, 4, 23
Posterior lie, 6, 13, 14, 20, 35
Postmaturity, 11, 12, 16
Postpartum bleeding, 13, 19, 22
Pushing, 3, 5, 7, 10, 12, 17, 20, 21, 23, 33,
   42, 44

Repeat cesarean, 7, 10, 15, 16, 17, 18, 31,
   42, 47, 49, 50
Repeating indications, 10, 11, 13, 21, 40
Resuscitation, 19, 23, 24
Risks of cesarean 3, 7, 17, 18
Rotation and descent, techniques to
   encourage, 7, 21, 35, 44, 49
Rupture of membranes, 3, 5, 6, 7, 10, 11,
   19

Safety of VBAC, 4, 7
Scalp sample, *See* Fetal scalp sample
Scopalomine, 22
Sedation of labor, 6, 11, 12, 19, 23, 44

Serum glucose, *See* Diabetes
Short, wrapped cord, 24
Shoulder dystocia and shoulders needing
   assistance, 12, 14
Soft-tissue dystocia, 42
Sonagram, 11, 12, 13, 17, 18, 19, 31
Spinal anesthesia, *See* Anesthesia
Spinal tap, *See* Infection
Staph infection, *See* Infection
Station, *See* Descent of the baby
Strep infection, *See* Infection
Stripping membranes, 16, 23
Supine position, 10, 13, 19

Toxemia, 4, 18
Transverse arrest, 11
Transverse lie, 15, 17
Triplets, *See* Multiple gestation
Twins, *See* Multiple gestation

Urinating, labor and postpartum, 5, 9, 12
Uterus: exploration of, 16, 26; rupture of,
   4, 9, 16, 17, 18, 19

Vacuum extractor, 21, 34
Vaginal birth, importance to health of
   newborn, 18
VBAC: after classical cesarean, 2, 3, 10,
   15, 26, 27, 47; after multiple
   cesareans, 10, 15, 17, 42, 47
Version, of breech, oblique, or transverse
   baby, 16, 17, 36
Vertical incision, *See* VBAC after classical
   cesarean
Vomiting in labor, 16

Weight gain in pregnancy, 4, 22

X-ray pelvimetry, 7, 18, 19, 26

Environmental Factors

Assertiveness with practitioners, 6, 12, 13,
   16, 18

Baby moving down, coping with the
   sensation, 14, 17, 21, 42
Bach Flower Remedies, 17
Back labor, 11, 12, 13, 14, 16, 19
Birth plan, 6, 13, 14, 16
Bringing the baby down, coping with
   pressure from the practitioner 5, 7,
   44, 49

Choices of the future, 49
Choices where there appear to be none, 7, 10, 12
Choosing: childbirth educator, 9, 10, 14, 18; practitioner, 4, 6, 10, 11, 17, 18, 51; *See also* Home birth, unattended
Cooption of husband by doctor, 13, 33, 49, 51
Court-ordered cesarean, 7

Dancing in labor, 8, 49
Deceiving the patient, 3, 12, 16, 18, 36, 49
Decision making, 3, 4, 6, 7, 9, 12, 14, 21, 27, 44, 45, 46
Disruption of labor, 6, 9, 10, 11, 16, 49
Drinking and eating in labor, 5, 6, 9, 14, 16, 19, 33

Father catching his own baby, 14, 29, 46, 51
Father-centered cesareans, 9, 10, 44
Following my body, 5, 6, 9, 10, 12, 14, 22, 33, 42

Grandmothers at birth, 18, 51
Guilt, *See* Scare tactics

Health care in a foreign country, 19
Home birth, unattended, 4, 7, 15, 19, 21, 29
Home labor, hospital birth, 5, 9, 12, 21, 33, 44, 49
Home VBAC, 6, 13, 14, 15, 16, 17, 18, 19, 20, 21, 22, 24, 29
Hospitals: planned transport to, 3, 5, 9, 12, 33, 49, 51; policy, 5, 9, 10, 16, 18, 19, 22, 25, 46, 49, 51; treatment of newborns, 15; unplanned transport to, 15, 21, 44
Husband's (father's) role in labor, 7, 11, 12, 13, 14, 18, 21, 44, 46, 51

Iatrogenic (doctor-caused) complications, 5, 10, 13, 17, 19, 22, 23
Informed consent, 7, 10, 12, 19, 46, 49
Integrating labor into everyday life, 12, 13, 14, 20, 41
Internal exams, 5, 10, 18, 49
Interventions to avoid cesarean, 10, 21
Isolation/separation: from the baby, 4, 7, 9, 10, 11, 12, 14, 17, 18, 19; from husband (father), 4, 7, 10, 11, 12, 18, 51

Labor bed delivery, 4, 44
Labor support: from husband (father), 5, 6, 7, 11, 12, 14, 18, 19, 21, 23, 46, 51; from women, 5, 7, 9, 10, 16, 17, 22, 33, 49
Laboring alone, feeling alone in labor, 5, 6, 8, 9, 10, 13, 41
Lack of preparation for birth, 14
Lack of support for VBAC, 5, 6, 7, 9, 12, 33, 51
LaMaze education, *See* "Natural" childbirth
Legal issues in birth, 5, 7, 10, 17, 19, 46, 49, 51
Lip service to VBAC, 7, 13

Mothering the mother, 10, 14
Mother support groups, 6, 9

"Natural" childbirth, 4, 7, 12, 13, 22, 51
Needs, getting them met, 6, 10, 14, 42, 44

Optimum birth letter, *See* Birth plan

Pediatrician, interviewing and choosing, 13
Positive doctor, negative partner, *See* Practitioners, conflicts within a practice
Postcesarean support, 10, 12, 14
Postpartum support, 14, 18
Post-VBAC recovery, 10, 11, 12, 18
Practitioners: choosing by interview, 4, 6, 10, 11, 17, 18, 51; condescending attitudes, 3, 6, 7, 12, 13; conflicts among, over VBAC, 26, 52; conflicts within a practice, 5, 7, 9, 11, 13, 23; pressuring women to perform, 5, 6, 7, 10, 12, 19, 21, 46, 49; responsibility of, 15; support of bonding, 4, 11, 20, 22, 24, 44, 45; support of VBAC, 3, 28, 32, 35, 42, 48; support of women, 4, 5, 9, 10, 11, 12, 13, 14, 16, 17, 21, 23, 24, 27, 28, 29, 30, 33, 34, 35, 36, 37, 40, 41, 42, 45, 47, 48; training of, 13, 23, 26, 38; unsupportive, 4, 5, 6, 7, 9, 11, 13, 18, 19, 21, 22, 46, 49, 51
Pregnancy as illness, 7, 13
Preparation for labor support, 13, 14
Protecting the patient, *See* Deceiving the patient

Relaxation, baths and showers for, 12, 13, 16, 19

Refusing medical procedures, 6, 8, 15, 16, 46, 51

Safe place for labor and birth, 5, 9, 13, 17, 19, 23, 24, 44, 49

Scare tactics, 5, 7, 9, 13, 14, 16, 22, 49

Set-up for repeat cesarean, 13, 49

Sexual abuse: its effect on labor, 21; in labor, 7

Siblings at birth, 13, 14, 16, 18, 20

Single mothers, 15

Support of VBAC during pregnancy, 4, 5, 6, 7, 9, 10, 11, 12, 13, 14, 16, 17, 18

Techno-birth, 14

Technology as decision maker, 10

Time and space for birthing, 5, 6, 7, 12, 19, 22, 29, 34, 35, 40, 44, 45, 46, 47, 49

Timing of labor; 11, 21, 41, 49; management of, 5, 12, 21, 31, 33, 42, 47, 49, 51

Traveling for a VBAC, 9, 20, 47

Uninvolved or unsupportive husband (father), 14, 33, 44, 49, 51

Usurping women's power in birth, 5, 7, 17, 19, 22, 44, 49

VBAC education, 5, 7, 9, 10, 13, 14, 16, 42, 49

VBAC management, 4, 9, 10, 12, 13, 14, 15, 16, 17, 18, 21, 28, 32, 33, 34, 36, 40, 42

Feelings

After-birth awe, 16, 24

Alone, 6, 7, 14, 19

Anger, 4, 9, 11, 12

Asking for a cesarean, 43, 45

Avoiding cesarean by ending childbearing, 4, 14, 16, 51

Birth: bridge between pregnancy and motherhood, 16, 44; and death, 10, 11, 14, 15, 19, 23, 24; as healing, 4, 14; memories, Introduction, 22, 24; as microcosm of the world, 10, 19; as reflection of ourselves, 14, 18, 44

Birth days, 19

Bonding, 6, 7, 10, 11, 14, 18, 19, 23

Buried alive, 14

Cesarean: a decision I could understand, 13, 14; need for attention and support, 14, 44; rescue from pain, 6, 13; and sterilization, 19

Changing attitudes, 13, 16, 52

Cheated, 18

Concern about baby's health, 4, 7, 9, 10, 19, 22, 23

Confronting emotional issues in labor, 21, 22, 44, 45

Determination to have a VBAC, 4, 9, 12, 13, 17, 42, 43

Disappointment, 7, 10, 11

Doctor as "God," 7, 14, 17, 18; See also Loving the doctor

Doctors' wives in labor, 33, 34

Emotional pain of cesarean, 6

Escaping from labor, 43, 44

Failure, 3, 4, 9, 11, 13, 42, 50

Fathers' feelings, 4, 12, 13, 14, 44, 46, 49

Fears: of the hospital, 13; of labor, 5, 6, 13; in pregnancy, 7, 14, 23, 43, 51

Feelings about abortion, 45

Frustration, 12

Getting stuck, See Hurdles in labor; Disruption of labor, in Index of Environmental Factors

Going backwards, 9

Grieving, 6, 9, 13, 16, 19, 23

Guilt, 9, 22

Having a cesarean is not really giving birth, 3, 7, 12

Healing: our children, 16, 19; the couple, 9, 13, 14; ourselves, 9, 13, 17, 18

Helplessness, 4

Herpes feelings, 9

Holding the baby up, 9, 21, 44

Hoping the VBAC will happen magically, 10

Hurdles in labor, 6, 10, 21, 22, 44, 45, 47, 49

Ideal birth, 10, 12

Ignorance, 7, 14

Intuition, 6, 10, 12, 14, 17, 19, 24, 51
Is this baby mine? 4, 17

Less-than-perfect baby, 19
Letting go, 9, 13, 14, 21, 42, 44, 45; of the placenta, 16, 22
Loss of control, 6, 9, 14, 19
Loving the doctor, 9, 18, 21; *See also* Doctor as "God"

Making labor happen, 14
Maternal feelings, postcesarean and post-VBAC, 3, 4, 6, 10, 14, 18, 19, 51
Moment of choice, 24
Mystical closeness with the baby, 16, 17, 23, 24, 45

Natural birth as an operation, 14, 19
Normal, 3
Nurses' attitudes, 16

Paternity, 45
Perfection, 10, 19, 42
Permission to fail, 42
Personal growth, 6, 9, 10, 14, 16, 18, 19, 22, 42, 44, 49
Personal power in pregnancy, labor, and birth, 7, 9, 12, 19
Planting seeds, 5, 7, 10, 14, 18, 42, 47
Positive cesarean experience, 10, 13, 17, 18, 21
Postpartum depression, 6, 11, 14, 22, 51
Powerlessness, 19
Practitioners' feelings, concerns, and beliefs, 3, 4, 6, 7, 13, 17, 18, 19, 23, 24, 26, 42, 44, 48, 50
Pressure to perform, 7, 19, 21
Pride, 7
Priorities for birth, 23
Protecting the baby by not letting it be born, 22

Proving I could do it, 11
Pure birth, 10

Questioning the necessity of a cesarean, 4, 5, 7, 9, 14, 16, 17, 18, 19

Relaxation and release, *See* Letting go
Removed from the birth process, 19
Repeating patterns, 10, 11, 13, 21, 40
Resignation to another cesarean, 6, 32, 43

Safe, 9
Self-worth, 3, 9
Sexual abuse, 21
Sexuality: in labor and birth, 9, 21; postcesarean, 9
Sibling bonding, 14, 18, 20
Single mothers, 15
Spiritual experience, 6, 13
Spiritual healing, *See* Healing ourselves
Spiritual preparation for VBAC, 6, 9, 15, 17
Strength and weakness, 6, 13, 14
Subsequent pregnancy and feelings about cesarean, 9, 13

Taking responsibility, 5, 6, 7, 9, 13, 14, 15, 17, 18, 42
Trapped in the hospital, 13
Trust and control, 7, 9, 10, 13, 14, 16, 18, 21, 22, 23, 33, 41, 49

VBAC labor and previous labor, 7, 12, 13, 14, 16, 17
Victory, 2, 3, 4, 5, 6, 9, 10, 11, 12, 13, 14, 16, 17, 18, 19, 21, 23, 24, 28, 29, 32, 33, 36, 40, 41, 42, 47, 48, 51, 52
Violated, 7, 19, 21

Waiting to be ready, 14

VBAC: Very Beautiful And Courageous

A woman birthing her baby into her own hands is a symbol of the primal experience of woman power in awe of the miracle of the soul's new life.

A moment without time, space, or personality, it matters not where or with whom the birth takes place. What matters is simply the knowledge that the power to birth is within—that the woman could give birth anywhere, anytime, with anyone—in the hospital, at home, in the car, all alone in the wilderness, or at Yankee Stadium with thousands of fans applauding.

Through the courage from within, pain is transformed into a beautiful gift. As her baby descends, as she feels her own body opening to the life of her child, as she instinctively reaches down with her own hand and touches the emerging baby, her soul merges with the soul of the baby. Time stops. A moment of electricity, of awe, of tears, of indescribable joy. . . .

The mother's power melts into love for her child. Both mother and child have been beautifully transformed, but never severed from one another. The circle of union, letting go, and reunion is complete.

VBAC: VERY BEAUTIFUL AND COURAGEOUS is a process, not an outcome. We find the courage and beauty within ourselves, as we receive the most precious gift of our lives—our children.

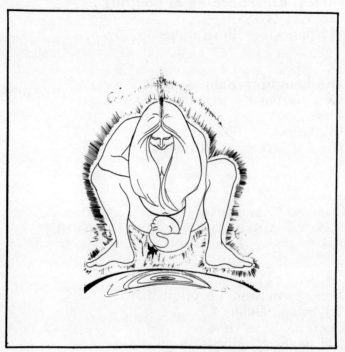

Illustration © 1987 Elizabeth Sundance

Related Books

Babies, Breastfeeding & Bonding
INA MAY GASKIN
240 pages   Illustrations

The Laughing Baby
Remembering Nursery Rhymes & Reasons
ANNE SCOTT
160 pages   Illustrations
Musical Scores   Rhymes

Silent Knife
Cesarean Prevention & Vaginal Birth After Cesarean
NANCY WAINER COHEN & LOIS J. ESTNER
464 pages   Illustrations

Transformation Through Birth
A Woman's Guide
CLAUDIA PANUTHOS
208 pages   Illustrations

Immaculate Deception
A New Look at Women and Childbirth
SUZANNE ARMS
416 pages   Illustrations

Ended Beginnings
Healing Childbearing Losses
CLAUDIA PANUTHOS & CATHERINE ROMEO
224 pages   Photographs

Other Books of Interest

Academic Women
Working Towards Equality
ANGELA SIMEONE
176 pages

Women Teaching For Change
Gender, Class & Power
KATHLEEN WEILER
240 pages

Women's Work
Development & the Division of
Labor by Gender
ELEANOR LEACOCK,
HELEN I. SAFA
& CONTRIBUTORS
320 pages   Photographs

Women & Change in Latin America
New Directions in Sex & Class
JUNE NASH, HELEN I. SAFA
& CONTRIBUTORS
384 pages   Photographs

The Trials & Tribulations of Little Red Riding Hood
Versions of the Tale in
Sociocultural Context
JACK ZIPES
320 pages   Photographs

Other Books of Interest

Unequal Access
Women Lawyers in a Changing America
RONALD CHESTER
160 pages

The Psychology of Spiritual Growth
Channelled from the Brotherhood by
MARY ELIZABETH CARREIRO
160 pages
A Gentle Wind Book, Volume I

Modern Religion & The Destruction of Spiritual Capacity
Channelled from the Brotherhood by
MARY ELIZABETH CARREIRO
160 pages
A Gentle Wind Book, Volume II